Psychiatry Reborn

International Perspectives in Philosophy and Psychiatry

Series editors: Bill (K.W.M.) Fulford, Lisa Bortolotti, Matthew Broome, Katherine Morris, John Z. Sadler, and Giovanni Stanghellini

Volumes in the series:

Psychiatry Reborn
Biopsychosocial psychiatry in modern medicine

Edited by

Julian Savulescu
Uehiro Chair in Practical Ethics, University of Oxford

Rebecca Roache
Senior Lecturer in Philosophy, Royal Holloway, University of London

Will Davies
Associate Professor and Tutorial Fellow in Philosophy, St Anne's College, University of Oxford

Consulting Editor

J. Pierre Loebel
Clinical Professor Emeritus, Psychiatry and Behavioral Sciences, School of Medicine, University of Washington

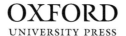
OXFORD
UNIVERSITY PRESS

OXFORD
UNIVERSITY PRESS

Great Clarendon Street, Oxford, OX2 6DP,
United Kingdom

Oxford University Press is a department of the University of Oxford.
It furthers the University's objective of excellence in research, scholarship,
and education by publishing worldwide. Oxford is a registered trade mark of
Oxford University Press in the UK and in certain other countries

© Oxford University Press 2020

The moral rights of the authors have been asserted

First Edition published in 2020

Impression: 2

Published in the United States of America by Oxford University Press
198 Madison Avenue, New York, NY 10016, United States of America

British Library Cataloguing in Publication Data

Data available

Library of Congress Control Number: 2020938132

ISBN 978–0–19–878969–7

Printed and bound by
CPI Group (UK) Ltd, Croydon, CR0 4YY

Foreword

Since the 1990s, there has been a burgeoning interest in psychiatry as clinical practice, as policy, and as research endeavour, by not only philosophers and ethicists, but researchers across disciplines. Psychiatry is messy, vague, complex, and yet crucially important. For those of us who teach medical students, or who act as supervisors for trainee psychiatrists who have recently switched from acute medicine, seeing the acculturation of practitioners who enter psychiatry can remind one of both its difference and its excitement. Medicine is caricatured as becoming largely operationalized with clear clinical guidelines for intervention. There are protocols and flowcharts to follow, investigations to perform, and evidence-based treatments to provide. Patients are grateful for their care, by and large, fulfil the sick role, and are able to refuse the treatment on offer. There are ethical dilemmas and differences in values, but these appear starkly and often as the exception rather than the rule. For the clinician entering psychiatry, the perceived difference in practice can be marked. Uncertainty and ambiguity can be stressful—trainees can feel more fulfilled when their patients have a physical health issue, when a blood test comes back with an abnormality. They are doing 'real' medicine. But with time, rather than seeing psychiatry reduced to a narrow conception of medicine ('We are just the same as other doctors, we diagnose and treat illnesses'), I hope that our students and trainees come away with a conception of medicine that is enriched by psychiatry—they begin to see psychiatry as 'medicine-plus', as medicine as it could be. They learn skills in managing chronic conditions and comorbidity; in working with large interdisciplinary teams and with diagnostic uncertainty; in keeping development, families, culture, and society in mind; in combining pharmacological, psychotherapeutic, and social interventions; and in advocating for patients and working with them to coproduce knowledge and understanding. What one sees in skilled physicians from other disciplines—particularly in areas such as paediatrics, palliative care, diabetes, rheumatology, neurology, and geriatrics—is an envy of psychiatry, an envy of our awareness of the complexity of our clinical work, of the structures that help us practise in such a space, and the humanism and pluralism of our work.

One of the areas which psychiatry can, on occasion, pride itself in is the 'biopsychosocial model', the topic of this edited volume. This can be used as a means of distinguishing psychiatry from other areas of medicine and as a means of demonstrating that psychiatry isn't purely in the business of reductive biomedicine. However, despite this, psychiatrists are often criticized, by psychologists, social scientists, philosophers, service users, and others, of being locked in 'the medical model' and in a form of naïve positivistic empiricism, where despite gestures to society and psychological causation, neuroscience and genetics are the defining disciplines. In turn, when psychiatrists point to the biopsychosocial model in defence, they can draw on vague and inchoate ideas of how different models of causation can interact and be used both scientifically and ideographically to understand and help *this patient here*. This volume takes the biopsychosocial model seriously, and the contributors engage with a variety of ways in which the model can be cashed out and understood. These include considering it as a causal, explanatory, and pluralist approach (Roache), as a means of capturing the complex multiframeworks causal structures that underlie psychiatric illness (Kendler and Gyngell), and in appraising how social causation and construction have a coherent role in a physicalist conception of psychiatric illness (Levy), and if not able to define illness, being a useful way to think about explanation and causation (Sinnott-Armstrong and Summers). Similarly, if there are certain problems we find hard to answer, we may gain more traction on thinking about harm rather than the onset of particular conditions when asking causal questions (Cooper). Pluralism is a key element of the biopsychosocial model, and hence the model can serve as a defence against monist reductionism, with values-based practice being a potentially ally in its implementation (Fulford). Other contributors have stressed the richness of causal accounts of psychiatric illness (Haller and Cohen Kadosh; Viding; McCrory; Cecil), examining development, both neurologically and socially, alongside adverse events and epigenetics. Bayesian approaches to psychopathology may serve as rich means to understand resilience and vulnerability and as a means of reconciling the components of the biopsychosocial model, and the relationship of the individual with their environment (Dayan, Roiser, and Viding). The biopsychosocial model is a useful lens through which to examine how psychiatry may develop in the future, and whether with any possible 'paradigm shift' comes the risk of loss our common sense understanding of mental life and ourselves (Thornton), and caution that with important mechanistic, neuroscientific understanding of mental illness, the human and interpersonal should not be effaced (Hyman and McConnell), and how perhaps neuroscience may enrich our self-understanding and save clinicians and their patients from alternating between folk psychology and science (Glover).

The Loebel Lectures and Research Programme, supported by Pierre and Felice Loebel, was one of the most fulfilling, intellectually exciting, and pleasurable activities I was able to be involved with while at the University of Oxford. This edited book is one of many outputs from the programme, the backbone of which was the annual Loebel Lectures. For the programme, we were fortunate to have Ken Kendler, Steven Hyman, and Essi Viding as our lecturers who very generously gave up their time to speak, but also to engage in workshops with wider delegates. Many of the discussions from the lectures and workshops have now been collated and masterfully edited by Will Davies, Julian Savulescu, and Rebecca Roache. This book is a testament to the passion of Pierre Loebel towards the development of a humanistic, pluralistic, and scientifically rigorous, psychiatry and is a call to all of us as trainers, supervisors, and teachers to develop clinicians of the future to listen to its lessons and to improve the care and understanding of those suffering from mental distress.

Matthew Broome
Chair in Psychiatry and Youth Mental Health and Director of the
Institute for Mental Health, University of Birmingham, Birmingham, UK,
and Distinguished Research Fellow, Oxford Uehiro Centre for Practical
Ethics, University of Oxford, Oxford, UK

Acknowledgements

Julian Savulescu, on behalf of the editors

This volume arises from the Oxford Loebel Lectures and Research Programme, generously funded by Pierre and Felice Loebel from 2014 to 2017. Pierre Loebel's commitment to advancing philosophical and clinical delineation and understanding of biopsychosocial psychiatry, his openness to debate, and his appreciation of the value of interdisciplinary endeavours in addressing its complexities have driven this project over many years.

The project centred around three series of Loebel Lectures, held in Oxford. The Loebel Lecturers were each selected for their groundbreaking work in illuminating our understanding of an aspect of biopsychosocial psychiatry: Professor Kenneth Kendler (2014), Professor Steven Hyman (2015), and Professor Essi Viding (2016). Each lecturer gave generously of their time and talents not only to the public lectures, but to an intensive workshop around the themes of their lectures. These lecturers and workshops formed the basis of the chapters within this volume. We would like to thank all of our lecturers, and all those who participated in the workshop, both those who went on to contribute chapters to this volume, and those whose contribution illuminated, elucidated, or challenged the lecturers in the course of the programme.

We benefitted from the expertise of many, including an International Advisory Board, and in particular fellow project leaders Dr Edward Harcourt and Professor Glyn Humphreys. We were deeply saddened by the death of Glyn Humphreys in 2016, and dedicate this book to the memory of a thoughtful, collegiate, and kind colleague who supported the project amidst his own hugely influential and groundbreaking research in psychology, cognition, attention, and neuropsychology, and his duties as head of department.

Finally, I wish to express my personal gratitude to the Uehiro Foundation for Ethics and Education for their support for my chair, the Uehiro Chair in Practical Ethics, and to the Oxford Uehiro Centre for Practical Ethics. The Foundation's support provides what I believe is a unique and unparalleled research environment that is an ongoing source of inspiration.

As Pierre would say, *The Eagle has Landed.*

Pierre Loebel

Professor J. Pierre Loebel was born in Romania, schooled in Palestine and England, studied philosophy and experimental psychology at Oxford University, followed by medical school in South Africa, and psychiatry at The Bethlem Royal and Maudsley Hospitals, London. Influenced by the teaching and training of Alwyn Lishman,

Michael Shepherd, and Isaac Marks and influenced by their wide-ranging formulations of patients, he acquired his interest in bio-psycho-socially oriented clinical practice. While on the Faculty of the University of Washington, Seattle, School of Medicine, Department of Psychiatry and Behavioral Sciences, and specialized in geriatric psychiatry, he emphasized the use of bps principles in the development of integrated care in Long Term Care institutions. Keeping a multi-authored compilation like this one on course is to the credit of Julian Savulescu, with his assistant Miriam Wood, mine Deborah Logan, and our OUP editors Martin Baum and Janine Fisher who were involved throughout the process. Working with contributors from many countries and time zones presented an unusually challenging task. I also want to thank Julian and the many persons, especially Professors Kenneth Kendler, Steven Hyman, and Essi Viding, who contributed to the Oxford Loebel Lectures and Research Programme from which this book developed, and Nicholas Rawlins who played a vital part in spurring on the project. Valuable inspiration and help were provided by friends and colleagues Nassir Ghaemi and John Wynn, and, in the past, by Professor Alwyn Lishman at the Maudsley Hospital and Institute of Psychiatry in London, and Professor Carl Eisdorfer at the University of Washington, Seattle. Finally, I cannot overstate the value of the support and encouragement received from my wife and our children, Antony, Nicolas, Justine, and Louise.

Contents

Abbreviations

ADHD	attention deficit hyperactivity disorder		GE	gene–environment
			GPI	general paresis of the insane
ALSPAC	Avon Longitudinal Study of Parents and Children		GWA	genome-wide association
			GWAS	genome-wide association study
ASD	autism spectrum disorder		HPA	hypothalamic–pituitary–adrenal
BDT	Bayesian decision theory		IPOMDP	interactive partially observable Markov decision process
BPS	biopsychosocial			
CBPS	constitutive biopsychosocial		LG	licking and grooming
CP/HCU	conduct problems and high levels of callous–unemotional traits		MRI	magnetic resonance imaging
			NIMH	National Institute of Mental Health
CP/LCU	conduct problems and low levels of callous–unemotional traits		NIMHE	National Institute for Mental Health England
CpG	cytosine–guanine dinucleotide		NMDA	N-methyl-D-aspartate
CSIP	Care Services Improvement Partnership		OCS	obsessive–compulsive disorder
			PD	psychotic disorder
CU	callous–unemotional		PE	psychotic experience
DNAm	DNA methylation		PFC	prefrontal cortex
DSM	*Diagnostic and Statistical Manual of Mental Disorders*		POMDP	partially observable Markov decision process
EBPS	explanation biopsychosocial		PTSD	post-traumatic stress disorder
EMP	empirically based pluralism		RDoC	Research Domain Criteria
fMRI	functional magnetic resonance imaging		rGE	gene–environment correlation
			SAD	social anxiety disorder
G×E	gene–environment interactions		US	United States

Contributors

Charlotte A.M. Cecil
Assistant Professor, Department of
Child and Adolescent Psychiatry,
Erasmus Medical Centre, Rotterdam,
Netherlands, and Department of
Psychology, King's College London,
London, UK

Jan Christoph Bublitz
Researcher, University of Hamburg,
Hamburg, Germany

Kathrin Cohen Kadosh
Senior Lecturer in Developmental
Cognitive Neuroscience, School of
Psychology, University of Surrey,
Guildford, UK

Rachel Cooper
Professor of History and Philosophy
of Science, Lancaster University,
Lancaster, UK

Will Davies
Associate Professor and Tutorial Fellow
in Philosophy, St Anne's College,
University of Oxford, Oxford, UK

Peter Dayan
Director, Max Planck Institute for
Biological Cybernetics and Professor,
University of Tübingen, Tübingen,
Germany

K.W.M. (Bill) Fulford
Fellow of St Catherine's College, Member
of the Philosophy Faculty, and Director
of the Collaborating Centre for Values-
based Practice, St Catherine's College,
Oxford, UK, and Emeritus Professor
of Philosophy and Mental Health,
University of Warwick, Coventry, UK

S. Nassir Ghaemi
Professor of Psychiatry, Tufts University
School of Medicine, Boston, MA, USA

Jonathan Glover
Professor of Ethics, King's College
University of London, London, UK, and
Distinguished Research Fellow, Oxford
Uehiro Centre for Practical Ethics,
University of Oxford, Oxford, UK

Christopher Gyngell
Research Fellow, Murdoch Children's
Research Institute, University of
Melbourne, Melbourne, Australia

Simone P.W. Haller
Department of Experimental
Psychology, University of Oxford,
Oxford, UK

Richard Holton
Professor of Philosophy, University of
Cambridge, Cambridge, UK

Steven E. Hyman
Harvard University Distinguished
Service Professor of Stem Cell and
Regenerative Biology, and Director
of the Stanley Center for Psychiatric
Research, Broad Institute of MIT and
Harvard, USA

Kenneth S. Kendler
Professor, Virginia Institute for
Psychiatric and Behavioral Genetics,
Department of Psychiatry, Virginia
Commonwealth University, Richmond,
VA, USA

Neil Levy
Professor of Philosophy, Macquarie
University, Sydney, Australia, and
Senior Research Fellow, Oxford Uehiro
Centre for Practical Ethics, University of
Oxford, Oxford, UK

J. Pierre Loebel
Clinical Professor Emeritus, Psychiatry
and Behavioral Sciences, School of
Medicine, University of Washington,
Seattle, WA, USA

Doug McConnell
Research Fellow, Oxford Uehiro Centre
for Practical Ethics, University of
Oxford, Oxford, UK

Eamon J. McCrory
Professor of Developmental
Neuroscience and Psychopathology,
University College London, London, UK

Matthew Parrott
Associated Professor, University
of Oxford and Fellow and Tutor
in Philosophy, St Hilda's College,
Oxford, UK

Rebecca Roache
Senior Lecturer in Philosophy, Royal
Holloway, University of London,
London, UK

Jonathan P. Roiser
Professor of Neuroscience and
Mental Health, Institute of Cognitive
Neuroscience, University College
London, London, UK

Julian Savulescu
Uehiro Chair in Practical Ethics,
University of Oxford, Oxford, UK

Walter Sinnott-Armstrong
Stillman Professor of Philosophy, Duke
University, Durham, NC, USA

Graeme C. Smith
Emeritus Professor of Psychiatry,
Monash University, Clayton, Victoria,
Australia

Jesse S. Summers
Academic Dean and Department of
Philosophy, Duke University, Durham,
NC, USA

Tim Thornton
Professor of Philosophy and Mental
Health, University of Central Lancashire,
Preston, UK

Essi Viding
Professor of Developmental
Psychopathology, Division of Psychology
& Language Sciences, University College
London, London, UK

Part 1

Introduction

Chapter 1

Introduction

J. Pierre Loebel and Julian Savulescu

Introduction

Psychiatry suffers from the lack of a unifying theory. Psychiatrists are physicians with specialist training in mental illness. However, no generally accepted theory of mental illness exists, in part because there is little agreement on what the concepts 'mental' and 'illness' entail. Lacking such a theory, the profession has experienced internal divisiveness (Clare, 1976), uncertainty among applicants for training (Choudry and Farooq, 2017), and attacks from outside (Szasz, 1984). Since the decline of nineteenth- and twentieth-century paradigms (psychoanalysis, behaviourism), psychiatrists have been in search of one that acknowledges what is universally recognized, that is, that human beings function in a nexus comprising the psyche, the soma, and the social surround, and that each domain requires consideration when drawing up a psychiatric formulation and treatment plan. The biopsychosocial (BPS) paradigm proposed by George L. Engel (Engel, 1977) was adopted without much enquiry into details. Challenges force advocates into the embarrassing position of having to acknowledge that modern psychiatry is operating in a theoretical vacuum (McLaren, 2002) (or what has been referred to as an absence of 'an overarching conceptual framework' (Kendler, 2012b)). Another outcome has been fragmentation of professional orientation (Gabbard and Kay, 2001) such that some clinicians subscribe primarily to the psychoanalytic model of the mind, its discontents and disorders; others to a neuropsychopharmacological one; while many march to the uneasy eclecticism of the BPS model. This has been challenged vigorously (Ghaemi, 2010, Chapter 20, this volume) for its philosophical difficulties and lack of diagnostic (nosological) and prescriptive (therapeutic) power. In its weak form, BPS does not justify the term 'model', being merely a simplistic reference to the fact that the three domains should each be considered when constructing a formulation and treatment plan.

This book, however, presents a nascent, stronger version of the concept based on a growing body of genetic, epigenetic, and other evidence that encompasses a central, overlapping component to the Venn diagram description of the BPS conceptualization. To adapt an aphorism (Stein, n.d.), there *is* a there there. Want of evidence about the mechanisms of interaction between the bio-, psycho-, and the social realms is being replaced by discoveries of the relationships between psychiatric disorders and genetic factors, life events, and rearing (Caspi et al., 2003; Nemeroff, 2016; Kendler et al., 2018); how to characterize mental illness in BPS terms (Kendler, 2012a); the neurochemical and anatomical changes that occur during psychotherapy (Cozolino,

2002); and how experience alters neurotransmitters during learning and memory functions (Kandel, 1998).

While the biomedical approach will always continue to be useful, philosophical difficulties are addressed (Davies and Roache, 2017; Roache, Chapter 2, this volume) and the mechanisms elucidated of the interactions between the domains envisaged in the BPS concept (Kendler et al., 2005; Viding, Chapter 10, this volume). As important is the need 'to adopt and maintain a personal perspective while tending to presumed brain function … [T]he challenge for psychiatry is to embrace the advancing views provided by neurobiology … while resisting the temptation to trivialize the role of human interpersonal engagement and an interpersonal perspective in the clinical encounter' (Hyman and McConnell, Chapter 17, p. 269, this volume).

Other contributors expand the field by finding room in the BPS conceptualization for a values component (Fulford, Chapter 8, this volume) and a discussion of formulation (Smith, Chapter 9, this volume) that references diagnosis and the *Diagnostic and Statistical Manual of Mental Disorders* (American Psychiatric Association, 2013), resistance and resilience, propensity and vulnerability, risk factors, and the potential not only of recovering from an ailment but the attainment of wellness (Bolton, Chapter 13, this volume).

As such, the BPS approach serves Hippocrates' aphoristic injunction 'to understand not only the illness the patient has, but the patient the disease has'. Early explorers and cartographers wrote that beyond the margins of their discoveries 'Here Be Dragons'. The contributors to this book shed light on the dragons of psychic function with the result that no apologies need any longer to be made for seeking BPS conceptualization which now gains the heuristic and clinical traction that has been lacking. Practitioners marching under the BPS banner can have increasing confidence that they may now apply a combinatorial approach that looks at 'causes, mechanisms, consequences and the most-likely-useful interventions' (J. Wynn, personal communication) in the confidence that this stems from an evidence-based, scientific underpinning. This book provides the multifaceted foundation for a comprehensive, modern psychiatry that until now has been a slogan 'more honoured in the breach than the observance' (Shakespeare, 1604).

References

American Psychiatric Association (2013). *Diagnostic and Statistical Manual of Mental Disorders*, 5th ed. Washington, DC: American Psychiatric Association.

Caspi, A., Sugden, K., Moffitt, T.E., Taylor, A., Craig, I.W., Harrington, H., McClay, J., Mill, J., Martin, J., Braithwaite, A., and Poulton, R. (2003). Influence of life stress on depression: moderation by a polymorphism in the 5-HTT gene. *Science*, **301**(5631), 386–389.

Choudry, A. and Farooq, S. (2017). Systematic review into factors associated with the recruitment crisis in psychiatry in the UK: students' trainees and consultants' views. *British Journal of Psychiatry Bulletin*, **41**(6), 345–352.

Clare, A. (1976). *Psychiatry in Dissent*. London: Tavistock Publications.

Cozolino, L. (2002). *The Neuroscience of Psychotherapy: Building and Rebuilding the Human Brain*. New York: W.W. Norton and Co.

Davies, W. and **Roache, R.** (2017). Reassessing biopsychosocial psychiatry. *British Journal of Psychiatry*, **210**(1), 3–5.

Engel, G. (1977). The need for a new medical model: a challenge for biomedicine. *Science*, **196**(4), 129–136.

Gabbard, G. and **Kay, J.** (2001). The fate of integrated treatment: whatever happened to the biopsychosocial psychiatrist? *American Journal of Psychiatry*, **158**(12), 1956–1963.

Ghaemi, S. (2010). *The Rise and Fall of the Biopsychosocial Model*. Baltimore, MD: Johns Hopkins University Press.

Kandel, E. (1998). A new intellectual framework for psychiatry. *American Journal of Psychiatry*, **155**(4) 457–469.

Kendler, K. (2012a). Levels of explanation in psychiatric and substance use disorders: implications for the development of an etiologically based nosology. *Molecular Psychiatry*, **17**(1), 11–21.

Kendler, K. (2012b). The dappled nature of causes of psychiatric illness: replacing the organic-functional/hardware dichotomy with empirically based pluralism. *Molecular Psychiatry*, **17**(4), 377–388.

Kendler, K., **Kuhn, J.W.**, **Vittum, J.**, **Prescott, C.A.**, and **Riley, B.** (2005). The interaction of stressful life events and a serotonin transporter polymorphism in the prediction of episodes of major depression. *Archives of General Psychiatry*, **62**(5), 529–535.

Kendler, K., **Ohlsson, H.**, **Sundquist, K.**, and **Sundquist, J.** (2018). Sources of parent-offspring resemblance for major depression in a national Swedish extended adoption study. *JAMA Psychiatry*, **75**(2), 194–200.

McLaren, N. (2002). The myth of the biopsychosocial model. *The Australian and New Zealand Journal of Psychiatry*, **36**(5), 701–703.

Nemeroff, C. (2016). Paradise lost: the neurobiological and clinical consequences of child abuse and neglect. *Neuron*, **89**(5), 892–909.

Shakespeare, W. (1604). *Hamlet*. Act 1:4.

Stein, G. (n.d.). Whenever you get there, there is no there there. Goodreads. https://www.goodreads.com/quotes/339785-whenever-you-get-there-there-is-no-there-there. Accessed 26 November 2018.

Szasz, T. (1984). *The Myth of Mental Illness*. New York: Harper.

Chapter 2

The biopsychosocial model in psychiatry: Engel and beyond

Rebecca Roache

Introduction

Psychiatry uncomfortably spans biological and psychosocial perspectives on mental illness. As a branch of medicine, psychiatry is under pressure to conform to a biomedical model, according to which diseases are characterized primarily in biological terms (e.g. genetic influence, molecular changes in the body's organs, abnormalities detectable via blood tests, magnetic resonance imaging scans, etc.). As well as being a branch of medicine, however, contemporary psychiatry draws on psychotherapeutic approaches—particularly, at least in the US, on the psychoanalytic tradition—which make no reference to the biological underpinnings of mental life. Instead, they explain patients' mental distress in terms of life experience.

These different approaches ought to inform and complement each other—after all, each aims at understanding the mind, and each contributes something unique and important to this understanding. However, historically, this has not happened. With no theory creating global, systematic links between the two approaches, psychiatry is divided between those clinicians who adopt a psychotherapeutic perspective; those who take a biomedical approach by conceiving mental illness in terms of somatic disorder, on a par with the rest of medicine; and those who subscribe to the eclecticism of the *biopsychosocial* approach. The latter often involves little more than an acknowledgement that biological, psychological, and social factors are all relevant to understanding mental illness. It does not give guidelines for how these factors should be combined, nor for how to formulate and understand explanations of mental illness that refer to biological, psychological, and social factors. It has been criticized both for failing to specify how mental illnesses may be diagnosed and characterized in biopsychosocial terms and for failing to provide directions for treatment (McLaren, 2006, 2007; Ghaemi, 2009, 2010).

Psychiatry's tripartite division—between biomedical approaches, psychotherapeutic approaches, and 'eclectic' approaches that try to combine elements of both—is not a recent phenomenon. S. Nassir Ghaemi remarks that it is a common (if overly simplistic) view that 'nineteenth-century European psychiatry was predominantly biological and twentieth-century American psychiatry was mostly psychoanalytic, and now the pendulum is swinging back in the biological direction' (Ghaemi, 2010, p. 3). Even in recent years, adherents to each approach have had a variety of motivations: the biomedical approach, for example, was supported by behaviourism in the early twentieth century, by advances in psychopharmacology around the mid-twentieth century, and by the more recent rise of neuroscience from the end of the century. What emerges from this picture is that psychiatrists are yet to find a way to slot together the biological, the psychological, and the social contributors to mental illness. They are yet to agree on how these three perspectives combine and relate to produce mental illness. What is still needed in psychiatry is a conceptual scaffolding: a way of arranging these different perspectives on mental illness in order to enhance understanding and effective treatment of it.

History

The term 'biopsychosocial' is most strongly associated with George Engel, whose most famous article on the biopsychosocial model was published in 1977. The origins of the term are somewhat unclear: Ghaemi claims it was coined by Roy Grinker in a 1954 lecture (unpublished until decades later (Grinker, 1994)), yet Edward Shorter notes that Engel spoke of interactions between biological, psychological, and social levels as early as 1951 (Shorter, 2005). Grinker was less ambitious than Engel about the scope and relevance of a biopsychosocial approach, and most contemporary discussion of the biopsychosocial model focuses on Engel. I, too, will focus mainly on Engel, returning to consider Grinker's position towards the end of this chapter.

Engel was an internist who was strongly influenced by, and trained in, psychoanalysis. Historically, Engel's views on the importance of a biopsychosocial approach drew on a holistic approach that can be traced back to Hippocrates; on the patient-centred approach to treatment popularized by Adolf Meyer (1917); and on the influence of William Osler, who is quoted as saying, 'The good physician treats the disease but the great physician treats the patient who has the disease' (Shorter, 2005, p. 3). Engel (1977) drew upon general systems theory—according to which the various 'levels' of conceptualizing illness (biological, psychological, social) form a hierarchy with some laws and principles applying only within a level and others applying to the system as a whole—to envisage a holistic way of understanding and scientifically studying the mind, and of conceptualizing patients and their treatment. It is this approach that he termed the biopsychosocial model, and he argued that it should be adopted not only by psychiatry, but by medicine in general. Here, however, we focus on the biopsychosocial model in the context of psychiatry.[1]

In one sense, the idea that we should take a biopsychosocial approach to understanding mental illness is so obvious as to be trivial: of course a patient's condition can be influenced by biological, psychological, and social factors. As Edward Shorter remarks in his historical account of the biopsychosocial model:

> It has always been apparent to physicians, in an insight that different generations gain in their own ways, that the body, the patient's personal history, and their current social circumstances all play a role in the pathogenesis of illness and in the patient's interpretation

---

[1] The wider historical motivations of Engel's view will not be explored here. For more, see Pilgrim (2002), Shorter (2005), and Ghaemi (2010).

> of their symptoms. This is the implicit biopsychosocial model: the recognition that ma-
> terial lesions, life experiences, and current social situation all matter in the presentation of
> illness; they influence what the physician sees in the consulting room. ... Holistic concepts
> go back to Hippocrates and these Hippocratic notions represent an implicit recognition
> of what much later generations would begin to articulate as 'models'. (Shorter, 2005, p. 2)

What more, then, does the biopsychosocial model add to the uncontroversial acknowledgement that biological, psychological, and social factors all have roles to play
in 'what the physician sees in the consulting room'? One plausible answer is that, in
advancing the model, Engel aimed to make explicit how the biological, the psychological, and the social all had a place in conceptualizing mental disorder, and to systematize and enshrine this recognition in the way in which psychiatry is practised.
Engel was, after all, writing in the wake of a division in psychiatry, to which he was
responding. On the one hand, there was the 'exclusionist' view of Thomas Szasz, who
argued that mental disorder—given its lack of basis in biological pathology—is not
really disease in the sense that somatic (i.e. non-psychiatric) disease is, and that so-
called mental illness should be reclassified as 'problems of living', and treated outside
of medicine (Szasz, 1960, 1961). On the other hand was what Engel called the 'medical
model': the reductionist view that mental illness should be conceived as brain dysfunction; that is, as somatic disease. Any purported mental illness that cannot be so
reduced and conceived should not, according to the medical model, be the concern
of the medical subdiscipline of psychiatry. This reductionist view was advanced in
Arnold Ludwig's 1975 paper, 'The psychiatrist as physician'.

A common strand to both the exclusionist view and the medical model was the idea
that all disease must be understood in *biological* terms: any condition that cannot be
characterized in such terms has no place in medicine. Engel explicitly acknowledged
this division in psychiatry. His argument for the biopsychosocial model proceeded
first by demonstrating that the 'biology only' view of psychiatry and of medicine is
inadequate, and then by demonstrating how psychosocial factors can be incorporated into psychiatry and medicine in order to improve it. As we have seen, critics of
the biopsychosocial model are not convinced by the second step in Engel's argument.
Engel does not, for example, set out in detail *how* the three perspectives—biological,
psychological, and social—should be combined to improve psychiatry. In addition,
while Engel initially conceives the biopsychosocial model as a scientific model for the
study of mental illness that is comparable to a Kuhnian paradigm,[2] he goes on to describe it as much more than this; as something more akin to a way of life. He writes,
for example, of the model's relevance in understanding the different social roles of the
patient and the physician (Engel, 1977, p. 132), and the diverse social roles of different
medical staff (1978, p. 160); and he argues (speculatively) that conceptualizing patients
in biopsychosocial terms—by attending to their fears and expectations, for example,
rather than merely their biological symptoms—will lead to better patient outcomes
(1978, 1980). Ghaemi has criticized Engel's approach, arguing that its holistic, patient-
centred aspects are not novel, and can be found in Osler's medical humanist approach.

---

[2] See, especially, Engel (1977, p. 130).

Ghaemi observes, moreover, that one can acknowledge the relevance of biological, psychological, and social perspectives without thereby endorsing Engel's biopsychosocial model; Ghaemi himself argues that these perspectives are better combined in an approach, inspired by Karl Jaspers, whereby psychiatrists engage in reflection on the methods they use and why they use them. Ghaemi calls this approach 'methodological consciousness' (Ghaemi, 2009, 2010).

We can argue about what sort of view Engel was advancing with his biopsychosocial model, and about the extent to which acknowledging the importance of biological, psychological, and social factors commits one to Engel's view or is compatible with some other approach. Addressing such conceptual issues is a task for another paper, however. Here, I wish to survey some of the evidence for the relevance of biological, psychological, and social perspectives on mental illness, and to consider what they tell us about the manner and the extent to which psychiatry should be biopsychosocial. Since I propose to set aside conceptual questions relating to how the biopsychosocial model should best be conceived, I will dispense with the term 'model' and write instead of a biopsychosocial *approach*. Adopting a biopsychosocial approach to psychiatry involves acknowledging the relevance of biological, psychological, and social factors to understanding and treating mental illness, yet it need not commit one to endorsing the biopsychosocial model, nor to endorsing any particular account of how that model should be conceived.

The relevance of empirical research

Empirical studies that elucidate, in various ways, why our minds work the way they do are peppered with references to biopsychosocial interactions: to psychological outcomes of biological events, to social and biological factors combining to produce psychosocial outcomes, to the biological underpinnings of psychological processes, and so on. Advocates of a biopsychosocial approach to psychiatry may view such empirical work as evidence of the value of this approach. But how, exactly, do such studies illustrate the value of a biopsychosocial approach? In the following paragraphs, I divide empirical studies that identify biological, psychological, and social contributors to mental illness and its treatment into two rough categories, corresponding to two ways in which attending to a full range of biopsychosocial considerations in empirical work enhances the way in which mental illness is understood and treated. These categories are not mutually exclusive; indeed, it may be that the studies mentioned have something to add to each category.

The first category contains studies that *enhance our understanding of how and why mental disorders arise*. It often happens that a comprehensive causal explanation of mental disorders refers to a combination of biological, psychological, and social considerations. This should be unsurprising: as persons, we have psychological experiences and are involved in social relations, yet we are also biological systems. Given that mental disorders are characterized in terms of their psychosocial features (see Broome and Bortolotti (2009) for more on this), which in turn are realized in our biology, attending to biological, psychological, and social considerations is prudent if we wish to maximize our understanding of the aetiology of mental disorders.

One of the most famous examples of an empirical study that considers a combination of biopsychosocial features to enhance our understanding of the mind is Eric Kandel's Nobel Prize-winning work to explain how the brain changes at the cellular molecular level (that is, biologically) when we remember (that is, when we undergo a psychological change) (Kandel, 2001). Kandel, a psychiatrist trained in the psychoanalytic tradition, reports that he became interested in studying the biology of memory as a result of coming to feel that the psychoanalytic approach was 'limiting because it tended to treat the brain, the organ that generates behaviour, as a black box' (Kandel, 2001, p. 1030). He goes on to explain that studying memory from both psychological and biological perspectives might yield insights not available when studying memory from either perspective alone:

> My purpose in translating questions about the psychology of learning into the empirical language of biology was not to replace the logic of psychology or psychoanalysis with the logic of cellular molecular biology, but to try to join these two disciplines and to contribute to a new synthesis that would combine the mentalistic psychology of memory storage with the biology of neuronal signaling. I hoped further that the biological analysis of memory might carry with it an extra bonus, that the study of memory storage might reveal new aspects of neuronal signaling. Indeed, this has proven true. (Kandel, 2001, p. 1030)

Kandel, then, notes that memory is a process with both psychological and biological aspects, and hypothesizes that studying its psychological aspects together with its biological ones, along with the interactions between these, will enhance our understanding beyond that which can be gleaned from studying either aspect in isolation. This is a lesson that advocates of a biopsychosocial approach to psychiatry might argue could be applied more widely: people, their minds, and their mental disorders, are biopsychosocial, and so studying their biological, psychological, and social aspects together may reveal more than the sum of studying any one of these aspects in isolation.

The importance of this lesson is illustrated by a famous study that takes a biopsychosocial approach to explaining the aetiology of mental disorder. Avshalom Caspi and his colleagues showed that childhood maltreatment combined with a certain genotype (that is, a psychosocial phenomenon combined with a biological feature) predisposes males to antisocial behaviour in adulthood. Prior to this work, it was known that '[a]lthough maltreatment increases the risk of later criminality by about 50%, most maltreated children do not become delinquents or adult criminals' (Caspi et al., 2002, p. 851). The results of Caspi and colleagues' study 'may partly explain why not all victims of maltreatment grow up to victimize others, and they provide epidemiological evidence that genotypes can moderate children's sensitivity to environmental insults' (Caspi et al., 2002, p. 851). The psychosocial insight with which Caspi began—viz. that childhood maltreatment increases the risk of later criminality—tells us only part of the story about the link between maltreatment and criminality. Far more of the story emerges when we also consider relevant biological factors, because considering these factors enables us to identify the subgroup in which the effect is seen: it is not merely that childhood maltreatment increases the risk of later criminality, but that childhood maltreatment *given a particular genotype* increases the risk of later criminality. Caspi and colleagues' work shows us that, in attempting to understand the aetiology of mental illness, we risk missing important insights by considering only parts of the biopsychosocial picture.

A third example of empirical work that falls within the first category is that of Charles Nemeroff and Wylie Vale. Their work follows the same format as that of Caspi and colleagues in that it shows how genetic and psychosocial factors combine to increase the risk of mental disorder. Nemeroff and Vale begin with the observation that it is widely accepted that depression results from a combination of genetic factors and stressful experiences. They go on to identify the specific neurobiological mechanisms by which stressful experiences cause depression. Throughout their paper, they emphasize the relevance of these observations for the development of treatments, and they conclude with the following remarks:

> Clearly, this work contributes to the identification of sub-populations of neurobiologically distinct forms of depression, which will likely lead to prediction of treatment response, reduced heterogeneity of study populations in clinical trials, and identification of a novel class or classes of antidepressants and anxiolytics. This is necessary because current rates of response (55% to 65%) and remission (35% to 50%) after 8 to 10 weeks of treatment with SSRIs or related antidepressants are unacceptably low. (Nemeroff and Vale, 2005, p. 12)

These comments from Nemeroff and Vale highlight an important point about psychiatry, which is worth bearing in mind as we consider the merits of a biopsychosocial approach. Psychiatry is a goal-directed discipline; it aims to prevent, cure, or manage mental disorders. Efforts to understand the aetiology of mental processes and mental disorders are important to psychiatrists only in so far as they help them achieve this goal. If we were to discover an obscure plant that, when eaten, could cure every type of mental disorder without any adverse side effects, then there would no longer be any need for psychiatrists to try to understand how and why mental disorders arise. (Indeed, if this plant could be made abundant and easily accessible, the skills of the psychiatrist would be rendered wholly obsolete.) In the absence of such a shortcut to successful treatment, however, attempting to understand how and why mental disorders arise remains our best chance of finding out how to treat them successfully.

The studies just mentioned in connection with the first category, and others like them, demonstrate that a biopsychosocial approach is important for achieving such understanding. The lesson from these studies can be that, in attempting to uncover the aetiology of mental disorders, we should be alert to the possibility that this aetiology may be spread over biological, psychological, and social categories. Kenneth Kendler, drawing on Nancy Cartwright's terminology, has made precisely this point in noting that the causes of psychiatric disorders are *dappled* (Kendler, 2012).

Uncovering the dappled aetiology of mental illness does not only help us learn more about the mental disorders that we have already identified. Sometimes, a multilevel understanding of mental disorders facilitates new, more nuanced distinctions between different disorders, or between their different subtypes. We saw, in the remarks quoted earlier, that Nemeroff and Vale take their work to help enable 'the identification of sub-populations of neurobiologically distinct forms of depression', which in turn would enable a more tailored, targeted approach to studying and treating these different forms. As a result, while depression (like other mental disorders) is diagnosed on the basis of psychosocial considerations, such as the patient's subjective experiences and clinical observation, in the future the subtype of depression could then be specified with reference to biological considerations.

In a similar vein, Oliver Howes and Shitij Kapur propose a new classification of schizophrenia into two subtypes, depending on whether or not the patient's symptoms can be attributed to abnormally high levels of dopamine. Howes and Kapur outline the advantages of attending to biological considerations in addition to psychosocial ones when reclassifying schizophrenia:

> The proposed subtyping has several potential advantages over the current phenomenological classification or the move to dimensions. First, it is based on a neurobiological mechanism with implications for treatment choice—and thus can unite academic classification and clinical utility. Second, it has clear implications for treatment: type A (hyperdopaminergic) schizophrenia will respond to dopamine-blocking drugs, whereas type B, where there is no elevation in dopamine, will not. Third, by focusing on mechanisms over phenomenology it provides a sound basis for research that has the potential to lead to new treatment options. For example, research into type B could potentially identify new targets that would be effective for patients whose illness responds poorly to current antipsychotics, offering better-tolerated alternatives to clozapine, the only drug currently licensed for this indication. Fourth, it could lead to tests that guide treatment choice at illness onset—this could enable type B patients, who we predict will not respond to conventional antipsychotics, to be fast-tracked to clozapine or new treatments as they emerge. … This has the potential to greatly improve treatment[.] (Howes and Kapur, 2014, p. 2)

To summarize, then, the first category of empirical studies that identify biological, psychological, and social aspects of mental illness comprises those that highlight the value of a biopsychosocial approach to psychiatry by enhancing our understanding of how and why mental disorders arise. These studies do this by detailing the dappled biopsychosocial aetiology of mental disorders, and sometimes also by enabling us to identify subtypes of mental disorders according to their distinct biological aetiologies.

Whereas studies in the first category elucidate the aetiology of mental disorders, the second category contains studies that *enhance our understanding of how mental disorders are best treated*. It is important to separate questions about the relevance of a biopsychosocial approach to *understanding* mental disorders from questions about the relevance of a biopsychosocial approach to *treating* mental disorders. The importance of separating these two sets of questions can be illustrated by considering the possibility that there may be some mental disorders whose aetiology can only be fully understood by attending to a complicated interplay of biological, psychological, and social considerations, yet which can be treated with a relatively simple, 'single level' intervention. This might be the case if it were discovered that depression—a condition that, as Nemeroff and Vale demonstrate, can arise from a range of complex biopsychosocial interactions—could be successfully treated with a new type of brain surgery; that is, with a biological intervention. ('Biological' in that it acts directly on the brain, rather than via the patient's psychological experiences and/or social interactions.) In such a case, while a biopsychosocial approach might be important to *understanding* depression, it would not be relevant at all to *treating* depression once the successful treatment has been identified.

Studies that enhance our understanding of how mental disorders are best treated include the work of Julian Leff and colleagues, who showed that the social environment of schizophrenics who are in remission and on neuroleptic drugs has a direct effect on relapse rates (Leff et al., 1982, 1985). Specifically, they found that '[r]elapse of schizophrenia is more likely if patients live with relatives who are excessively critical and/or over-involved. Such relatives are designated as high EE ["expressed emotion"]' (Leff et al., 1982, p. 121). Leff and colleagues discovered, moreover, that relapse rates could be significantly reduced via a programme of social interventions aimed at reducing the relatives' EE and/or reducing patients' social contact with the EE relatives. Here, then, is an example of a study that identifies psychosocial factors that undermine the effectiveness of schizophrenic patients' biological treatment (that is, their drugs), and recommends psychosocial measures to promote recovery.

Other work that takes a biopsychosocial approach to evaluating treatment options includes a review by Shanaya Rathod and colleagues of the effectiveness of cognitive behavioural therapy at managing medication-resistant symptoms in schizophrenics who are also taking antipsychotic medication (Rathod et al., 2008); Shaila Misri and colleagues' assessment of biopsychosocial factors affecting the success of treatment of mood and anxiety disorders in postpartum women (Misri et al., 2012); and Gerald Hogarty and colleagues' findings that whether or not personal therapy promotes positive outcomes for schizophrenics depends on whether or not patients live with family (Hogarty et al., 1997a, 1997b).

A more general investigation into the effectiveness of different treatment methods along the biopsychosocial spectrum is conducted by Glen Gabbard and Jerald Kay. They consider whether combining psychotherapy with pharmacotherapy—that is, a psychosocial intervention with a biological intervention—is more effective than either therapy alone. They note that, while it often is more effective to combine treatments, further research is needed to answer some important questions, such as:

> When should psychotherapy precede medication? When should it be added to pre-existing pharmacotherapy? Are some forms of psychotherapy more effective for understanding compliance problems [i.e. patients failing to take prescribed medication]? Is it possible that some forms of psychotherapy work better with specific medications than others? What are the limits of brief integrated treatment? Is the one-person or two-person treatment model [i.e. patient receives psychotherapy and pharmacotherapy from one person versus two people] more cost-effective in the long run? Does the fragmentation in the two-person treatment model lead to adverse outcomes more often than the one-person model? Are there different outcomes in treatment if the meaning of medications is addressed versus ignored? (Gabbard and Kay, 2001, p. 1961)

This approach by Gabbard and Kay illustrates that, in seeking the best treatment plans for patients, psychiatrists must be guided—other things being equal—by which plans produce the best outcomes in terms of increasing patient well-being.[3] This approach is

---

[3] 'Other things being equal' because issues such as cost, scarcity of resources, feasibility, etc. will also be relevant to decisions about treatment plans.

reflected in the other studies mentioned here too: the best treatment approach is the one that produces the best results, regardless of the extent to which it is fully biopsychosocial.

What lessons do studies in the second category have for advocates of the biopsychosocial approach? They reveal that—like the authors of the studies cited in this category—it is important to remain open to the possibility that the success of treatment plans for mental disorders may be determined by a mixture of biological, psychological, and social factors. Having explored these possibilities, we can choose treatments that, according to the available evidence, will promote the best outcomes. The best outcome may be one that works through a biological mechanism (e.g. drugs, surgery) alone, a psychological mechanism (e.g. psychotherapy) alone, a social mechanism (e.g. changes to a patient's living conditions) alone, or any combination of these. Commitment to a biopsychosocial approach, then, should not involve dogmatic insistence that any treatment intervention should incorporate a biological, psychological, and social aspect. As such, a biopsychosocial approach is relevant to the search for the best treatment, in that it reminds us to consider all possible options, but it is not relevant to the treatment itself, once the best treatment has been identified.

Biopsychosocial psychiatry, then and now

In the previous section, I outlined some ways in which empirical studies underline the importance of a biopsychosocial approach to psychiatry. I argued that a biopsychosocial approach is relevant for two main reasons. First, it reminds us that, in attempting to understand mental illness, we should bear in mind that the *causes* of mental illness may be a combination of biological, psychological, and social. Neglecting any one of these perspectives may result in our neglecting important aspects of a disorder's aetiology. Second, it reminds us that in comparing and evaluating *treatment* plans, we may have available biological, psychological, and social options for intervention. To produce the best results, we should compare these and—other things being equal—choose the one that promotes the best outcome in terms of patient well-being.

These observations should be unsurprising. That we should consider biological, psychological, and social aspects when trying to understand a patient's condition, and when deciding upon the best treatment, is not a controversial or outlandish proposal. After all, in trying to understand everyday, familiar, non-psychiatric behaviour, and in considering how to respond to it, we frequently consider biological, psychological, and social options. Imagine, for example, that I am slightly late for a lunch date with a friend, and that when I arrive she is very annoyed with me—*disproportionately* annoyed, it seems to me. How might I explain her behaviour? Well, I can take into account that people prefer their friends to be reliable, and that being kept waiting makes people annoyed. These observations go some way to explaining my friend's annoyance, but they do not explain why she is *disproportionately* annoyed. In order to explain that, I might entertain various hypotheses, such as the psychological explanation that perhaps she has had a stressful morning, or the social explanation that perhaps she has some additional reason for being annoyed with me, or the biological explanation that—since I know that my friend is diabetic and sometimes skips breakfast—perhaps low blood sugar has made her irritable. It could be that *all* of these explanations are correct. Ignoring any one of them will result in my having only a partial understanding of her behaviour. Note, moreover, that the fact that my friend's behaviour has a fully biopsychosocial explanation—that is, an explanation that makes reference to biological, psychological, *and* social factors—does not itself tell me how I might best respond to it. Perhaps my friend will be most effectively placated by eating something, or by my apologizing for my lateness, or by my sympathizing with her about her stressful morning, or by a combination of all of these. It may not be clear which of these is the best option, but what does seem clear is that none of them can antecedently be ruled out as obviously less promising than the others.

In other words, then, even in an everyday, familiar sort of scenario like the one just described, ignoring any part of the biopsychosocial spectrum would lead to an impoverished understanding of the subject's condition; moreover, even with a fully biopsychosocial understanding of the subject's (undesirable) condition, it may not be obvious how—that is, whether by biological, psychological, or social means, or a combination of these, or by something else entirely—that condition might best be alleviated. Taking a biopsychosocial approach to understanding and responding to my friend's behaviour, in this scenario, amounts simply to an acknowledgement of these observations. And, given that a biopsychosocial approach seems sensible and prudent in the scenario I have just described—indeed, it reflects the way in which we generally do try to make sense of, and respond to, other people's behaviour—we might view it as the natural starting point for trying to make sense of, and respond to, the far more complex behaviour that arises from mental disorder.

In considering what recent empirical research into mental illness tells us about the relevance of attending to biological, psychological, and social factors, what I have described is *a* biopsychosocial approach to psychiatry. How does this compare to *the* biopsychosocial model described by Engel? Well, it seems that Engel's view changed over time. In his 1977 paper he remarks that '[w]hether [the biopsychosocial model] is useful or not remains to be seen' (Engel, 1977, p. 135), which suggests that he took the merits of the biopsychosocial model to depend on the evidence. By contrast, in his later work (Engel, 1978, 1980) he argues on speculative, a priori grounds that adopting the biopsychosocial model is preferable to adopting the biomedical model. This latter approach was, in Kendler's terminology, 'a priori—driven by a theoretical commitment to pluralism' (Kendler, 2012, p. 383).

In part, Engel's conception of the biopsychosocial model resembled a Kuhnian paradigm. In the 1977 paper in which he introduced the model, Engel tells us that 'a model is nothing more than a belief system utilized to explain natural phenomena, to make sense out of what is puzzling or disturbing'. A *scientific* model, in addition, 'involve[s] a shared set of assumptions and rules of conduct based on the scientific method and constitute[s] a blueprint for research' (Engel, 1977, p. 130). The biopsychosocial model is, according to Engel, a scientific model, as is the competing biomedical model which views disease as 'fully accounted for by deviations from the norm of measurable biological (somatic) variables' (Engel, 1977, p. 130); and his conception of scientific models is close to Kuhn's conception of paradigms.

Yet Engel also viewed the biopsychosocial model as more than a Kuhnian scientific paradigm. Drawing on the language of sociology, in places he seems to be proposing the model as a medical world view, or as a way of life for medical staff: he writes that the model is a 'blueprint for research, a framework for teaching, and a design for action in the real world of health care' (Engel, 1977, p. 135). Not only does he recognize that patient outcomes depend partly on the relationship between the patient and medical staff, he also expresses views about what sorts of behaviours by medical staff will improve patient outcomes. Referring to both psychiatric and somatic treatment, he writes:

> [T]he physician's role is, and always has been, very much that of educator and psychotherapist. To know how to induce peace of mind in the patient and enhance his faith in the healing powers of his physician requires psychological knowledge and skills, not merely charisma. (Engel, 1977, p. 132)

In a later paper, he argued that the often antagonistic roles adopted by doctors, nurses, and other health professionals according to the biomedical model fail to maximize patient outcomes, and he called for a reconceptualization of these roles:

> But the care of the sick calls for collaboration and smooth interaction between professionals, with complementary roles to fulfil and tasks to perform. This is impossible as long as the dominant model is one which philosophically denies the application of science to the care of the patient, places science and humanism in opposition, and divides health professionals into a 'superior' group who treat disease and a 'lesser' breed who care for the sick. (Engel, 1978, p. 160)

Engel took the biopsychosocial model to provide the key to a better way of doing things. He described an example of a cardiac patient who was treated (Engel tells us) according to the biomedical model. He argued that this approach exacerbated the patient's symptoms, whereas a biopsychosocial approach would have ensured an improved outcome. He remarks that:

> It is hoped the example ... will indicate how adoption of a biopsychosocial model can contribute to the unity of the health professions and render collaboration, communication, and complementarity a reality rather than mere sloganeering. Through sharing basic knowledge and a common way of looking at Man, from the organisation of his body to the determinants of his behaviour to the social structures of which he is an integral part, health professionals would have in common the languages essential for communication and cooperation and for the complementarity inherent in the need for the special knowledge and skills required for the many varied activities involved in providing high-level health care. (Engel, 1978, p. 164)

Engel's commitment in his 1978 paper to a global, way-of-life sort of biopsychosocial approach may strike us as unpalatably evangelical, yet it has to some extent made its way into mainstream medical and psychiatric practice in the guise of so-called biopsychosocial history forms: checklists that are used by medical professionals to help them ensure they have considered all relevant aspects of a patient's history.

When the biopsychosocial model is criticized, criticism generally targets the more sweeping claims made by Engel. For example, Ghaemi, who has perhaps been the model's most vocal critic, writes:

> The model's claim, in the words of its founder Engel, is that 'all three levels, biological, psychological, and social, must be taken into account in every health care task'. No single

illness, patient or condition can be reduced to any one aspect. They are all, more or less equally, relevant, in all cases, at all times. (Ghaemi, 2009, p. 3, quoting Engel, 1978)

In essence, Ghaemi's view is that those aspects of Engel's biopsychosocial model that are plausible and sensible are not original—Engel's view that psychiatrists should consider different perspectives can be found in Jaspers' work, while his emphasis on holism and attending to the person rather than merely to the disease reflects Osler's medical humanism—and the rest is implausible and should be rejected. Let us consider his reasons for rejecting the biopsychosocial model.

Ghaemi ascribes to Engel an implausible view that he terms 'additive eclecticism':

> The basic idea is that 'more is better': truth is achieved by adding more and more perspectives, getting closer and closer to a highly complex reality. This is common sense, perhaps, but not scientific sense. Reductionism is not always wrong; peptic ulcer disease, long considered a classic psychosomatic illness, proves to be caused by *Helicobacter pylori*. In a hallmark of science, the apparently complex proved to be simple. (Ghaemi, 2009, p. 4)

One might defend the biopsychosocial model against this criticism of Ghaemi's by remarking that while it may not be the case that truth is achieved by *adding* more and more perspectives—after all, sometimes certain perspectives turn out to be irrelevant, as Ghaemi notes—it may nevertheless be the case that truth is achieved by *considering* more and more perspectives; that is, by entertaining them and either assimilating them into one's view of the subject in question or rejecting them, depending on whether they advance understanding. This takes us away from Engel's a priori commitment to pluralism, and is the lesson we drew from the first category of empirical studies considered in the previous section: sometimes we find causes of mental disorders in unexpected places, so it would be a mistake antecedently to rule out a biological, a psychological, or a social explanation. However, Ghaemi has an answer ready in response to this point:

> Another conceptual defence sees the biopsychosocial model heuristically, reminding us to pay attention to three aspects of illness. Then the question becomes: how do we choose? How do we prioritise one aspect versus another? Some might propose that evidence-based medicine provides the mechanism of choice, but often evidence is limited or absent. The biopsychosocial model, as classically advanced, does not guide us on how to prioritise. Consequently, prioritisation happens on the run, with each person's own preferences, and the model devolves into mere eclecticism, passing for sophistication. (Ghaemi, 2009, p. 4)

What is wrong with eclecticism? Ghaemi explains:

> [B]iopsychosocial advocates really seek eclectic freedom, the ability to 'individualise treatment to the patient', which has come to mean, in practice, being allowed to do whatever one wants to do. This eclectic freedom borders on anarchy: one can emphasise the 'bio' if one wishes, or the 'psycho' … or the 'social'. But there is no rationale why one heads in one direction or the other: by going to a restaurant and getting a list of ingredients, rather than a recipe, one can put it all together however one likes. This results in the ultimate paradox: free to do whatever one chooses, one enacts one's own dogmas (conscious or unconscious). (Ghaemi, 2009, p. 3)

Throughout his criticism, Ghaemi switches between conceiving of the biopsychosocial model as a tool for understanding mental illness and as a tool for deciding on a treatment plan. He criticizes the model on the ground that it does not tell us how to prioritize one aspect of a mental disorder—biological, psychological, or social—over another when deciding on a treatment plan. But, in this case, there is an easy answer for the advocate of a biopsychosocial approach. Other things being equal, we prioritize whichever sort of intervention we have reason to believe (based on the available evidence) will promote the best outcome. The biopsychosocial model does not tell us which treatment to choose; it reminds us only to consider all the options.

Ghaemi takes advocates of the biopsychosocial model to oppose the idea that, when choosing treatments, we should select those that produce the best outcomes:

> An empirical defence of 'the more is better' philosophy sometimes is made based on the eclectic biopsychosocial intuition that medications and psychotherapy are always, and inherently, more effective than either alone. Empirically, sometimes this is so, sometimes not. Using one method or treatment purely often produces better results or is more valid than using multiple approaches together. (Ghaemi, 2009, p. 4)

Did Engel really believe 'that medications and psychotherapy are always, and inherently, more effective than either alone'? Ghaemi ascribes this view to Engel, apparently on the basis of Engel's claim—quoted by Ghaemi—that 'all three levels, biological, psychological, and social, must be taken into account in every health care task' (Engel, 1978, p. 164, cited in Ghaemi, 2009, p. 3). Yet it is far from clear that Ghaemi's interpretation of Engel is correct in this respect. Engel's claim that biopsychosocial factors 'must be taken into account in every health care task' appears in the conclusion of an argument for *conceptualizing* patients and their conditions according to biological, psychological, and social factors, rather than according to biological factors alone (Engel, 1978, pp. 161–162). It does not, then, relate to the treatment methods that one selects. Engel remarks that in selecting the appropriate treatment for the clinical case discussed in the paper, 'differences between the [biomedical] reductionist and [the biopsychosocial] systematist temporarily vanish' (1978, p. 162), with adherents to each approach choosing 'identical' treatments.

Engel did not—as I have done here—explicitly distinguish between a biopsychosocial approach to *understanding* mental illness and a biopsychosocial approach to *treating* it. As a result, it is not always clear whether and how he might conceive of and apply the biopsychosocial model differently in each case. This confusion is compounded by the fact that he speculates that conceptualizing patients in biopsychosocial terms will translate into better outcomes, as when he argues—based on speculation about how a clinical case might have gone had it been approached according to the biopsychosocial model rather than according to the biomedical model—that patients fare better when medical staff take a biopsychosocial approach than when they take a biomedical approach (Engel, 1978, 1980).[4] In other words, Engel expects better patient outcomes to emerge straightforwardly from adopting a biopsychosocial *understanding* of patients and their conditions; he does not consider at all how a biopsychosocial approach might affect decisions

---

[4] Engel's conviction that the biopsychosocial model is better for patients marks a point of departure from his 1977 article, in which he cautiously remarked that '[w]hether [the biopsychosocial model] is useful or not remains to be seen' (Engel, 1977, p. 135).

about treatment. Indeed, given that he views the biopsychosocial and biomedical clinicians as likely to choose identical treatments, he seems not to view a biopsychosocial approach as influencing treatment decisions at all. Instead, he views the patient's more positive outcome on the biopsychosocial model as arising from factors other than treatment choices, such as the way in which medical staff relate to the patient.

There are, then, improvements that we can make to Engel's account of the biopsychosocial model. We can be clear about distinguishing between what adopting a biopsychosocial approach entails for understanding mental illness—that is, for research into the causes of mental disorders—and what it entails for treating it. We can also consider the extent to which we want to buy wholesale into Engel's view of the model as a way of life: we may decide not to adopt a biopsychosocial approach as a 'blueprint for research, a framework for teaching, and a design for action in the real world of health care', but instead to cherry-pick those aspects of it that have been shown to produce the best results, or that best reflect the most plausible conceptual framework for understanding mental illness.

Ghaemi, as mentioned previously, argues that we should reject the biopsychosocial model in favour of a Jaspers-inspired 'methodological consciousness', in which 'we need to be aware of what methods we use, their strengths and limitations, and why we use them' (Ghaemi, 2009, p. 4), and an Osler-inspired approach in which:

> Where disease is present, one treats the body; where disease is ameliorable but not curable, one still treats with attention to risks; and where no disease exists (some patients have symptoms or signs, but no disease, e.g. cough, rather than pneumonia) one attends to the human being as a person. (Ghaemi, 2009, p. 4)

Ghaemi focuses here on the *treatment* of mental illness; as such, his characterization of methodological consciousness resembles the biopsychosocial approach to treatment for which I have argued, in which we consider biological, psychological, and social approaches, and—guided by empirical evidence—choose whichever of these produces the best patient outcomes. As such, Ghaemi's position might be conceived not as attacking a progressive, post-Engelian biopsychosocial approach, but as improving on it. Ghaemi acknowledges that Engel's biopsychosocial model can be improved upon, but objects to the use of the term 'biopsychosocial' to describe improved versions, and advocates instead using the Jaspersian term 'methodological consciousness' (Ghaemi, 2010, p. 212). In this case, however, disagreement between Ghaemi and advocates of an improved biopsychosocial approach is merely terminological. The important issue is how we might best understand and treat mental illness, not how we might best name our approach.

As a concluding reflection, it is interesting to note that while I have argued for a modified, updated version of Engel's biopsychosocial approach to psychiatry, the biopsychosocial position that I have advanced bears some resemblance to that adopted by Grinker. In explaining his biopsychosocial approach, Grinker writes:

> I have little use for the pleas to utilize holistic approaches operationally. The scientist has to focus, with a particular frame of reference and from a specified position, on a part of the world of man. Yet unified or holistic concepts in general are important as organizing principles for the understanding of general processes. (Grinker, 1966, cited in Ghaemi 2010, p. 35)

Grinker, then, views taking a 'unified or holistic' biopsychosocial view as important to understanding—but he does not advocate a holistic approach to treatment. That the latter is true emerges more clearly elsewhere, as when he remarks that the biopsychosocial psychiatrist 'freely selects from a wide variety of sources what is available and appropriate' (Grinker, 1965, cited in Ghaemi, 2010, p. 32). Ghaemi, based on his admirably extensive reading of Grinker's work, interprets 'available and appropriate' to mean pragmatic and empirically verified. As such, Grinker's biopsychosocial approach is closer to the position for which I have argued here than is Engel's: Grinker believes that taking a biopsychosocial ('unified or holistic') view of mental illness is useful in achieving understanding, but when selecting treatment methods, one must choose—based on empirical evidence—the best of what one has available.

Conclusion

Consistent with the way in which we attempt to understand and respond to other people even in everyday, familiar, non-pathological contexts, adopting a biopsychosocial approach to psychiatry should be viewed as involving an approach to understanding mental illness, and an approach to treating it. In trying to *understand* mental illness, adopting a biopsychosocial approach should be taken to consist in remaining open-minded to the possibility that the causes of a patient's condition, or of a particular type of condition, may (but need not) consist of a combination of biological, psychological, and social factors. In making decisions about how to *treat* mental illness, or a given patient, adopting a biopsychosocial approach should involve keeping in mind that the most effective treatment may involve a solely biological intervention, a solely psychological one, a solely social one, or a combination of these. A useful and effective biopsychosocial approach reminds us to consider all of these possibilities, and select the most promising one, based on the available empirical evidence.

References

Broome, M.R. and Bortolotti, L. (2009). Mental illness as mental: in defence of psychological realism. *Humana Mente*, 3(11), 25–43.

Caspi, A., McClay, J., Moffitt, T.E., Mill, J., Martin, J., Craig, I.W., Taylor, A., and Poulton, R. (2002). Role of genotype in the cycle of violence in maltreated children. *Science*, **297**(5582), 851–854.

Engel, G. (1977). The need for a new medical model: a challenge for biomedicine. *Science*, **196**(4286), 129–136.

Engel, G. (1978). The biopsychosocial model and the education of health professionals. *Annals of the New York Academy of Sciences*, **310**, 169–181; reprinted in *General Hospital Psychiatry*, 1979, **1**(2), 156–165.

Engel, G. (1980). The clinical application of the biopsychosocial model. *American Journal of Psychiatry*, **137**, 535–544; reprinted in *Journal of Medicine and Philosophy*, 1981, **6**(2) 101–124.

Gabbard, G.O. and Kay, J. (2001). The fate of integrated treatment: whatever happened to the biopsychosocial psychiatrist? *American Journal of Psychiatry*, **158**(12), 1956–1963.

Ghaemi, S.N. (2009). The rise and fall of the biopsychosocial model. *British Journal of Psychiatry*, **195**(1), 3–4.

Ghaemi, S.N. (2010). *The Rise and Fall of the Biopsychosocial Model: Reconciling Art and Science in Psychiatry*. Baltimore, MD: Johns Hopkins University Press.

Grinker, R.R. (1994). Training of a psychiatrist-psychoanalyst. *Journal of the American Academy of Psychoanalysis*, *22*(2), 343–350.

Grinker, R.R. (1966). "Open-system" psychiatry. *American Journal of Psychoanalysis*, *26*(2), 115–128.

Hogarty, G.E., Greenwald, D., Ulrich, R.F., Kornblith, S.J., DiBarry, A.L., Cooley, S., Carter, M., and Flesher, S. (1997). Three-year trials of personal therapy among schizophrenic patients living with or independent of family, II: effects on adjustment of patients. *American Journal of Psychiatry*, **154**(11), 1514–1524.

Hogarty, G.E., Kornblith, S.J., Greenwald, D., DiBarry, A.L., Cooley, S., Ulrich, R.F., Carter, M., and Flesher, S. (1997). Three-year trials of personal therapy among schizophrenic patients living with or independent of family, I: description of study and effects on relapse rates. *American Journal of Psychiatry*, **154**(11), 1504–1513.

Howes, O.D. and Kapur, S. (2014). A neurobiological hypothesis for the classification of schizophrenia: type A (hyperdopaminergic) and type B (normodopaminergic). *British Journal of Psychiatry*, *205*(1), 1–3.

Kandel, E. (2001). The molecular biology of memory storage: a dialogue between genes and synapses. *Science*, *294*(5544), 1030–1038.

Kendler, K.S. (2012). The dappled nature of causes of psychiatric illness: replacing the organic-functional/hardware/software dichotomy with empirically based pluralism. *Molecular Psychiatry*, **17**, 377–388.

Leff, J., Kuipers, L., Berkowitz, R., Eberlein-Vries, R., and Sturgeon, D. (1982). A controlled trial of social intervention in the families of schizophrenic patients. *British Journal of Psychiatry*, **141**, 121–134.

Leff, J., Kuipers, L., Berkowitz, R., and Sturgeon, D. (1985). A controlled trial of social intervention in the families of schizophrenic patients: two year follow-up. *British Journal of Psychiatry*, **146**(1), 594–600.

Ludwig, A.M. (1975). The psychiatrist as physician. *Journal of the American Medical Association*, **234**(6), 603–604.

McLaren, N. (2006). Interactive dualism as a partial solution to the mind-brain problem for psychiatry. *Medical Hypotheses*, *66*(6), 1165–1173.

McLaren, N. (2007). *Humanizing Madness*. New York City: Future Psychiatry Press.

Meyer, A. (1917). Progress in teaching psychiatry. *Journal of the American Medical Association*, **69**, 861–863.

Misri, S., Albert, G., Abizadeh, J., Kendrick, K., Carter, D., Ryan, D., and Oberlander, T.F. (2012). Biopsychosocial determinants of treatment outcome for mood and anxiety disorders up to 8 months postpartum. *Archives of Women's Mental Health*, *15*(4), 313–316.

Nemeroff, C.B. and Vale, W.W. (2005). The neurobiology of depression: inroads to treatment and new drug discovery. *Journal of Clinical Psychiatry*, **66**(Suppl 7), 5–13.

Pilgrim, D. (2002). The biopsychosocial model in Anglo-American psychiatry: past, present and future? *Journal of Mental Health*, **11**(6), 585–594.

Rathod, S., Kingdon, D., Weiden, P., and Turkingdon, D. (2008). Cognitive-behavioral therapy for medication-resistant schizophrenia: a review. *Journal of Psychiatric Practice*, **14**, 22–33.

Shorter, E. (2005). The history of the biopsychosocial approach in medicine: before and after Engel. In: P. White (Ed.), *Biopsychosocial Medicine* (pp. 1–20). Oxford: Oxford University Press.

Szasz, T. (1960). The myth of mental illness. *American Psychologist*, **15**, 113–118.

Szasz, T. (1961). *The Myth of Mental Illness*. London: Paladin.

Part 2

Multilevel Interactions

Chapter 3

Multilevel interactions and the dappled causal world of psychiatric disorders

Kenneth S. Kendler and Christopher Gyngell

Introduction

Despite substantial advances in our understanding of many somatic diseases, the nature of many psychiatric disorders remains elusive. This has contributed to debates within psychiatry regarding how best to understand and model psychiatric science. In this chapter, based on the inaugural Loebel Lectures given by one of us (KSK), we show how an appreciation of the multilevel causal nature of psychiatric disorders can move these debates forward. In Part 1, we review empirical evidence, taken nearly exclusively from Kenneth Kendler's own work, which show causal mechanisms in psychiatric disorders operate over multiple causal levels. We first examine the ways in which genetic risk factors interact with environmental factors in the aetiology of depression and substance use disorders. We then discuss the phenomenon of genotype–environment correlation, where certain environmental risk factors are influenced by genetic risk factors. We then briefly discuss examples of 'top-down' causation, in which factors at one causal level impact the risk factors at lower levels.

In Part 2, we discuss the implications of these findings for philosophical debates about the nature of psychiatry. Again drawing on the published work of Kendler, we argue that the non-additive relationship between risk factors at different causal levels provides good reasons to resist hard reductionist models of psychiatric disorders. Similarly, we argue that psychiatry should resist attempts to base classification schemes on a hard medical model, which sees mental illness as resembling Mendelian diseases with discrete causal explanations. We argue that the causes of psychiatric disorders are 'dappled' across multiple levels, making classification based on standard reductionist medical models difficult. Instead, psychiatry should embrace the fuzzy and complex causal picture that research suggests reflects the true nature of mental illness. We end by charting a path forward for psychiatric research, based on a rich multilevel framework.

Part 1: multilevel interactions

Causal levels

It has long been thought that psychiatric disorders/illness could be caused by a wide variety of factors. The *Anatomy of Melancholy*, first published in 1621, lists a huge number of causes of depression, including the following: terrors or frights, loss of liberty, poverty, all possible accidents, death of friends, clot blood in the brain, God, the Devil, diseases and fumes arising from the stomach, the heat of the sun, a blow to the head, garlics, hot baths, overmuch waking, overmuch hot wine, solitariness, old age, overmuch study, nature passions, water unclean, filth, herbs, cabbage, garlic, rough-roots, disorders of eating, etc. (Burton, 1638).

Today, psychiatrics still recognize that many different factors contribute to mental illness. These causal factors are often grouped into different 'causal levels'. These levels include:

- Molecular genetic variants—such as known allele variants.
- Latent genetic risk factors—genetic risk factors revealed by statistical models applied to twin, family, and adoption studies.
- Individual-level environmental risk factors—such as traumatic life events.
- Family-level environmental risk factors—such as parenting practices.
- Community-level environmental risk factors—such as social deprivation.
- Cultural-level environmental risk factors—such as attitudes towards smoking.
- Latent environment risk factors—environmental risk factors shared by people who share similar environments, but where the exact variables are not known.

One key question regarding the aetiology of mental illness is how risk factors at different levels relate and interact with each other. If I have a molecular genetic variant and an individual-level environmental factor that both increase my risk of depression, what will their combined influence be? The simplest way risk factors at different causal levels can act with each other is by adding their risk together. For example, assume that by itself a gene variant increases my risk of depression by 10%, and the environmental factor increases my risk by 5%. If the presence of both factors together increased my risk of depression by 15%, then these factors have an additive relationship with each other. When risk factors are additive, the magnitude of their influence is not affected by risk factors at other levels.

However, some risk factors add together in more complex ways. Suppose again that by themselves a gene variant increases my risk of depression by 10%, and the environmental factor increases my risk by 5%. However, when they occur together, my risk of depression is increased by 50% rather than 15%. In this case the risk factors are doing more than just simply adding together. They have a synergistic or multiplicative, rather than just an additive, relationship with each other.

Our focus in this chapter will be on risk factors that interact with each other in non-additive ways, such as in the previous example. When risk factors have non-additive relationships, the amount of risk they add depends on the presence of risk factors at other levels.

Gene–environment interactions

Individual-level environmental risk factors

One of the first examples of risk factors for psychiatric disorders having a non-additive relationship with each other was demonstrated between latent genetic risks and individual-level environmental risks for depression (Kendler et al., 1995). In a population-based study of twins from Virginia, one of us (KSK) along with co-authors examined how the risk of depression was influenced by traumatic life events including the death of a close relative, being assaulted, and having serious marital problems. We found that how much each of these events increased one's risk of depression was heavily influenced by their latent genetic risk. Individuals who had a monozygotic co-twin with depression (and thus had high latent genetic risk) were more likely to develop depression in response to these traumatic events than individuals with dizygotic twins who had depression (who had a lower genetic risk). This showed that how sensitive individuals are to adverse life events depends on their genes. These results are depicted in Figure 3.1.

This study provides a clear example of risk factors at different levels which have a non-additive relationship with each other. For individuals with a high latent genetic risk of depression, the effect of this risk is dependent on whether their lives include traumatic life events. In the absence of these events, the latent genetic risk does not add much to one's total risk of depression; in the presence of these events, the increased risk is substantial. Likewise, the influence of a traumatic life event on one's risk of depression depends on underlying genetic risks. Looking at just one risk factor in isolation is therefore insufficient.

Another important thing to make note of in this study is the shape of the curve shown in Figure 3.1. The effect of latent genetic risk on depression *fans out* when we move from the absence to the presence of traumatic life events. In the absence of adverse life events, it was hard to distinguish those with high latent genetic risk of depression with those with low latent risk of depression. However, once individuals start to experience adverse life events, the difference between them becomes very obvious.

Family-level environmental risk factors

Similar interactions have been observed between latent genetic risk and family-level environmental risks for drug abuse (Kendler et al., 2012). In a large adoption study, Kendler and co-authors showed that a latent genetic risk of drug abuse affected how sensitive individuals were to environmental risks in their adoptive environment. Genetic risk was estimated by looking at the history of drug abuse and related pathologies in an individual's biological family, and environmental risks were estimated by looking at the same histories in an individual's adoptive families. Individuals with a low genetic risk of drug abuse were relatively resistant to risk factors in their adoptive environment. The total risk of drug abuse rose by approximately 1% as these individuals moved from the least risky to the most risky adoptive environments. In contrast, individuals with the highest genetic risk were very sensitive to these risks. The risk of drug abuse in these individuals increased by 5% as they moved from the lowest to

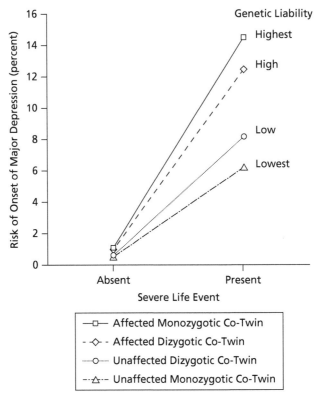

Figure 3.1 Risk of major depression per month as a function of genetic liability and stressful life events.
Reproduced with permission from Kendler K.S. et al. Stressful life events, genetic liability, and onset of an episode of major depression in women. *Focus*, 8(3), 459–470. Copyright © 2010 American Psychiatric Association Publishing.

highest environmental risk category, a fivefold difference compared to those with a low genetic risk. This is shown in detail in Figure 3.2.

Figure 3.2 provides another example of the *fan-shaped* pattern we saw in Figure 3.1. The total risk of drug abuse for individuals with different latent genetic risks fans out as they are exposed to more pathogenic environments. This seems to be a fundamental feature of many gene–environment interactions in psychiatric syndromes. Individuals with particular genotypes are relatively insensitive to risks in their environment, whereas others are much more susceptible.

This study provides another example of when genetic and environmental risk factors for psychiatric disorders have a non-additive relationship with each other. The amount of increased risk that latent genetic factors add for drug abuse is dependent on whether an individual is exposed to particular individual-level risk factors. Similarly, the effect of environmental risk factors is dependent on the level of genetic liability of the individuals experiencing them.

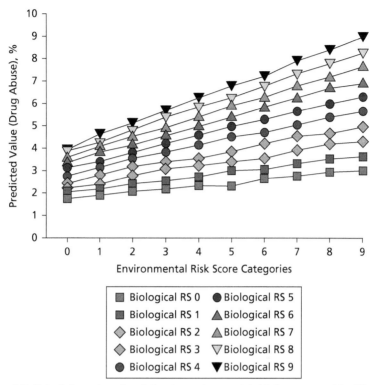

Figure 3.2 Risk of drug abuse in relation to environmental risk for groups with different latent genetic risks. RS, risk score.

Reproduced with permission from Kendler K.S. et al. Genetic and familial environmental influences on the risk for drug abuse: A National Swedish Adoption Study. *JAMA Psychiatry*, 69(7), 690–697. Copyright © 2012. American Medical Association.

Community-level environmental risks

This fan-shaped pattern of gene–environment interaction is seen again when looking at the interactions between latent genetic risk and community-level environmental factors on alcohol consumption. Genetic risks for externalizing disorders (such as attention deficit hyperactivity disorder) are known to increase alcohol consumption in adolescence. However, this effect is heavily moderated by certain environmental factors such as alcohol availability and peer-group deviance. The now familiar fan-shaped interaction between genetic risk for externalizing disorders and alcohol availability is shown in Figure 3.3, which outlines data on alcohol consumption in a study of male twins in Virginia (Kendler et al., 2011).

Figure 3.3 shows that for individuals in environments with relatively low levels of alcohol availability, genetic risks make little difference to how much alcohol they consume. In contrast, in environments with high alcohol availability, there is a dramatic difference between those with high and low genetic risk.

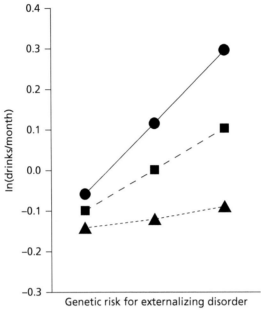

Figure 3.3 The prediction of the maximal yearly alcohol consumption from ages 12–14, as measured by standardized monthly intake, by the genetic risk for externalizing disorders, alcohol availability, and their interaction. The results, from a best-fit regression model, are depicted for three hypothetical individuals with a moderately high level of alcohol availability [–●–, values 1 standard deviation (S.D.) above the mean], an average level of alcohol availability (– –■– –, mean value), and a moderately low level of alcohol availability (- -▲- -, values 1 S.D. below the mean). Maximal yearly alcohol consumption is expressed by the average monthly alcohol consumption in that year, standardized so that, at the mean level of genetic risk and the mean level of alcohol availability, the score is approximately zero. The y-axis then depicts this mean score in standard deviation units. Reproduced with permission from Kendler K.S., Gardner C., and Dick D.M., Predicting alcohol consumption in adolescence from alcohol-specific and general externalizing genetic risk factors, key environmental exposures and their interaction. *Psychological Medicine*, 41(7), 1507–1516. Copyright © 2010 Cambridge University Press.

A very similar relationship is found between the genetic risk factors for alcohol use disorders and peer-group deviance. Peer-group deviance is a measure of how likely one's friends are to engage in a range of deviant behaviours including smoking, drinking, stealing, skipping school, cheating on tests, using illicit drugs, and breaking the law (Kendler et al., 2007). Using the same data from the Virginia twin study, Kendler and co-authors estimated peer-group deviance by getting individuals to self-report how likely their friends were to engage in deviant behaviours. The study showed that in environments of low peer deviance, one's genetic predisposition towards drinking was effectively silenced. There is little or no difference between individuals who have a high genetic predisposition to high alcohol consumption and those that do not have a genetic predisposition. In contrast, differences in genetic risk have very large effects on alcohol consumption once individuals are in environments with high rates of peer deviance.

The moderating effect of peer deviance on genetic risk of substance abuse has been replicated in a different model with a much larger sample size. Rather than using self-reports to estimate peer-group deviance, one of us (KSK) and co-authors generated an objective measure of peer deviance, using data from multiple Swedish nationwide registries and healthcare data (Kendler et al., 2014). The peer-group deviance score for a given individual was calculated as the proportion of people born within 5 years of them, in the same small geographic area, who eventually developed drug abuse problems (close relatives were excluded). Genetic risk of drug abuse was estimated using the same registries, by looking at rates of drug abuse in an individual's relatives. The interactions between genetic risks of drug abuse and peer deviance are shown in Figure 3.4.

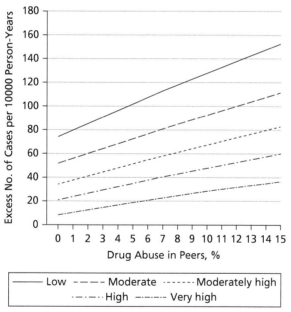

Figure 3.4 Interactions between genetic risk and peer deviance on risk of drug abuse. The lines represent five levels of genetic risk for drug abuse: low (no affected relative), moderate (only mother affected), moderately high (all siblings affected), high (father and 50% of siblings affected), and very high (monozygotic co-twin affected). The y-axis represents risk of drug abuse and the x-axis represents a measure of peer deviance.

Reproduced with permission from Kendler K.S. et al. Peer deviance, parental divorce, and genetic risk in the prediction of drug abuse in a nationwide Swedish sample: evidence of environment-environment and gene-environment interaction. *JAMA Psychiatry*, 71(4), 439–445. Copyright © 2014. American Medical Association.

This model confirms the observation from the Virginia twin study that low peer deviance moderates high genetic risk of drug abuse. In environments of low peer-group deviance, genetic risk for drug abuse is effectively downregulated, and has little effect on one's absolute chances of drug abuse. In environments of high peer deviance, this genetic risk is much more likely to be expressed.

Cultural-level environmental risks

The ability of certain environmental factors to impact the phenotypic expression of genetic risk factors is also found when looking at interactions between genetic risk factors and cultural risk factors. Using the data from the Swedish Twin Registry, one of us (KSK) and co-authors examined the lifetime history of tobacco use in members of 778 male–male and female–female twin pairs, raised together and apart, born from 1890 to 1958. Looking at smoking rates in monozygotic and dizygotic twins, an estimate was made of the role latent genetic risk factors were playing in differences in tobacco consumption, and how this changed over time. For males, the prevalence of regular tobacco use was stable over this time period at around 65–70%. Around 50% of the variation observed in tobacco consumption in males was explained by latent genetic factors, and this remained relatively constant between 1910 and 1958 (Kendler et al., 2000). However, in females, tobacco use was quite rare for those born early in the twentieth century and became much more common later. Interestingly, the role of latent genetic factors in females also increased very significantly over this time. In the 1910–1924 cohort, there was no evidence that genetic factors played any role in the difference in female tobacco consumption. In the 1940–1958 cohort, genetic factors were explaining more than 60% of the observed variation. This dramatic rise is seen is Figure 3.5.

The large increase in the heritability of tobacco use in females can be easily explained by cultural factors. In 1910, there was a tight social control over female smoking. Smoking was seen as a male activity and there was strong social pressure on females not to smoke. This is reflected in the low smoking prevalence scores for this cohort. In these conditions, any genetic factors that may affect tobacco consumption were effectively silenced. As we move to the 1925–1939 and 1940–1958 cohorts, this social control of female smoking begins to be lifted, thanks partly to the women's rights movement. Women began to see themselves as having a right to smoke and indeed smoking may have become a symbol of their new social liberation. This explains why the prevalence of smoking in females rose rapidly though these cohorts. In these new social conditions, latent genetic factors related to tobacco consumption were finally expressed. In the final cohort, the heritability of tobacco use matches that of males. Genes that were previously silenced have now become unleashed.

Environment–environment interactions

In 'Gene–environment interactions' we saw that genetic and environmental risk factors for psychiatric disorders often interact with each other in non-additive ways. However, it is important to note that non-additive interactions can occur between different risk factors of any class. One example of this is the relationship between early life severe events and acute proximate stress—two different environmental risk factors.

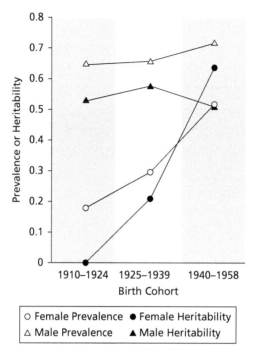

Figure 3.5 The prevalence and estimated heritability of regular tobacco use in three historical birth cohorts of Swedish male and female twins reared together and reared apart.

Reproduced with permission from Kendler K.S. et al. Tobacco consumption in Swedish twins reared apart and reared together. *JAMA Psychiatry*, 57(9), 886–892. Copyright © 2000. American Medical Association.

Using a population-based sample of 1404 female adult twins, one of us (KSK) and co-authors investigated the relationship between early life sexual abuse and stressful live events for the risk of depression (Kendler et al., 2004). The subjects were divided into three classes, those that had no history of sexual abuse, those with a history of moderate sexual abuse (such as genital touching with no intercourse), and those with a history of severe sexual abuse (sexual intercourse without consent). Stressful live events were divided into four different classes depending on their severity. Classes one and two represented relatively minor events such as being involved in a car crash or having legal problems, class three represented significant life events such as divorce or losing one's job, and class four represented very serious life events, such as the death of a loved one. The results are seen in Figure 3.6.

As we can see, the effect of early sexual abuse on one's risk of getting depression depends heavily on whether one's life contains proximate causes of stress. In the absence of a recent stressful life event, early childhood sexual abuse makes only a modest difference to an individual's risk of depression. However, once individuals start to experience stressful life events, their early abuse shows its influence. This is another

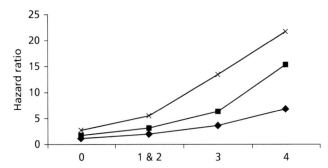

Figure 3.6 The hazard ratio for onset of an episode of major depression as a function of level of exposure to a stressful life event and prior history of childhood sexual abuse. Reproduced with permission from Kendler, K.S., Kuhn, J.W., and Prescott, C.A. Childhood sexual abuse, stressful life events and risk for major depression in women. *Psychological Medicine*, 34(8), 1475–1482. Copyright © 2004 Cambridge University Press.

example of a fan-shaped interaction that we saw in the gene–environment interactions in Figures 3.1–3.4—however, in this case genes play no role.

Genotype–environment correlation

So far we have been discussing the way risk factors at different causal levels interact with each other in the development of psychiatric disorders. Another very important type of interaction can occur between levels when genetic risk factors actually influence which environmental risk factors an individual is exposed too. This is an example of genotype–environment correlation.

The tendency of certain genes to affect the environments they are expressed in has been studied extensively in other species. Beavers, for example, have genes which predispose them to build dams. Once these dams are built, they act as the environments in which the other beaver genes are expressed. This is a case of genes 'having feet'—going out into the world and effecting things. In a similar way, certain genes possessed by humans may lead them to create certain social environments for themselves.

Importantly, these 'genes with feet' may vary between different individuals. Just as variations in the beaver genotype will cause individuals to build different kinds of dams, variations in human genes can cause them to create different social environments for themselves. Some individuals are more prone to create environments which contain stressful life events, or deviant peer groups, for example.

This effect was seen from data from 55 independent studies looking at heritability of 35 different environmental factors. The weighted heritability for all environmental measures in all studies was 27% (Kendler and Baker, 2007), with most environmental factors having a heritability of between 15% and 35%. This means differences in genes explain between 15% and 35% of the observed variation in environmental factors such as divorce, maternal warmth, and peer-group deviance.

Further examples of heritable environmental measures were discovered by Kendler and co-authors looking at the causal mechanisms which underlie depression (Kendler et al., 2006). As noted in 'Individual–level environmental risk factors', both genetic risk factors and stressful life events contribute to depression. However, these factors are often correlated with each other. Genetic difference helps explain why some people suffered more stressful life events than others. This is intuitive in a way. Those with genetic predispositions to poor impulse control, for example, might be more likely to suffer adverse life events than those with good impulse control. Their genetic tendencies to give into temptation may make it difficult for them keep a job or remain faithful in a marriage. Conversely, those with more stable personalities are more likely to have larger and more supportive social networks. This is just two examples of the types of genes which might to contribute to individuals creating certain social environments for themselves.

Another environmental risk factor which is acted on by genes is peer-group deviance. People with certain genetic propensities are more likely to find themselves in deviant peer groups than others. Again this is in some ways intuitive. People have different natural inclinations, and we may expect those with similar inclinations to seek each other out because they tend to like to do the same things. Those who are naturally thrill-seeking may be more drawn to deviant lifestyles than those who have other inclinations. This can partly explain why peer deviance is modestly heritable.

One interesting thing to note about the heritability of peer-group deviance is that it is heavily influenced by age. A study by Kendler and co-authors looked at heritability of peer deviance in boys across five age cohorts (8–11, 12–14, 15–17, 18–21, and 22–25 years) (Kendler et al., 2007). In the youngest cohort, the heritability of peer deviance was below 30%, but this rises to over 50% in the oldest cohort. Again, this makes intuitive sense. At young ages, the ability of individuals to influence their peer group is low. There is a tight social control exerted on them by their parents. As they age, this control is loosened. Youths have increasing control over their peer groups and they become more mobile. As this process happens, individuals begin to sort into groups that have similar interests. By adulthood, those who are naturally inclined towards a deviant group have had the opportunity to find one, while those who don't want to join such a group have found alternatives.

A final example of genes influencing environmental risk factors is seen in the case of smoking. One of the most robust links between a gene and behaviour is the link between variants of the *CHRNA3* gene and tobacco consumption. People with a variant of the *CHRNA3* gene smoke on average over 700 more cigarettes per year than smokers without this variant (Thorgeirsson et al., 2008). The *CHRNA3* gene codes for a nicotine receptor in the brain, which helps provide a simple explanation of this result. People with some variants of the *CHRNA3* receptor are less sensitive to nicotine and therefore need to smoke more cigarettes in order to get the same effect. Further, because these individuals are consuming more cigarettes and ingesting more nicotine, their bodies become more addicted to this molecule and they have a harder time giving up.

Not surprisingly, people with the *CHRNA3* gene variant are also at greater risk of lung cancer. *CHRNA3* can therefore be seen as an oncogene—albeit it one with a much more complicated causal mechanism than other oncogenes. Most oncogenes have their effect through '*inside the skin*' pathways. They typically control cell division but have no effect on which environmental variables an individual is exposed to. However,

CHRNA3 is a clear example of an '*outside the skin*' pathway. Rather than just impacting cellular proliferation, this gene variant actually causes greater exposure to an environmental risk variable. The *CHRNA3* gene variant causes people to go out and buy more cigarettes which subsequently exposes them to more carcinogens, which creates an increased risk of cancer. It is another example of a gene which has feet.

The importance of development

As we saw in 'Genotype–environment correlation', the relative importance of different causal factors for an individual's risk of developing a psychiatric disorder changes as they age. Another example from the tobacco-use literature helps makes this point explicit. When looking at the relative importance of individual-level environmental factors, shared environmental factors, and genetic factors on tobacco consumption on twins, we see a very significant age-dependent effect (Kendler et al., 2012). In early adolescence, genes play nearly no explanatory role in why twins have similar smoking behaviour. Shared environmental factors, such as peer-group exposures, are by far the most important predictors of smoking. However, as individuals age, the importance of these shared environmental influences diminishes, and by the time individuals are in their thirties, shared environmental factors perform nearly no causal role in explaining why twins have similar smoking behaviours. In contrast, the role played by genetic factors steadily increases, to the point where they are the most significant causal factors when individuals are in their 30s. This is seen in Figure 3.7.

Similar age-dependent effects are seen in the relationship between genetic risks for conduct disorders and peer deviancy. Conduct disorders (associated with a prolonged pattern of antisocial behaviour) and peer deviancy are often correlated with each other. However, there are at least two different models to explain this correlation. In a *social influence model*, conduct disorders are caused by peer-deviance. Individuals may find themselves in a social situation which contains a high proportion of deviants. These

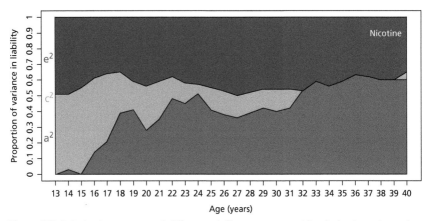

Figure 3.7 Relative importance of difference influences on smoking behaviour through time. Genetic factors = a^2 (red); shared environmental factors = c^2 (green); and e^2 = individuals-level environmental factors (blue).

deviants then corrupt this individual, who develops a conduct disorder as a result of being with deviant peers and seeking their approval. A *social selection model* sees the causal direction in the other way. People who are predisposed to conduct disorders actively try and seek out deviant peer groups. Which of these models tends to be more correct depends very much on the age at which we look at individuals. In a 2008 study, one of us (KSK) and co-authors looked at rates of peer deviance and conduct disorders in 746 adult male–male twin pairs at ages 8–11, 12–14, and 15–18 years—which separated out the effects of genetic predispositions, shared environmental risk factors, and individual-level risk factors (Kendler et al., 2008). The study indicates that both the social selection and social influence models play a large role in explaining the correlation between conduct disorders and peer deviance. However, the relative strength of each of these processes changes over time.

In the age 8–11 years cohort, there was strong evidence that peer deviance was causing conduct disorders in individuals through environmental risk factors. However, this effect appeared to diminish overtime, and in the 15–18 years age group there appeared to be no influence of peer deviancy on conduct disorders. In contrast, conduct disorders appeared to be causing peer-group deviance in a relatively stable manner through the three cohorts. The study shows that the while both the social influence and social selection models are important, the relative importance of these models is dependent on the development stage we examine. This suggests that if we are looking to implement environmental measures to reduce conduct disorders, we need to intervene early. While individuals are amenable to environmental influence while very young, this becomes less the case as they get older.

Top-down causation

The final type of between-level interactions we will examine involves the phenomenon of top-down causation. Top-down causation describes a process in which a causal factor operating at an upstream position on a causal pathway loops back to influence factors at much earlier stages. In many cases this phenomenon is highly specific to individuals, and as such is not as amendable to detailed study as other causal factors. However, intuitively many psychiatrists know at least one example of when a top-down explanation was the most appropriate for the presence or absence of a psychiatric disorder.

Take this story from the interview notes of one of us (KSK) from a study on alcoholics in Ireland. This story comes not from an alcoholic, but a sibling of alcoholics—we will call him Mick. At least two of his male siblings had alcohol dependency, and his father had been alcohol dependent. He told the following story:

> 'It was really hard Doctor, especially on Friday nights there would be an argument. Dad was meant to come home with his paycheck. Mum needed money for groceries, to pay for the light bill. And sometimes he wouldn't and he'd come home drunk. And I'd hear her yelling and I hear my dad hitting her and my mom screaming. I was the oldest and I was little, I couldn't do anything, I'd hide behind the door, crying. … And there was this time. It still gives me chills. I couldn't stand it.' At this point Mick describes how he tried to get between the father and the mother. And of course his dad grabbed him, threw him against the wall, slammed his mother, and he was nearly knocked unconscious. He then

said 'I was bleeding and I looked at them and my reaction was that I prayed to God. Please never let me become like him'. And he said at that point, 'I was never going to let alcohol cross my lips'.

When he was interviewed for the study, Mick remained true to this pledge—he had been a life-long abstainer. He had seen the ravages of alcoholism in his brothers. While we cannot know for sure that the reason Mick was able to overcome his predisposition to alcoholism was because he had this experience, it certainly seems plausible. We recognize that sometimes individuals can make decisions which override their genetic predispositions. People can choose to leave a deviant peer group, choose to quit smoking, and resist the temptation of alcohol. Hence, psychiatric and substance use disorders can also be seen to have a distinct class of top-down influences. People can choose to avoid environmental risk factors; they can resist their genetic inclinations.

Part 2: the dappled causal nature of mental illness

In Part 1 of this chapter, we reviewed evidence from genetic epidemiological studies of mental illness showing how risk factors at several different causal levels are important. Further, risk factors at different levels can interact with each other in non-additive ways. This means that we often cannot know the effect of a risk factor by looking at it in isolation—we also need to know what is happening at other causal levels.

We will now discuss how these findings relate to broader debates within psychiatry about the nature of psychiatric disorders and the best way to structure psychiatric science. Again, this will draw heavily on the previous published works of one of us (KSK) in the philosophy of psychiatry. We first look at implications for debates about the relative status of different causal explanations in psychiatric disorders. Some reductionists claim that psychiatric disorders are *social* diseases in essence that don't have an underling biological contribution, while others claim that psychiatric disorders are fundamentally *genetic* and/or *biological* in nature. Evidence of non-additive interactions between genetic and environmental levels shows the difficulties of holding such reductionist views. We argue we should resist reductionisms, and the associated view that psychiatric classification schemes should be based on a hard reductionist medical model.

To explain psychiatric disorders we need to adopt a multilevel framework. We need an approach that recognizes multiple independent causal mechanisms for psychiatric disorders that operate over several causal levels. While current multilevel frameworks, such as the biopsychosocial approach to psychiatry, provide a useful perspective on which to base these models, they have not been developed to the point where they can guide research and treatment of psychiatric illness. We end this chapter by outlining an approach that can help fill this theoretical gap—empirically based pluralism.

Resisting hard reductionism

As noted in 'Causal levels', the idea that psychiatric disorders had many distinct causal pathways used to be embraced by the medical community. The 1621 edition of the *Anatomy of Melancholy* lists a staggering number of potential causes of depression. During this time it was thought that there were numerous ways to get depression and the disease didn't have a single aetiology. However, this started to change around the late nineteenth century. Around this time, other areas of medicine had great success in explaining many seemingly complex diseases in terms of simple aetiologies. Tuberculous was found to be caused by a single pathogen, scurvy was found to be caused by a single vitamin deficiency, and cystic fibrosis was described as a recessive genetic disease. This imbued great optimism in the psychiatric community that many complex psychiatric disorders would also be able to be explained by single clear aetiologies. Initially this project met great success. In 1913, Hideyo Noguchi and J.W. Moore demonstrated that a common type of psychiatric illness, known then as *general paresis of the insane*, was in fact caused by prior infection by the syphilis bacterium. Subsequent treatment with penicillin virtually wiped out the illness from all Western countries. This provided fodder for a reductionist charge to find definitive aetiologies for all psychiatric disease.

However, after the initial success with general paresis of the insane, the quest has largely been a failure. Despite extensive attempts to find single root causes for disorders such as schizophrenia, major depression, and alcoholism, none have been found. The more we learn about the nature of these diseases, the more it appears there are multiple independent causal pathways. Causal factors are *dappled* over many different levels.

The research presented in Part 1 of this chapter provides further reason to believe that hard reductionist models are likely to fail to explain psychiatric disorders. Attempts to find causal mechanisms by looking solely at one level are likely to overlook important information. For example, take the claim that all psychiatric disorders are ultimately genetic.[1] This implies that once we have a complete understanding of the genetics underlying psychiatric disorders we will have a complete understanding of psychiatric illness itself. However, the interactions between genetic and environmental risk factors that we observed in Part 1 suggests this view is problematic. The causal effects of genes on psychiatric disorders appear in many circumstances to depend on the environment in which they are expressed. The same set of genes will have a different effect if they are expressed in an environment in which an individual is exposed to stressful life events, than if they are expressed in an environment free of stressful events. Because we can't know what environment a set of genes will be expressed in just by studying the genes themselves, we need to look beyond just genes when explaining psychiatric illness.

The converse applies for any arguments that attempt to privilege environmental-level risk factors when explaining psychiatric disorders. Whether particular environmental events increase one's chance of developing a psychiatric disorder depends on particular facts about the individual experiencing the events, including their genetic makeup. Accordingly, to understand mental illness we can not only look at environmental contributors.

This suggests we should not attempt to reduce psychiatric disorders to diseases with single clear aetiologies. We should embrace the possibility that psychiatric disorders have many independent causal mechanisms.

---

[1] Kandal (2005) embraces a view very similar to this type of genetic reductionism.

Resisting hard medical models

One area where reductionist ideas have influenced psychiatry is in the classification of psychiatric disorders. The later iterations of the *Diagnostic and Statistical Manual of Mental Disorders* have operationalized a *soft* medical model of psychiatric illness. This classifies psychiatric disorders according to a number of factors including symptoms, signs, and course of illness. Many in psychiatry are unhappy with this approach and believe classifications should follow a 'hard medical model', where illnesses are linked to a single clear aetiological mechanism.

However, for consistency, a move to a hard medical model would typically require that explanations for psychiatric disorders be derived from single causal levels. Such a move is not supported by the current state of psychiatric research. It is unlikely that a single causal level will provide us with the necessary power to provide a good explanation of psychiatric illness. To make this point explicit, one of us (KSK) listed seven criteria that a good explanation could be expected to meet (Kendler, 2012). These are:

♦ *Strength*—which reflects the magnitude of the association between the explanatory variable and disease risk.

♦ *Causal role*—which reflects the degree to which the risk factors identified in the explanatory process truly alter the probability of disease as opposed to being associated through non-causal mechanisms.

♦ *Generalizability*—which reflects the degree to which an explanation applies across a wide range of differing background conditions.

♦ *Specificity*—which refers to the degree to which that explanation applies only to the disorder under consideration versus other disorders.

♦ *Manipulability*—which reflects the degree to which an explanation (1) identifies risk factors can be altered through intervention and (2) provides interventions which impact the risk of illness.

♦ *Proximity*—which reflects the location of the risk factor in the causal chain to the disease. An explanation with high proximity sits close to the disease process in a causal chain. If, by contrast, many steps intervene between the explanation and the disease, then that explanation would have low proximity. Low proximity in no way implies that such distal risk factors reflect 'ultimate' causes.

♦ *Generativity*—which reflects the probability that the explanatory variables identified would have the potential to lead to further fruitful aetiological understanding of the disease.

Kendler then compared how the explanation of the disease cystic fibrosis in terms of a mutation in the *CFTR* gene satisfies the above-listed criteria for explanation, and did the same for several different explanations of alcohol dependence. The results are seen in Table 3.1.

As we can see, the *CFTR* mutation hypothesis provides a very good explanation of cystic fibrosis. It satisfies all the criteria of a good explanation. By contrast, none of the proposed explanations of alcohol dependence provide good explanations of this illness across the board. For example, while childhood sexual abuse is a strong predictor of alcohol dependence, it is not specific. This environmental variable predisposes people

Table 3.1 An evaluation of selected explanations for cystic fibrosis and alcohol dependence by seven criteria

Disorder/level	Strength	Causal role	Generalizability	Specificity	Manipulability	Proximity	Generativity
Cystic fibrosis							
CFTR mutations	++	++	++	++	+	++	++
Alcohol dependence							
Latent genetic risk	++	++	+	–	––	––	0
ALDH variants	++	++	––	++	++	0	–
GABA receptor variants	––	++	+	+	0	+	++
Childhood sexual abuse	++	+	+	–––	–––	–––	0
Frontal lobe dysfunction	+	+	0	–––	–	–	+
Impulsivity	++	+	+	–––	–	–	+
Peer deviance	++	0	+	–––	+	+	+
Social norm expectations	+	+	0	+	++	–	–
Taxation	+	+	++	+	++	–––	–––

CFTR, cystic fibrosis transmembrane conductance regulator gene.

Scores: ++ high; + moderate; 0 intermediate or unknown; – low; –– very low.

Reproduced with permission from Kendler, KS. 'Levels of explanation in psychiatric and substance use disorders: implications for the development of an etiologically based nosology'. *Molecular Psychiatry*. Volume 17, Issue 1, pp. 11–21. Copyright © 2012 Springer Nature Publishing AG. DOI: 10.1038/mp.2011.70

to a wide range of pathologies. Conversely while *ALDH* genetic variants are specific to alcohol dependence, they are not generalizable, many people with alcohol dependence do not have these mutations. Models of other psychiatric disorders, such as depression, would yield very similar results.

When we look at psychiatric disorders, then, no one causal level provides all the explanatory power we seek in clear aetiologies. This makes the move to a hard medical model in psychiatry difficult. One option is for the field to pick one level of causation to focus on, and exclude all others. For example, psychiatry could stipulate that all psychiatric classifications need to be based on genetic contributors and ignore all other potential causes. However, such a move is not supported by science, and would be a value-based decision. An alternative move is to abandon the hard medical model, and instead embrace the 'fuzzy, cross-level mechanisms, which may more realistically capture the true nature of psychiatric disorders' (Kendler, 2012, p. 11).

Empirically informed pluralism

How should we structure psychiatric science if we abandon the march towards reductionism and hard biomedical models of mental illness? Once we embrace the multiple-level causal picture of mental illness, we need to develop new research frameworks that can help orient research and treatment in beneficial ways. This requires the development of multiple-level perspectives on psychiatry such as the biopsychosocial approach. The essential claim of the biopsychosocial approach is that all mental illness is the result of the biological, psychological, and social influences, and that no one of these influences has any special causal privilege over the other. The biopsychosocial approach views mental illness as the result of a process which occurs over multiple causal levels.

One key area that needs to be addressed in psychiatry is the implications of multi-level frameworks for research and treatment. Just because biological, psychological, and social factors are all part of a process which causes mental illness doesn't mean they are equally important in explaining why some people get psychiatric disorders and others don't. Similarly, knowing that all three levels are part of an interlinked process doesn't tell us how best to reduce rates of mental illness.

In this section, we will outline one broad way to structure research under a multi-level framework called empirically based pluralism (EMP). EMP embraces neutrality about different causal levels and mechanisms originally, but then focuses in on factors that empirical studies have shown have a clear causal influence. EMP operates through three paradigms, which will be explained in the following subsections.

Populate the major levels and sublevels with validated risk factors

Rather than just assuming which factors will be important for any particular mental illness, we need to investigate them with rigorous research methodologies. We need to look for multiple forces across a variety of causal levels. EMP embraces an 'interventionist' view of causation as guide in this paradigm. Anything that when manipulated makes a difference to an outcome is considered 'a cause' under an interventionist model. This view has the advantage of being completely agnostic about different causal levels—none are excluded a priori. When applied to psychiatry we need to look for factors which, when manipulated, predict or prevent psychiatric illness regardless of whether they are biological, psychological, or social.

Evidence suggests that much current psychiatric research is directed at identifying single-level risk factors. In a survey of articles in 12 leading psychiatric journals, 69% of research articles were examining single-level predictors. This was divided relatively equally between causal mechanisms at biological, psychological, and social causal levels (Kendler, 2014). This suggests that researchers are already engaging in the first paradigm of EMP—populating causal space with validated risk factors across multiple levels.

Clarification of causal mechanisms

Knowing which causal levels are important is just the first step of EMP. As we showed in Part 1 of this chapter, knowing that both genes and environmental factors are important means very little if you don't understand how they together impact the risk for disease. This is addressed in the second paradigm of EMP. After we know what factors have causal influence, we need to determine how these relate to each other. When looking for causal mechanisms that explain psychiatric disorders, we need to look for mechanisms capable of operating over multiple levels which have non-additive interactions and explain top-down causal effects. Research needs to be aimed at providing explanations for how the various underlying influences of mental illness come together to produce a unified whole.

Tracing causal pathways back up into the mental

The third paradigm to guide research under EMP is to work back up from science-driven *explanations* of mental illness to an empathy-based *understanding* of mental illness. This draws on a distinction famously articulated by Jaspers with origins back to Dilthy and Weber (Jaspers et al., 1997), on which we *explain* mental illness by providing an in-depth account of the biological and social factors which give rise to its occurrence, and *understand* mental illness when we can imagine what it is like to have experiences of it. To understand depression, we need more than just knowledge of its underlying causal factors, but rather the capacity to imagine feeling alone, helpless, etc. This is vital for psychiatrists to be able empathize with their patients in treating psychiatric disorders.

Jaspers thought that some psychiatric disorders were un-understandable in that the experiences people had when suffering from them were so unlike anything people normally experience, it was impossible for a person who is well to imagine it. Take this description of a reference delusion that is often reported in schizophrenics:

> Everybody is in the street because of him; each gesture of these people has some significance for him; newspaper advertisements refer to him.

Most people would find such a state of mind very difficult to comprehend. However, one of us (KSK) and Campbell, have shown how sometimes epidemiological research can help expand the realm of the understandable. This is what we call explanation-aided understanding. As an example, the finding that schizophrenia is associated with misfiring of the midbrain dopamine neurons could help people imagine what it is like to have some schizophrenic delusions. One of the roles of the dopamine system is to tag information we encounter in our environment as important. When we see something, and our dopamine neurons fire, it acts as signal for us that this thing is important and we should focus our attention on it.

Many of us have experienced these neurons misfiring before on a small scale. Here is one example:

> You are waiting at an airport for a loved one. You see, in a crowd of passengers, a person in the distance who seems to be her. You jump to your feet and, with a rush of emotion, move toward her to embrace. As you get closer, you realize you were wrong. There was some similarity in body size, gait or clothing that caused you to think this person was your loved one. Your emotional response was misattributed. Through an error in your perceptual system, meaning was placed where it did not belong. (Kendler and Campbell, 2014, p. 3)

Now imagine what would happen if our dopamine neurons were misfiring all the time, so that everything we saw become marked with significance. Would we start to see everything in the world as being there just for us? This may be similar to what it is like for a schizophrenic to experience delusions.

This is an example of 'explanation-aided understanding'. This type of bottom-up work, which allows us to derive a picture of what it is like to have a mental illness from an intricate understanding of the underlying causal mechanisms, is the final paradigm to guide research under a empirically informed pluralist model.

Conclusion

The more we understand about mental illness, the more it becomes clear that it cannot be understood through simple causal models. Psychiatric illness is unlike infectious disease or simple Mendelian disorders. The risk factors for psychiatric disorders are sprinkled across multiple causal levels and don't coalesce into a single clear mechanism. The dappled causal nature of mental illness shows the need for psychiatric medicine to move away from the seductive simplicity of reductionism and hard medical models. The structure of psychiatric science needs to embrace multiple-level causal frameworks, such as that provided by the biopsychosocial approach. We have outlined the first steps of an approach, EMP, which helps provide structured guidance for psychiatric research under a multilevel framework.

References

Burton, R. (1638). *The Anatomy of Melancholy.* Oxford: Henry Crisps.

Jaspers, K., Hoenig, J., and Hamilton, M.W. (1997). *General Psychopathology.* Baltimore, MD: Johns Hopkins University Press.

Kandel, E. (2005). *Psychiatry, Psychoanalysis and the New Biology of Mind.* Arlington, VA: American Psychiatric Publishing.

Kendler, K.S. (2012). Levels of explanation in psychiatric and substance use disorders: implications for the development of an etiologically based nosology. *Molecular Psychiatry*, **17**(1), 11–21.

Kendler, K.S. (2014). The structure of psychiatric science. *American Journal of Psychiatry*, **171**(9), 931–938.

Kendler, K.S. and Baker, J.H. (2007). Genetic influences on measures of the environment: a systematic review. *Psychological Medicine*, **37**(5), 615–626.

Kendler, K.S., and Campbell, J. (2014). Expanding the domain of the understandable in psychiatric illness: an updating of the Jasperian framework of explanation and understanding. *Psychological Medicine*, **44**(1), 1–7.

Kendler, K.S., Chen, X., Dick, D., Maes, H., Gillespie, N., Neale, M.C., and Riley, B. (2012). Recent advances in the genetic epidemiology and molecular genetics of substance use disorders. *Nature Neuroscience*, **15**(2), 181–189.

Kendler, K.S., Gardner, C., and Dick, D.M. (2011). Predicting alcohol consumption in adolescence from alcohol-specific and general externalizing genetic risk factors, key environmental exposures and their interaction. *Psychological Medicine*, *41*(7), 1507–1516.

Kendler, K.S., Gatz, M., Gardner, C.O., and Pedersen, N.L. (2006). A Swedish national twin study of lifetime major depression. *American Journal of Psychiatry*, **163**(1), 109–114.

Kendler, K.S., Jacobson, K.C., Gardner, C.O., Gillespie, N., Aggen, S.A., and Prescott, C.A. (2007). Creating a social world: a developmental twin study of peer-group deviance. *Archives of General Psychiatry*, **64**(8), 958–965.

Kendler, K.S., Jacobson, K., Myers, J.M., and Eaves, L.J. (2008). A genetically informative developmental study of the relationship between conduct disorder and peer deviance in males. *Psychological Medicine*, **38**(7), 1001–1011.

Kendler, K.S., Kessler, R.C., Walters, E.E., MacLean, C., Neale, M.C., Heath, A.C., and Eaves, L.J. (1995). Stressful life events, genetic liability, and onset of an episode of major depression in women. *American Journal of Psychiatry*, **152**(6), 833–842.

Kendler, K.S., Kuhn, J.W., and Prescott, C.A. (2004). Childhood sexual abuse, stressful life events and risk for major depression in women. *Psychological Medicine*, **34**(8), 1475–1482.

Kendler, K.S., Ohlsson, H., Sundquist, K., and Sundquist, J. (2014). Peer deviance, parental divorce, and genetic risk in the prediction of drug abuse in a nationwide Swedish sample: evidence of environment-environment and gene-environment interaction. *JAMA Psychiatry*, **71**(4), 439–445.

Kendler, K.S., Sundquist, K., Ohlsson, H., Palmer, K., Maes, H., Winkleby, M.A., and Sundquist, J. (2012). Genetic and familial environmental influences on the risk for drug abuse: a national Swedish adoption study. *Archives of General Psychiatry*, **69**(7), 690–697.

Kendler, K.S., Thornton, L.M., and Pedersen, N.L. (2000). Tobacco consumption in Swedish twins reared apart and reared together. *Archives of General Psychiatry*, **57**(9), 886–892.

Thorgeirsson, T.E., Geller, F., Sulem, P., Rafnar, T., Wiste, A., Magnusson, K.P., Manolescu, A., Thorleifsson, G., Stefansson, H., Ingason, A., et al. (2008). A variant associated with nicotine dependence, lung cancer and peripheral arterial disease. *Nature*, **452**(7187), 638–642.

Chapter 4

When answers are hard to find, change the question: Asking different causal questions can enable progress

Rachel Cooper

Introduction

This chapter argues that empirical progress can sometimes be enabled by a shift in the causal questions that researchers ask. The first section reviews the grounds for pessimism regarding current research programmes in psychiatry; the prospects that the causes of mental disorder will soon be found appear increasingly remote. I then move on to consider possible ways forward. The second section looks to the history of medicine. K. Codell Carter's (2003) *The Rise of Causal Concepts of Disease* argues that the late nineteenth century saw great gains in medical knowledge partly as a result of a change in the types of causal questions that researchers were disposed to ask. In the third section, I turn to philosophy. I employ the philosophical claim that causal explanation is contrastive to suggest that projects that seek 'the causes of disorder' might pursue this aim in multiple ways. Researchers must select which causal questions to ask, out of multiple possibilities. That there are multiple causal questions that can be asked is important because some causal questions will prove easier to answer than others. As researchers often have the option of pursuing multiple lines of enquiry, whenever a research programme encounters difficulties in trying to address causal questions that appear hard to answer, it can be worth considering whether a switch in the types of causal questions being asked might help make things easier. The final, fourth, section turns to details and examples. At present, the causal questions standardly asked by psychopathologists have the form 'Why do certain people have condition X as opposed to being neurologically and psychologically typical?' I will argue that in some cases an alternative question to ask would be 'Why are certain people with condition X harmed by it while for others it is harmless?' This alternative question might on occasion prove easier to answer.

Pessimism regarding current research programmes

A popular model has seen nosology, knowledge of the causal mechanisms of disorder, and therapeutics as being ideally linked in the following way. First, psychiatric disorders should be picked out by close attention to symptoms; patients with similar symptoms should be classified together. Hopefully, 'validators'—family studies, treatment response, natural history—will confirm these groupings. Then researchers can set about seeking the underlying mechanisms and causes of the disorder, by looking for abnormalities in neurotransmitters, and using brain imaging studies, and genetic studies, and so on. With luck, the causes of disorders will be discovered, and then, eventually, with more luck, treatments which act against the causes can be developed.

On this model, nosology, the discovery of the causes of disorders, and the development of treatments are tied together. Thus, those who want to be able to help patients should first seek valid classifications, and then seek to develop causal knowledge (see Ghaemi (2012) for a clear current-day advocate for this approach). In psychiatry, this model of progress enjoyed a notable early success with neurosyphilis (Blashfield and Keely, 2010). When it comes to most mental disorders, however, there has so far been less progress. Knowledge of the causal mechanisms that underlie disorders is patchy, and many conditions cannot yet be reliably and effectively treated. Optimists continue to hope that slow and incremental advances will eventually yield results. Many, however, are becoming impatient with the supposition that current research programmes will make steady, albeit slow, progress. There are multiple grounds for concern.

First, and most obviously, it has become increasingly plausible that the causes of many mental disorders are hideously complex. A few decades ago, researchers could dream of finding 'the gene' for schizophrenia, or the brain abnormality underlying depression. Now, however, hopes of finding simple necessary and sufficient causal mechanisms that underlie many common mental disorders have been largely abandoned. To give some indication of the complexity likely involved, consider Kendler and colleagues' (2002) article, 'Toward a comprehensive developmental model for major depression in women'. In this publication, Kendler and colleagues develop a fairly complex statistical model that can predict 52% of the variance in liability to episodes of depression. The article starts by setting out the causal factors known to be implicated in the development of major depression in women:

> Major depression is a prototypical multifactorial disorder. An individual's probability of suffering from an episode of major depression is affected by many factors including predisposing genetic influences, exposure to a disturbed family environment, childhood sexual abuse, premature parental loss, predisposing personality traits, early-onset anxiety or conduct disorder, dysfunctional self-schemata, exposure to traumatic events and major adversities, low social support, substance misuse, marital difficulties, a prior history of major depression, and recent stressful life events and difficulties. (Kendler et al., 2002, p. 1133 (bibliographic references removed))

Clearly many factors can be involved in the development of depression. The model developed by Kendler and colleagues is accordingly complex. Although a great achievement, the model is notably limited in a number of ways. Most obviously, the model can account for only 52% of the variance in episodes of depression; much variance is currently unexplained. The model also assumes that causal variables interact only additively. The authors acknowledge that this assumption is implausible, but comment that 'Although we could have included interactions in our model, the analysis and subsequent interpretation of the very large number of such possible interactions among these variables is daunting' (Kendler et al., 2002, p. 1139). Overall, the model developed by Kendler and colleagues makes it clear that although quite a lot is known about the causal factors involved in the development of depression, there is also a great deal that is not understood. In the years since this study, some progress has been made, but the overall picture remains the same (Kendler, 2013). The causes of common mental disorders are likely complex and multifactorial.

There are also grounds for pessimism regarding therapy. Many of the causal factors that are implicated in the development of mental disorders may not be amenable to intervention. Genetic factors and diffuse social factors, for example, may often be very difficult to do anything about. It may not be easy to develop effective preventative strategies in mental health, or to work out how to cure mental disorders when they do develop.

Pessimism regarding current research programmes that seek the causes of disorder is often linked with concerns about the current means of classifying mental disorders (Uher and Rutter, 2012; Insel, 2014). The suggestion is increasingly heard that current classifications may be leading research down false paths, and might need radical revision. As is well known, the *Diagnostic and Statistical Manual of Mental Disorders*, third edition (*DSM-III*), published in 1980, sought to avoid contestable theoretical assumptions and set out to be a purely descriptive classification (American Psychiatric Association, 1980, pp. 6–8). Producing a theory-free classification was a strategy adopted as a means of making the *DSM* acceptable to mental health professionals working within different theoretical frameworks. The *DSM-III* prioritized reliability, possibly at the expense of validity. The idea was that the classification would be revised in due course in line with developing research. The problem is that if the descriptive syndromes included in the *DSM* fall too far short of mapping onto 'natural' distinctions in the domain of psychopathology, then a research programme directed at incremental improvements may not be capable of correcting initial errors. If there are important causal factors that might be found in some subgroup of those with a particular *DSM* diagnosis, or in a population that cuts across current categories, these are likely to be missed by current research programmes. Some now think that a new approach to classification will be required for research to make headway.

Various groups have made different suggestions for dealing with these perceived problems. Notably, the Research Domain Criteria project, initiated by the US National Institute of Mental Health, aims to provide a framework for research such that researchers can more easily study subject populations that do not map on to *DSM* categories (Insel, 2014). While it should be hoped that the Research Domain Criteria project will meet with some success, it is a long-term project and success is by no means certain. Current difficulties with research into the causes of psychopathology are such that it is also worthwhile to consider other options.

Learning from history: asking different causal questions can enable progress

K. Codell Carter's (2003) *The Rise of Causal Concepts of Disease* argues that shifts in the causal questions that medical researchers asked were necessary for the great advances in medical knowledge seen in the late nineteenth century. Carter argues that the idea that one might seek to discover *the* cause of a disease is comparatively recent. At the start of the nineteenth century, few expected diseases to have unique causes. It was considered perfectly reasonable to think that the same disease might have different causes in different afflicted individuals. As a consequence, many and various causes were typically given for any disease. Those writing on puerperal fever, for example, might distinguish between 'predisposing' and 'exciting' causes and provide lists as follows:

> Predisposing causes included 'a soft and effeminate life, a milieu of luxury and abundance, the absence of exercise sufficient to induce physical vigor and complete vitality of the blood, … weakness produced by poverty, an unhealthy place of residence, a diet inadequately restorative, the abuse of spirituous liquors, various kinds of grief, debauchery, and excessive work. (Dubois, 1842, p. 348 cited in Carter, 2003, p. 40)

Exciting causes included:

> [T]he length of labour, an abundant uterine loss, a grave eclampsia, various maneuvers and surgical operations, something attendant on parturition or the accidents that complicate it, more or less serious genital lesions … the effect of cold air, the use of cold and humid linen, cold water lotions, departures from a [normal] regimen, exciting drinks ... the imprudence of some women who rise in the first days [after delivery] … and the emotional states of the newly delivered. (Dubois, 1842, pp. 348–349, cited in Carter, 2003, p. 40)

Carter notes that gradually, over the course of the nineteenth century, ideas about disease causation shifted. Long lists of multiple and various possible causes became less frequent and it became more usual to find claims which posited one cause per disease. Consider, for example, Semmelweis' view: 'I hold that every case of childbed fever, without a single exception, has only one cause, namely incorporation of decaying organic matter' (Györy, 1905, p. 94 cited in Carter, 2003, p. 49).

Carter explores how medicine moved from the idea that diseases have multiple causes (with different combinations of causes being involved in each case) to the idea that diseases have a universal cause. In Carter's telling, the shift in understanding came about for a number of reasons.

At the empirical level, the nineteenth century saw great advances in medical knowledge. The role played by parasites and bacteria came to be much better understood. For example, the parasitic cause of scabies was discovered in 1835, and that of trichinosis in 1860. In 1882, Robert Koch set out his postulates for demonstrating disease causation, based on his work on cholera, wound infections, and tuberculosis. Though important, these empirical advances will not be discussed further here. For my argument, the relevant part of Carter's narrative concerns conceptual and definitional changes.

First, the revolution in understandings of disease was partly constituted by a shift in the type of causal question that medics asked: 'Nineteenth-century physicians were more interested in questions like "Why does this person now have mumps?" than in questions like "How does mumps come about?"' (Carter, 2003, p. 22).

Explaining how it is that any individual gets a disease at a particular time can legitimately require a consideration of unique and individual causes. Suppose, for example, we ask 'Why has Max got mumps this week?' Our answer might legitimately consider why it is that Max has mumps, as opposed to, say, his siblings, or why it is that Max has mumps now, rather than developing it at some other time. We might say something like 'Max was exposed to the mumps virus two weeks ago because he goes to nursery, and a child at nursery had mumps and passed it on when their drinking bottles got mixed up. His siblings also went to nursery, and drank from the bottle, but their immune system was more robust because they were not as tired as Max'. We might then fairly say that the cause of his mumps was a lack of hygiene, or nursery care, or tiredness. On the other hand, if we ask 'How does mumps come about?' the implicit contrast is between the group of people who have mumps and some group of people who are healthy. In this case we need to search for some factor that is universally present in those who get mumps, but not in those who stay healthy. We will conclude that the cause of mumps is the mumps virus. By the end of the nineteenth century, the causal questions asked by physicians had shifted. Rather than asking why a particular individual got a disorder at a particular time, they shifted to asking what in general distinguishes people with a particular disorder from those without a disorder.

The second change required for revolution in causal understanding of disease was definitional. At the start of the nineteenth century diseases were defined in terms of symptoms; by the end of the century defining them in terms of causes became conceivable.

When diseases are defined in terms of symptoms, this opens up the possibility that different cases of the same disease might have radically different causes. As Carter explains:

> [A]s diseases were typically characterized they simply did not have universal necessary causes. If hydrophobia is an extreme inability to swallow, it really can be caused by blows to the throat, by psychological factors, or by the bites of rabid dogs ... As long as diseases were defined in terms of symptoms, different episodes of any one disease simply did not share a common necessary cause. (Carter, 2003, p. 36)

On such a picture, when different cases of the same disease have very different causes, it is only to be expected that they might also require different treatments. In the early nineteenth century, we thus see a different approach to disease. Given the then-dominant conceptions of disease causation and disease definition there was no straightforward link between nosology, the discovery of causal knowledge, and the discovery of effective treatments.

In contrast, when diseases are defined in terms of causes, the links between classification, causation, and treatment become quite different. It is no longer possible to think that cases of childbed fever can have many and various causes. Only those cases that are caused by *the* common cause of childbed fever count as genuine cases of the disorder: 'The definitions excluded from consideration all cases that failed to have the one common cause, and that cause became, thereby, universal and necessary' (Carter, 2003, p. 54).

Carter sees the shift to adopting the aetiological account of disease as a great advance. With diseases defined in terms of causes, a shift in causal questions from the individual to the general, and improvements in experimental methodologies, rapid progress could be made. It became possible for researchers to set out to discover the cause of a disease, and to then seek to develop a specific therapy that would cure it by attacking the cause.

The aetiological account of disease has worked well in some areas of medicine. But its successes in psychiatry have been modest. Carter's work shows that in the past, medical progress has been enabled by a shift in causal questions. This opens up the possibility that a further change in the causal questions asked might now permit further progress in areas of medical research that are struggling (such as psychiatry). Carter shows that when we ask what causes a disease we can ask a range of questions. Some questions will be easier to answer than others, and so progress can sometimes be facilitated by altering the causal questions that a research programme asks.

Turning to philosophy: multiple causal questions can be asked

In the philosophical literature, it has become widely accepted that 'seeking the causes' might be interpreted in multiple ways. Causal relations as they are in the world are messy and complex. When events occur there are many prior happenings in the world that are causally implicated; every event has multitudinous causes. Take a simple example, such as a wall collapsing. When it was originally built, the bricks were never placed as neatly as they might have been. One builder was inexperienced, the other short-sighted. The slight gaps in the mortar in the walls allowed water in, which froze on occasions, gradually breaking down the mortar. A child climbing on the wall caused further damage. Finally, a car swerved to avoid an oncoming bicycle (with brakes that, for multiple reasons, were more worn than they might have been) and knocked the wall over. This causal history, tedious as it already is, could, of course, be greatly expanded. Infamously, ultimately, the Big Bang is part of the history of every event. But of course referring to the Big Bang as a cause is very rarely informative. In giving an explanation, we select only a few events from a complex causal history and label them 'causes'.

Depending on our interests, different elements of the causal history will be of importance. How do we hone in on some particular part of the complex causal web? A number of philosophers have argued that causal explanations are at least implicitly contrastive (van Fraassen, 1980; Garfinkel, 1981; Lipton, 1990; Hitchcock, 1996). We don't simply explain 'why this' simpliciter, but rather 'why this rather than that'. Each fact to be explained has (at least implicitly) a foil—a relevant way in which things might have been different. In his classic article on contrastive explanation, the philosopher Peter Lipton gives the following example:

> We may not explain why the leaves turn yellow in November tout court, but only, for example, why they turn yellow in November rather than in January, or why they turn yellow in November rather than turning blue. (Lipton, 1990, pp. 248–249)

Generalizing, he claims that:

> To explain why P rather than Q, we must cite a causal difference between P and not-Q, consisting of a cause of P and the absence of a corresponding event in the history of not-Q. (Lipton, 1990, p. 256)

Asking different contrastive questions leads us to focus on different elements in the complex causal histories of events.

We can apply this thinking to consider the sorts of questions that are asked by researchers in psychopathology. The philosopher of psychiatry, Dominic Murphy, notes that multiple explanations of 'the cause' of some disorder may be possible:

> In studying eating disorders, for example, we find that the explanations we need in a given case depend on the relevant question: social factors may explain particular epidemiological patterns, such as variance in eating disorder levels across populations. Social factors alone, however, don't tell us why, out of all the girls in a family within an at-risk group, only one daughter develops an eating disorder. To explain her case, her membership in a class of people who share a particular brain chemical or childhood trauma may be more relevant than her membership of a specific culture. (Murphy, 2008, pp. 109–110)

In Murphy's example, we can think of researchers engaged in various explanatory projects as implicitly asking different contrastive causal questions. The researcher interested in epidemiological variation asks 'Why do girls in country X develop anorexia, while those in country Y do not?' The researcher interested in within-community differences asks 'Why is it that these girls in the community develop anorexia while those do not?', and so on. The take-home message is that there is not just one way to set about investigating 'the causes' of a mental disorder; there are multiple possible causal questions that can be asked.

Going forwards: concrete suggestions and examples

Plausibly, many current research programmes in psychiatry have become bogged down and are making slow progress. From the philosophical work that shows that the causal questions we might ask are multiple, and from Carter's work on the history of medicine, we can see that one way of accelerating progress might be to change the causal questions that are being asked.

In this section, I want to focus on one particular causal question that I think might fruitfully be asked more often: 'Why is it that some people with condition X are harmed by it, while for others it is harmless?'

First, a caveat. Asking 'Why is it that some people with condition X are harmed by it, while for others it is harmless?' is clearly a question that makes more sense in certain cases than others. Some psychiatric conditions are always nasty to have; depression, anxiety, and panic attacks are intrinsically unpleasant. But there are also conditions (here I avoid 'disorder' as some use 'disorder' only when there is harm) that sometimes cause no problems. Possible examples include tic conditions, asexuality, various types of fetish, hearing voices, Asperger syndrome, and mild learning disabilities. When it comes to such conditions, we might ask why it is that they cause harm in some cases but not in others.

We can make use of the idea that causal explanations are contrastive to see how this question is one way to interpret the demand to find 'the causes' of disorder. On Jerome Wakefield's popular account of disorder, for a condition to be a disorder it must be both a dysfunction and harmful (Wakefield, 1992). Wakefield offers an evolutionary account of function and of dysfunction. On his account, whether a condition is a dysfunction is a scientific, empirical matter; whether it is harmful is, of course, a value judgement. If we buy into such an account, then asking 'What causes disorder X?' is equivalent to asking 'What causes harmful dysfunction X?' Current research programmes have focused on explaining the dysfunction element of disorder, but it would be possible to switch emphasis and consider the causes of the harm element of disorder—and this is what I'm proposing. Rather than comparing those with a disorder with a contrast class made up of people with no dysfunction, we would instead compare them with a contrast class made up of people who share the dysfunction but who suffer no harm.

Of course, not everyone accepts Wakefield's account of disorder. Some take issue with his account of dysfunction (e.g. Lilienfeld and Marino, 1995; Cooper, 2002; Bolton, 2008), but agree with Wakefield that disorders are necessarily harmful. For such critics, and for all others who accept that being harmful is a necessary criteria for a condition to count as a disease (e.g. Nordenfelt, 1987; Reznek, 1987), one way of seeking the causes of disorder will be to consider what factors make it only sometimes the case that a condition produces harm.

Some theorists reject the claim that disorders need to be harmful (e.g. Boorse, 1977).[1] On accounts of disorder where harm is not a necessary constituent of disorder, finding out why it is that conditions only sometimes cause harm cannot be construed as a way of discovering the causes of *disorder*. Nevertheless, even on such accounts, discovering the causes of harm can still be construed as a way of discovering the causes of people's *problems*. As such, even those who reject the notion that harm is essential for disorder should be persuaded that investigating the factors that can render harmful symptoms harmless is worthwhile. Such research may lead to the development of interventions that reduce harm. Given that an ultimate aim of psychiatry must be to help people with mental disorders to live better lives, harm reduction is going to be an appropriate goal for psychiatric research regardless of the account of disorder that one holds.

With the rationale for investigating the causes of harm explained, to illustrate how such work might progress, I will consider its application to two examples; tic disorders and hearing voices. The examples are sketchy in so far as I have not attempted to comprehensively review the relevant literature. My aim is to illustrate the sorts of findings that might be hoped for (in the first example) and the sorts of problems that might be encountered (in the second). My aim is to show that seeking the causes of harm is worthwhile—although no panacea.

Example 1: what distinguishes harmful from harmless tics?

Some people with tics find them highly impairing; others have tics but do not mind. In a qualitative study, Andrew Buckser (2009) speaks to people with tic disorders to

---

[1] Within psychiatry, the most notable example of a definition of disorder where it is not essential that a disorder does harm is that included in the *DSM-5* (American Psychiatric Association, 2013, p. 20). In the *DSM-5*, mental disorders are only said to be 'usually associated' with harm. For discussion of this definition see Cooper (2015).

try and understand why it is that some tics are problematic and some are harmless. He finds that, in most cases, tics are only problematic in situations in which they can be viewed by others. It's the potential response of witnesses that makes tics embarrassing, and potentially impairing. If someone tics in their own home or in a private office they are unlikely to care.

Buckser shows that the problems caused by tic disorders vary radically with the opportunities for private ticcing that a social environment affords. Some social settings make it difficult for someone to tic unseen. For example, school classrooms are sometimes designed to make school children visible to teachers at all times. Other environments make it possible for tics to be discharged in private. In earlier work, Buckser (2008) had shown that in suitable environments many adults could develop techniques for managing motor tics that were so successful that their tics passed unnoticed by others. Buckser concludes that 'different institutional settings can produce radically different experiences of the disease' (Buckser, 2009, p. 293).

In this study, we see that depending on the causal question we ask about ticcing we get different answers. Ask 'Why is it that some people tic?', and the answer will be complex and contested. It will likely have something to do with neurological impairments, and these may well be hard to address. On the other hand, if we ask 'What is it that causes some tics to cause problems while others do not?', we get an answer that is fairly easy to obtain and suggests immediate and cheap possibilities for intervention. At least sometimes, the difference between problematic and unproblematic tics lies in the arrangement of furniture, and lives can be made easier by rearranging chairs and desks.

This example shows that in some cases questions of the form 'Why harmful symptoms rather than harmless symptoms?' are comparatively easy to answer. What's more, the answers to such questions can sometimes straightforwardly suggest ways in which people's lives might be made better.

Example 2: what distinguishes harmful voice hearing from harmless voice hearing?

My second example, though, suggests that progress will not always be so easy. Voice hearing (in the sense of hearing voices when no one is speaking) is a symptom associated with schizophrenia and other psychotic conditions, but there are also many people who would not fully satisfy the criteria for any psychiatric disorder who hear voices. Some voice hearers are tormented by their voices. For some voice hearers, however, hearing voices a positive experience; voices may offer helpful advice, or provide company, or be witty.

We can ask what makes the difference between voices that cause no problems and voices that cause harm. Although some work has addressed this question, unfortunately, as I shall show, it is somewhat unclear how the studies to date should be interpreted. There have been problems in selecting appropriate subject groups for research, the empirical results are hard to interpret, and their therapeutic implications are unclear.

Baumeister and colleagues (2017) review 36 studies that consider differences between 'clinical' and 'non-clinical' voice hearers. The inclusion criteria for the review leave it somewhat unclear whether the studies always examine 'non-clinical' voice hearers (i.e. voice hearers who have no history of engaging with mental health services for voice hearing) or are sometimes concerned with voice hearers whose voices cause no problems. This matters because the distinction between clinical and non-clinical voice hearers is not quite the same as the distinction between people who experience harmful voices and those who experience harmless voices. People who experience voices may be 'non-clinical', that is, they do not engage with mental health services, for a number of reasons. Some voice hearers will not be patients because their voices cause no problems—this is the population I'm suggesting we should be interested in. But among the 'non-clinical' there will also be individuals who experience voices that cause harm. Some 'non-clinical' voice hearers will experience harm but not enough harm for them to seek help. There may also be some 'non-clinical' voice hearers whose voices do cause problems, and who might benefit from clinical interventions, but who either avoid engagement with mental health staff or have been unable to access services. Still, while there might be some heterogeneity in the populations studied, the studies reviewed by Baumeister and colleagues can at least provide hints as to what the differences might be between those who experience voices that cause no problems and those that have harmful voices.

The studies reviewed typically compared clinical and non-clinical voice hearers on a number of measures. In a phenomenologically oriented study, Daalman and colleagues (2011) asked about the frequency, duration per hallucination, perceived location (inside or outside the head), loudness, explanation about the origin of the voices, emotional content (positive/ negative), degree of negative content, number of positive versus negative voices, controllability, total distress, age at onset, and number of voices. Other studies reviewed examined differences found on neuroimaging, trauma exposure, and cognitive measures. In the 36 studies reviewed by Baumeister and colleagues (2017), the most consistent findings were that clinical voice hearers heard voices more frequently, experienced more negative voice content, and tended to have an older age of onset. None of these differences look to be easily amenable to intervention. It is not clear how one might modify the frequency or emotional valance of voices, and age of onset clearly cannot be changed.

On some accounts, whether a voice hearer experiences a voice as negative or positive may be connected to their beliefs about the voice. Daalman and colleagues (2011) found that many of those who hear non-distressing voices attribute the voices to unspecific external or spiritual sources. In contrast, those who find their voices troubling are more likely to think that they come from some other living person, god, demons or devils, or an implanted device. The direction of causation is not entirely clear, but it is plausible that a person's beliefs about the source of a voice can affect how distressing it will be. Suppose one hears a voice saying 'Now you're going to go to church'. If one thinks that the voice stems from an implanted transmitter controlled by a critical priest then this will likely be experienced negatively, perhaps as a hectoring demand. On the other hand, if one thinks the voice is a spiritual guide offering advice, then the same message might be taken as a friendly suggestion. How someone responds to a voice may also make a difference to how the voice is experienced (although, again, here the direction of causation is somewhat unclear). Kråkvik and colleagues (2015) suggest that those who hear harmful voices are more likely to attempt to actively ignore them, or to try to understand them or to argue with them, while those with harmless voices are more likely to make no response. Some studies suggest that cognitive therapies might help those who are troubled by voices to alter their beliefs about voices, and/or ways of responding to them, and that this might help to reduce the extent to which voices cause distress (Thomas et al., 2014).

Whether the same causal mechanisms underlie voice hearing in the case of people who hear harmful voices and in the case of people who hear non-harmful voices is currently the subject of debate. The difference in age of onset between those who hear harmful and those who hear harmless voices might suggest that the causal mechanisms that underlie the voice hearing in the two groups differ. Daalman and colleagues (2011) comment:

> Patients were approximately 21 years when they first experienced AVHs [auditory verbal hallucinations, i.e. voices], compared to a mean age at onset of 12 in the nonpatients. This finding might be indicative of a difference in the etiology of AVHs in the psychotic and nonpsychotic subjects, as the onset of AVHs may be associated to aberrant synaptic connectivity. Synaptic density peaks during childhood, followed by an extensive decrease of neuronal connectivity (pruning) during adolescence, to reach normal levels in adulthood. Thus, the age of onset of AVHs in psychotic patients coincides with maximal synaptic density. In contrast, the age at onset of AVHs in psychotic patients coincides with synaptic elimination (pruning). (Daalman et al., 2011, p. 324)

The difference in age of onset might be explained by a difference in aetiology, but there are also other possible explanations for the correlation between younger onset and hearing non-harmful voices. It might be that children find it easier to adapt to hearing voices, and that those who start to hear voices when young thus have fewer problems with their voices as adults.

Overall, the studies that investigate differences between clinical and non-clinical voice hearers are disappointing. While cognitive therapies are being developed on the back of studies that suggest that beliefs about voices, and approaches to dealing with voices, may affect levels of distress, the studies do not suggest any *easy* ways whereby harmful voices might be rendered harmless. The possibility that clinical and non-clinical voice hearing may have a different aetiology makes the interpretation of the studies especially unclear. It is currently uncertain whether or not a clinical voice hearer has the same underlying condition as a non-clinical voice hearer.

In Carter's work on the development of the aetiological account of disease, he showed that asking new causal questions went hand-in-hand with defining the subject populations for research in new ways. Carter's work suggests that when a research programme takes on new causal questions, definitional changes are to be anticipated, as researchers who ask different causal questions will need to divide up the domain of interest to them in different ways. In the studies reviewed by Baumeister and colleagues (2017), it is noticeable that defining the populations of interest for research has been problematic. Ideally, it would be good to have studies that examine differences between harmless and harmful voice hearing, but current classifications and rating scales mean that selecting suitable subject populations for such research is difficult. At present, *DSM* diagnostic criteria often have built into them the idea that the condition must cause harm.[2] *DSM* criteria for schizophrenia mean that only people who are impaired by their condition can be diagnosed as having schizophrenia (American Psychiatric Association, 2013, p. 99). Flourishing voice hearers will thus automatically be excluded from any study that uses *DSM* criteria for schizophrenia to select a subject population. Elsewhere I have defended the idea that harm should be required as a criterion for a *DSM* diagnosis (Cooper, 2013). I think it is important that only people who are harmed by some condition are counted as having a disorder. However, if we want to investigate the differences between voice hearers who are harmed and those who are not harmed, it would be useful for researchers to be able to select a population of people such that it seems likely that all are affected by same sort of condition but where only a subpopulation are harmed by their condition. *DSM* diagnoses are poorly suited to this task.

Many studies do not rely on *DSM* diagnostic criteria, but rather try to select populations of non-clinical voice hearers on the basis of symptoms. Such methods can also sometimes exclude flourishing voice hearers. A number of the studies reviewed by Baumeister and colleagues (2017) collected subjects on the basis of their responses to the Launay and Slade Hallucinations Scale (LSHS), a self-report questionnaire designed to quantify the tendency to hallucinate in 'healthy' individuals. This scale includes two items related to voice hearing: item 8, 'In the past, I have had the experience of hearing a person's voice and then found that no-one was there' and item 12, 'I have been troubled by voices in my head'. A number of studies have used positive responses to these two items to select a population of non-clinical voice hearers. In such cases, I suggest the sampling method is problematic. Those who say that they have been *troubled* by voices in the past are more likely to have problems with their voices. People who have heard voices in the past but not been *troubled* by them will not be detected by this item.

Research into the causal factors that distinguish harmless from harmful symptoms requires it to be possible to pick out groups of people that experience 'symptoms' but for whom they are not problematic. To enable this, rating scales and definitions will need to be developed that do not presuppose that a 'symptom' is harmful. In Carter's historical study, a shift in the causal questions of interest went along with a reconceptualization of disorder definitions. Here, too, asking new causal questions will require new ways of defining subject populations to be developed. Researchers who want to investigate the causal factors that lead to symptoms being harmful will also need new ways to define the populations to be investigated.

---

[2] The general introduction to the *DSM* includes a definition of disorder. Between *DSM-IV* (American Psychiatric Association, 1994) and *DSM-5* (American Psychiatric Association, 2013) this definition was revised. It used to be that a condition could only be a mental disorder if it caused harm, now harm is not required. Nevertheless, many of the sets of diagnostic criteria for individual disorders continue to include the idea that the patient must be harmed by their condition for diagnosis. In many cases, such criteria have been inherited from the *DSM-IV*. The introductory definition of mental disorder included in the *DSM-5* was produced late in the revision process, and seems to have had little impact on the sets of diagnostic criteria (for fuller discussion, see Cooper (2015)).

I suggest that asking the question 'Why does condition X harm some people but not others?' will always be worthwhile in cases where some people with a condition are not harmed by it. The example of ticcing illustrates that sometimes asking this question might suggest simple interventions that might be hoped to render harmful instances of a symptom harmless. On the other hand, the example of voice hearing shows that even when some insight can be gained into the factors that make a symptom harmless, it will not always be straightforward to intervene. The question 'Why does condition X harm some people but not others?' is worth asking. Sometimes (although not always) this question will prove relatively easy to answer and will suggest ways to help people lead better lives.

Conclusion

In this chapter I have argued that empirical progress sometimes requires a change in the causal questions that researchers ask. I have used Carter's work in the history of medicine, and philosophical work on causation, to argue that projects that seek 'the causes of disorder' might pursue this aim in multiple ways. As there are multiple possible causal questions, researchers have a choice when it comes to selecting which causal questions to address. Some causal questions will turn out to be easier to address than others. This means that when research programmes stall, it is worth trying to re-start progress through switching the causal question. I considered one type of causal question—'Why do some people with condition X find it harmful and others harmless?'—that might plausibly be fruitfully addressed more often than at present.

References

American Psychiatric Association (1980). *Diagnostic and Statistical Manual of Mental Disorders* (3rd ed.). Washington, DC: American Psychiatric Publishing.

American Psychiatric Association (1994). *Diagnostic and Statistical Manual of Mental Disorders* (4th ed.). Washington, DC: American Psychiatric Publishing.

American Psychiatric Association (2013). *Diagnostic and Statistical Manual of Mental Disorders* (5th ed.). Washington, DC: American Psychiatric Publishing.

Baumeister, D., Sedgwick, O., Howes, O., and Peters, E. (2017). Auditory verbal hallucinations and continuum models of psychosis: a systematic review of the healthy voice-hearer literature. *Clinical Psychology Review*, **51**, 125–141.

Blashfield, R.K. and Keeley, J.W. (2010). A short history of a psychiatric diagnostic category that turned out to be a disease. In: T. Millon, R. Kreuger, and E. Simonson (Eds.), *Contemporary Directions in Psychopathology* (pp. 324–336). New York: Guilford Press.

Bolton, D. (2008). *What Is Mental Disorder?* Oxford: Oxford University Press.

Boorse, C. (1977). Health as a theoretical concept. *Philosophy of Science*, **44**(4), 542–573.

Buckser, A. (2008). Before your very eyes: illness, agency, and the management of Tourette syndrome. *Medical Anthropology Quarterly*, **22**(2), 167–192.

Buckser, A. (2009). Institutions, agency, and illness in the making of Tourette syndrome. *Human Organization*, **68**(2), 293–306.

Carter, K.C. (2003). *The Rise of Causal Concepts of Disease: Case Histories*. Aldershot: Ashgate.

Cooper, R. (2002). Disease. *Studies in History and Philosophy of Science Part C: Studies in History and Philosophy of Biological and Biomedical Sciences*, **33**(2), 263–282.

Cooper, R. (2013). Avoiding false positives: zones of rarity, the threshold problem, and the DSM clinical significance criterion. *The Canadian Journal of Psychiatry*, **58**(11), 606–611.

Cooper, R. (2015). Must disorders cause harm? The changing stance of the DSM. In: S. Demazeux and P. Singy (Eds.), *The DSM-5 in Perspective* (pp. 83–96.). Netherlands: Springer.

Daalman, K., Boks, M.P., Diederen, K.M., De Weijer, A.D., Blom, J.D., Kahn, R.S., and Sommer, I.E. (2011). The same or different? A phenomenological comparison of auditory verbal hallucinations in healthy and psychotic individuals. *The Journal of Clinical Psychiatry*, **72**(3), 320–325.

Garfinkel, A. (1981). *Forms of Explanation*. New Haven, CT: Yale University Press.

Ghaemi, N. (2012). Taking disease seriously: beyond 'pragmatic' nosology. In: K. Kendler and J. Parnas (Eds.), *Philosophical Issues in Psychiatry II: Nosology* (pp. 42–53). Oxford: Oxford University Press.

Hitchcock, C.R. (1996). The role of contrast in causal and explanatory claims. *Synthese*, **107**(3), 395–419.

Insel, T.R. (2014). The NIMH Research Domain Criteria (RDoC) Project: precision medicine for psychiatry. *The American Journal of Psychiatry*, **171**(4), 395–397.

Kendler, K.S. (2013). What psychiatric genetics has taught us about the nature of psychiatric illness and what is left to learn. *Molecular Psychiatry*, **18**(10), 1058–1066.

Kendler, K.S., Gardner, C.O., and Prescott, C.A. (2002). Toward a comprehensive developmental model for major depression in women. *American Journal of Psychiatry*, **159**(7), 1133–1145.

Kråkvik, B., Larøi, F., Kalhovde, A.M., Hugdahl, K., Kompus, K., Salvesen, Ø., Stiles, T.C., and Vedul-Kjelsås, E. (2015). Prevalence of auditory verbal hallucinations in a general population: a group comparison study. *Scandinavian Journal of Psychology*, **56**(5), 508–515.

Lilienfeld, S.O. and Marino, L. (1995). Mental disorder as a Roschian concept: a critique of Wakefield's 'harmful dysfunction' analysis. *Journal of Abnormal Psychology*, **104**(3), 411–420.

Lipton, P. (1990). Contrastive explanation. *Royal Institute of Philosophy Supplement*, **27**, 247–266.

Murphy, D. (2008). Levels of explanation in psychiatry. In: K. Kendler and J. Parnas (Eds.), *Philosophical Issues in Psychiatry: Explanation, Phenomenology, and Nosology* (pp. 99–124). Oxford: Oxford University Press.

Nordenfelt, L. (1987). *On the Nature of Health: An Action-Theoretic Approach*. Dordrecht: Kluwer.

Reznek, L. (1987). *The Nature of Disease*. London: Routledge.

Thomas, N., Hayward, M., Peters, E., van der Gaag, M., Bentall, R.P., Jenner, J., Strauss, C., Sommer, I.E., Johns, L.C., Varese, F., and García-Montes, J.M. (2014). Psychological therapies for auditory hallucinations (voices): current status and key directions for future research. *Schizophrenia Bulletin*, **40** (Suppl.4), S202–S212.

Uher, R. and Rutter, M. (2012). Basing psychiatric classification on scientific foundation: problems and prospects. *International Review of Psychiatry*, **24**(6), 591–605.

Van Fraassen, B.C. (1980). *The Scientific Image*. Oxford: Oxford University Press.

Wakefield, J.C. (1992). The concept of mental disorder: on the boundary between biological facts and social values. *American Psychologist*, **47**(3), 373–388.

Chapter 5

A developmental approach to understanding psychiatric disorders: Mapping aetiological pathways

Simone P.W. Haller and Kathrin Cohen Kadosh

Introduction

In the last two decades, advances in paediatric neuroimaging have provided us with a plethora of neuroimaging studies investigating how age-related changes in brain function and structure may contribute to changes in behaviour (Blakemore, 2008; Burnett et al., 2011). These results have deepened our appreciation of the dynamic neuro-maturational processes across the first decades of life. Yet, we are still a long way from turning brain evidence into strategies that could help with navigating specific developmental challenges more successfully (Cohen Kadosh et al., 2013b). In this chapter, we illustrate how charting developmental trajectories more continuously can inform our understanding of typical development and psychiatric aetiology, ultimately towards a goal long envisioned: using brain-based evidence to inform timing and efficacy of early intervention and prevention.

A paradigm shift towards mapping continuous trajectories of change over time

Adolescence is a transitional period, which begins with the onset of puberty and ends with the individual assuming a stable adult role (Lerner and Steinberg, 2004). Adolescence is marked by changes on many levels: changes in brain structure and function, genetic and hormonal innovations alongside puberty, as well as social–environmental changes. Concurrent with these developments are improvements in social–cognitive abilities (Blakemore, 2008; Burnett et al., 2011; Cohen Kadosh et al., 2013b; Linscott and van Os, 2013) linked to a stronger peer orientation during adolescence (Kloep, 1999; Rose and Rudolph, 2006) and increased participation in complex social networks (Steinberg and Silverberg, 1986). It has been suggested that the timing of these transformational processes could serve to multiply the risk for atypical development, particularly mental health disorders (Paus et al., 2008; Haller et al., 2014, 2015; Keshavan et al., 2014). Our current lack of a comprehensive understanding of typical developmental changes pre-puberty and across adolescence and risk trajectories is particularly problematic, as age-of-onset data suggest that many psychiatric disorders first emerge at the adolescent juncture or in young adulthood (Wittchen et al., 1999; Kessler et al., 2005). Early difficulties have also been shown to significantly increase the risk of long-term mental health problems during adulthood (Pine et al., 1996, 1999; Gregory et al., 2007; McGorry et al., 2011; Kaymaz et al., 2012a).

Mapping trajectories is critical for progress on mental health research and integrative models of psychiatric conditions for several reasons. First, delineating times of significant change will help us understand whether there are periods of significant and rapid maturation. While rapid change of a certain structure must not automatically mean that this structure and its function is particularly amenable to external influence at the time of change, it is plausible that early emerging functions will result in earlier brain specialization, thus likely leaving the cognitive/brain function in question less amenable to interventions at later time points (Johnson et al., 2015). Hence, differentiating changes that are unique to adolescence from those that are non-specific changes ongoing from earlier developmental stages, or adolescent-emerging changes that will mature at the later stage (Figure 5.1a), may prove very useful. Especially when mapping change in relation to external factors, we can move closer to understanding whether there are developmentally sensitive periods for certain functions and experiences. A second, related, key benefit of mapping developmental trajectories is that it would allow us to understand what constitutes typical variations and what represents a risk factor or risk trajectory. It is important to model factors on several levels to understand how a risk factor on one level may be conditional, interact, or find expression on another level of analysis. Understanding the pathways through which risk factors are expressed can elucidate individual differences in pathways to pathological outcomes. Specifically, it has long been recognized that there may be different aetiological pathways to the same psychiatric outcome (equifinality) and, vice versa, the same risk factors can result in different outcomes (multifinality). It is only when we understand the dynamic interplay between factors and developmental timing that we can understand aetiological paths to mental health conditions and are in a position to tailor intervention approaches appropriately and timely. An important step will be to move away from cross-sectional studies and to focus more on building comprehensive, continuous trajectories of cognitive and brain development in order to differentiate the type of developmental differences (i.e. developmental delay, lag, deterioration, or overall deficit) (Figure 5.1b) and changing risk correlates. Crucially, the broader these trajectories are, that is, the more cognitive skills, brain, hormonal, genetic, and environmental indices they encompass, the easier it would be to understand conditional, interactive, and cumulative effects of risk. This would allow us to tease apart the different pathways to a psychiatric outcome (e.g. where pathways diverge, the relative role of social experiences on different paths to disorder). Each type of developmental difference and pathway comes with its own implications for intervention approaches. For example, intervention programmes could be developed that target specific points of divergence from typical trajectories, or help to compensate for delay early on. No matter how these trajectories play out, getting a better handle on timing information, that

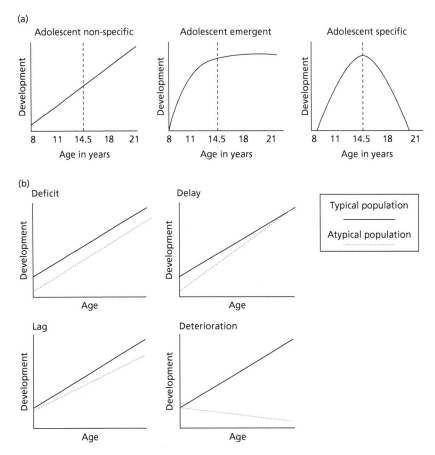

Figure 5.1 (a) Hypothesized patterns of cognitive and brain development during adolescence. For this chapter, adolescent-specific changes, which may indicate a period of increased plasticity, are of particular interest.
Reproduced from Casey, B.J. The teenage brain: an overview. *Current Directions in Psychological Science*, 22(2), 80–81. Copyright © 2013 SAGE Publications.
(b) Hypothesized developmental trajectories of neuropsychological functioning in healthy controls and psychotic disorder groups.
Adapted with permission from Reichenberg, A. et al. (In preparation).

is, understanding when and how risk factors are expressed in development, will be crucial if we are to devise interventions that target both brain function and behaviour before external influences are likely less impactful (Cohen Kadosh et al., 2013b; Johnson et al., 2015).

We will now discuss two examples of disorders that often first emerge at the adolescent juncture, psychosis and social anxiety, to illustrate the need for a developmental approach to understand psychiatric aetiology across groups of mental disorders with different genetic and environmental risk factor profiles.

Psychosis

With early-onset psychotic disorders (PDs) falling right into the transitional juncture from childhood to adolescence (Paus et al., 2008; McGorry et al., 2011), it is surprising that there is still relatively little research that examines different developmental factors that put youths at risk for the development of PDs during this period. A substantial body of genetic research has highlighted the heritability of PDs, and also the differential effects of genetic variants (Bacanu and Kendler, 2013). Recent data suggest that some of the genetic effects of risk for schizophrenia may be conferred via gene variants that are linked to postnatal pruning (Sekar et al., 2016). Hence, some genetic risks for psychosis may play out specifically in adolescence as a period of ongoing pruning of synapses (Burnett et al., 2011).

Another age-specific risk factor is early psychotic experiences (PEs). PEs such as delusions, hallucinations, or thought interferences are prevalent among the general population and particularly during childhood and adolescence (Cougnard et al., 2007; van Os et al., 2009; Kelleher et al., 2012). Persistence of PEs is a strong indicator of an increased risk for a later disorder, including psychosis (Kaymaz et al., 2012b). PEs have been linked with lower cognitive ability, poor psychosocial outcomes, general psychopathology, and self-harm (Barnett et al., 2012; Downs et al., 2013; Nishida et al., 2010; Polanczyk et al., 2010).

The effect of early psychotic experiences on cognitive functioning

In the adult PE literature, a substantial body of research has documented lower cognitive functioning in the domains of executive function, processing speed, and working memory (Simon et al., 2007; Fusar-Poli et al., 2012; Valli et al., 2012). These differences increase in severity through prodromal phases towards clinical psychosis (Simon et al., 2007; Meier et al., 2014) and greater deficits are found in those who do transition to psychosis (De Herdt et al., 2013).

In order to take a closer look at specific cognitive impairments in participants with PE, Reichenberg and colleagues (2010) investigated cognitive development in the Dunedin cohort, a longitudinal study of 1037 children in Dunedin, New Zealand, who were assessed regularly over 30 years. By comparing a schizophrenia case group and healthy controls from this sample, they found that those children who went on to develop adult schizophrenia exhibited early and relatively stable impairments in verbal and visual knowledge acquisition, reasoning, and conceptualization (i.e. developmental deficits). The schizophrenia case group also showed a developmental lag (i.e. growth that is slower relative to healthy children) in processing speed, visual–spatial problem-solving and working memory.

In a different study, Reichenberg and colleagues (in preparation) assessed the neuropsychological profiles of 4720 participants of the Avon Longitudinal Study of Parents and Children (ALSPAC). The ALSPAC cohort consists of originally 14,602 children who underwent comprehensive demographic, psychosocial, and clinical assessments through the ages of 4, 8, 11, 15, 18, and 20 years. Reichenberg and colleagues compared four groups of typically developing participants ($n = 4037$): a group diagnosed with depression (n = 251), a preclinical group with PEs (n = 358), and a group diagnosed with PDs (n = 74). Note that all groups were based on clinical assessments at age 18. They found evidence for a developmental language deficit in the PD group. With regard to working memory abilities, the PE group exhibited consistently lower abilities (i.e. a developmental deficit), whereas the PD group showed an increasing developmental delay in working memory abilities. Moreover, visuospatial abilities were consistently lower in the PE group. Last, processing speed impairments were subject to a developmental lag in both PD and PE groups, with the latter group exhibiting a smaller magnitude.

Dickson and colleagues compared the neuropsychological profiles of four groups of children aged 9–12 years: (1) children with high familial loading (i.e. more than one first-degree affected relative but less than two second-degree affected relatives (FHL)); (2) children with low familial loading (i.e. no more than one second-degree relative (FLL)); (3) children with well-replicated antecedents of schizophrenia (ASz); and (4) non-typically developing children (TD) (Dickson et al., 2014). They found that the FHL group exhibited worse performance on all measures, except for visual memory. Overall performance was ranked as follows: FHL < ASz < FLL < TD. When overall IQ differences were controlled for, only the group differences in executive functions (inhibition/switching) (FHL < all other groups) and visual memory survived (FLL < FHL). Their results also seemed to suggest that poor verbal memory is the best predictor for later conversion to diagnosis. The studies reviewed here highlight the important contribution that neuropsychological profiling, and especially longitudinal profiling can make to the risk assessment for PDs. In the next section, we will review how the research into the underlying brain bases can explain some of the observed developmental differences in cognitive functioning.

Brain development during adolescence and its relationship to psychotic experiences

A consistent body of neuroimaging research in recent years has revealed ongoing grey and white matter changes during adolescence (Giedd et al., 1999; Harris et al., 2011; Lebel and Beaulieu, 2011; Petanjek et al., 2011; Tamnes et al., 2013; Mills et al., 2014), along with increasing functional connectivity in default and resting state brain networks (Fair et al., 2007, 2008). All these changes affect not only the brain structure, but also the functional responsiveness and processing abilities of the developing brain. In the developing brain, prefrontal cortices are the last to reach structural maturity (Casey et al., 2005), a prolonged trajectory that is reflected in gradually developing executive functions and particularly working memory abilities (Casey et al., 2005; Blakemore, 2008; Dumontheil and Klingberg, 2012). In line with this, memory capacity increases continuously during typical development, with the underlying supporting brain network becoming increasingly localized to a predominantly frontoparietal network (Casey et al., 2005; Klingberg, 2006; Conklin et al., 2007). More advanced analysis techniques, such as dynamic causal modelling (Friston et al., 2003), have allowed us to pinpoint the underlying dynamics of this emerging network. Specifically, it has been shown that parietal regions are involved at an earlier stage of processing than frontal regions and that increasing memory load modulates parietal-to-frontal connectivity (Ma et al., 2012; Dima et al., 2014).

Taking into account the prolonged maturation of the prefrontal cortices may also go some way towards bringing together the hypofrontality theory of reduced prefrontal functioning in schizophrenia patients and the increased psychosis incidence rate in adolescence (Ingvar and Franzen, 1974; Kessler et al., 2007). The hypofrontality theory has received some support from a body of neuroimaging studies that have extended the profile of frontal lobe dysfunction to prodromal populations both in terms of elicited activation (e.g. Fusar-Poli et al., 2007; Corlett and Fletcher, 2012; Dutt et al., 2015) and structural differences (e.g. Thermenos et al., 2013; Alexander-Bloch et al., 2014). Yet, if adolescents are per se 'hypofrontal,' then it becomes even more critical to detect preceding differences in other brain structures, which exacerbate the fact that the pre-frontal cortex (PFC) does not step up to be more involved as in typically developing adolescents. More precisely, within the framework suggested by Casey (2013), it would be important to take into account the effect of non-specific adolescent-specific developmental changes, such as maturational changes.

One way of achieving this would be by looking at individual differences in the underlying neuroanatomy at different ages, that is, by looking at how the disorder affects the developmental process in affected, at-risk, and unaffected populations. For example, in a recent study, Alexander-Bloch and colleagues found abnormal non-linear growth processes in prefrontal and temporal brain areas in a longitudinal study of 106 participants with childhood-onset schizophrenia and 102 control participants aged 7–32 years (Alexander-Bloch et al., 2014).

Within the greater context of schizotaxia (the syndrome of brain dysfunction, expressed by negative symptoms and neuropsychological deficits), the most consistent finding of structural differences is a reduction in PFC volume (Thermenos et al., 2013). For example, in the Edinburgh longitudinal study (McIntosh et al., 2011) of 162 high-risk participants and 36 matched controls who were scanned repeatedly over 10 years, the bilateral PFC showed significant volume reduction in those participants who went on to develop schizophrenia. This was a significantly greater reduction in comparison to other groups that did not go on to develop schizophrenia. McIntosh and colleague also found reductions in temporal lobe volume and in whole brain volume for this sample. A key advantage of studying individual differences in brain development in a preclinical sample is that this approach avoids potential confounding variables such as the effects of treatment and medication, all of which are likely to shape behaviour and brain development. Ideally, building comprehensive developmental trajectories in both low- and high-risk preclinical samples would then allow us to determine biological markers of risk, such as the proposed lower PFC or temporal lobe volume, which may help predict a later progression to diagnosis more reliably. Such an approach was taken by Drakesmith and colleagues (2015). In the Avon Longitudinal Study of Parents and Children (ALSPAC) magnetic resonance imaging (MRI) study, a total of 4724 young adults, out of an initial cohort of 14,062 births, were assessed with the Psychosis-Like Symptom interview (PLIKSi) at age 18 years where 433 (9.2%) individuals were rated as having suspected or definite PE (Zammit et al., 2013). From this sample, 248 participants (125 controls and 123 suspected definite) were reassessed using the PLIKSi and underwent functional MRI at age 20 years. By combining these interview and brain data with a comprehensive cognitive assessment, the ALSPAC MRI studies were able to assess how changes in cognitive abilities relate to brain development, and vice versa, and, more importantly, how these relate to individual differences in PEs. With regard to differences in brain structure, Drakesmith and colleagues found evidence for structural differences in white matter connectivity, with reduced global and local efficiency in critical core network hubs (Drakesmith et al., 2015), as has been reported in previous work (Zalesky et al., 2011). Interestingly, they also found reduced density in the default mode network (DMN), a network of regions consistently found to be activating during rest when attention is turned inward and not cued by external stimuli. Lack of suppression of the DMN is associated with hallucinations and faulty self-processing (Anticevic et al., 2012; Whitfield-Gabrieli and Ford, 2012). Last, they reported reduced local efficiency in the posterior cingulate and parietal regions and left inferior frontal regions (all part of the DMN), with the efficiency reductions in the inferior frontal gyrus correlating negatively with the severity of auditory hallucinations. Notably, the reduced efficiency was only evident at the network level and not when looking at pair-wise comparisons for connections, suggesting that the observed differences were subtle, perhaps not a surprising finding given that this study examined individual differences in PE in a subclinical sample.

Functional brain responses

With regard to functional brain responses, much research has focused on comparing brain activation in the PFC during working memory tasks, such as the n-back task (Kirchner, 1958). In the n-back task, participants view a stream of consecutively presented stimuli. They are then asked to recognize a stimulus that was presented 0, 1, 2, or 3 trials previously. A meta-analysis of ten studies that used the n-back task with at-risk adult participants found decreased prefrontal activation (Fusar-Poli, 2012). The literature on clinical populations seems more complex, with a study in patients with schizophrenia and control participants showing that the simple hypothesis of hypofrontality may be indeed too simple (Callicott et al., 2003). For example, response times have been shown to vary greatly as a function of symptom severity and task difficulty and, importantly, within different areas of the PFC.

For example, Fonville and colleagues (2015) compared functional brain responses in a subset of participants from the ALSPAC study. They found no differences in brain response in core working memory brain regions, which contrasted with lower task performance in the 3-back condition. Similarly, Seidman and colleagues (2006) found increased activation in the dorsolateral PFC in a group of high-risk adolescents and young adults (aged 13–26 years), which remained significant when controlling for task performance, psychopathology, and IQ. In contrast, a study by Wolf and colleagues (2015) used a n-back task (0-, 1-, 2-back) and emotion categorization task in participants with PEs and without PEs aged 11–22 years. Testing a large sample, they found that the PE group exhibited less activation in the prefrontal regions for the n-back task, which went along with lower performance levels. At this point it is difficult to determine whether the lower performance levels resulted in decreased prefrontal response, or vice versa.

Last, Pauly and colleagues (2010) combined an *n*-back task with an emotion manipulation in at-risk adult participants and found that the participants did not exhibit any behavioural differences, but differed with regard to prefrontal activation. Specifically, they observed that the at-risk group did not show a prefrontal activation decrease, a group difference that they interpreted as an indication for compensatory network use in order to maintain task efficiency.

The interpretation that participants might use additional brain regions in order to compensate for non- or low-functioning brain networks is a long-standing assumption in the literature, where the same tasks are necessarily performed by different brain regions throughout development (Johnson et al., 2009, 2015). For example, in the face processing literature, it has been shown that with training and exposure, and as different brain regions mature, task recruitment patterns change as well (Cohen Kadosh and Johnson, 2007; Cohen Kadosh et al., 2011, 2013a).

An elegant way to differentiate changes in recruitment patterns is the use of dynamic causal modelling, which allows us to examine network responses and structure as a function of group membership (patients vs non-patients) or task requirement. In one study, Fonville and colleagues (2015) used this approach to uncover more subtle network differences in their sample of participants with and without PE, in spite of non-significant group differences in the functional analysis. Specifically, for their three groups of participants with persistent PEs, participants with transient PEs (which have disappeared from the first to the second assessment), and typical controls, they found that frontal-to-parietal modulation was the most likely configuration in the *n*-back task. However, the probability of best fit decreased from persistent PE to controls, with transient PE intermediate, which the authors interpreted as a predominant reliance on frontal network regions in the persistent PE group, whereas the control group relied on more mature, parietally driven networks during this task.

Interim summary: what can a developmental angle contribute to this psychotic experience research?

The work reviewed in the previous sections has provided a glimpse of how much could be gained by adding a developmental angle to our research into PEs and schizotaxia. That is, with most patients only being diagnosed in their early twenties (McGorry et al., 2011), it would appear negligent to ignore early developmental differences that can already be observed towards the end of the first decade of life (Beddington et al., 2008). One difficulty may be that these early risk indices appear quite different from the more established cognitive differences that we have come to expect in the adult literature. This may be due to the underlying brain structures that develop at different temporal time courses. For example, whereas early static deficits in verbal and visual knowledge (Reichenberg et al., 2010) could be due to structural differences in the temporal lobe (e.g. Alexander-Bloch et al., 2014), the more commonly reported hypofrontality differences may only emerge during adolescence, as a result of the prefrontal lobe failing to specialize in the same manner as in the typically developing adolescents. Indeed, it has been shown that the adolescence-specific delays and lags (Reichenberg et al., 2010; Casey, 2013) in processing speed or visuospatial problem-solving rely more heavily on slowly developing frontoparietal networks (Dumontheil et al., 2008; Dumontheil and Klingberg, 2012). Hence, whereas these differences are initially overlooked because the frontoparietal network is still developing in all participants, during adolescence, frontal lobe-dependent abilities will become more apparent as compensatory network configurations become unavailable. A developmental approach could help with bringing together how these individual variations in cognitive and behavioural factors contribute towards the different outcomes and ultimately, improve predictions as to whether some individuals are more at risk for making the transition from early PEs to an acute psychosis.

Social anxiety disorder

There is a pronounced increase of social anxiety symptomatology at the juncture of adolescence. In fact, the majority (75%) of cases have their onset in late childhood to mid-adolescence with very few new cases emerging after the mid-twenties (Wittchen et al., 1999; Kessler et al., 2005; Gregory et al., 2007). Since adolescence is generally associated with increased salience of (peer-related) social cues and heightened self-consciousness (Blakemore, 2008), it is maybe not surprising that social anxiety disorder (SAD) is one of the most common and impairing anxiety conditions in youth (Wittchen et al., 1999; Kessler et al., 2005). Since peer interactions are important socialization experiences for adolescents, avoidance of social exchanges, which is often linked to social anxiety, is likely particularly disabling and disruptive during this time (Miers et al., 2014).

Compared to PDs, adolescent SAD has a significantly weaker genetic component with the environment having a large impact, specifically unique environmental influences (Lau et al., 2007a, 2007b).

The cognitive aetiology of social anxiety disorder

Central targets of current psychological frontline treatments for SAD are cognitive biases in the processing social cues. Cognitive biases in attention allocation, in the interpretation of ambiguous social stimuli, and in core beliefs about performance in social situations are thought to give rise to a preferential processing of threatening over benign information (Clark and Wells, 1995). Hence, by increasing perceived social threat and negative social feedback in social interactions and performance situations, biases may maintain social fears and likely play a central role in shaping maladaptive patterns of social avoidance, which, in a vicious cycle, further reinforce social fears.

Compared to work in adults, significantly less work has focused on the presence and role of these biases in younger populations. This is problematic, given that current psychological treatments are based on the assumption that adolescent SAD has the same cognitive features as adult SAD. Additionally, little research has focused on describing how these clinically relevant processes change with time in typically developing youths.

Several studies have found some evidence for biased attention orienting in youths with SAD or with high trait levels of social anxiety relative to their non-socially anxious peers; however, a number of studies have found no evidence for biases in attentional orienting in anxious youths (Stirling et al., 2006; Roy et al., 2008). There are multiple sources from which these inconsistencies could arise: some of the most commonly used paradigms have poor reliability and investigations in youths may not have been systematic enough to discern more complex attentional patterns of hypervigilance–avoidance. There is also some recent work that suggests that there may be a general developmental heterogeneity of biases in anxious youths with changes in directionality of biases from childhood to adolescence (Gamble and Rapee, 2009), that is, there may be developmental effects in links between anxiety and attention capture by threat.

Ambiguity is inherent in social interactions, as interactions require individuals to continuously monitor and interpret dynamic and complex visual and verbal cues to make inferences about mental states of others. Skewed interpretations of these everyday ambiguous social experiences (e.g. a frown of an audience member during your presentation or a laugh behind you in the hallway) have also been suggested to play a central role in the maintenance of social anxiety. However, while adult studies have generally shown robust associations between social anxiety and interpretation bias (Amin et al., 1998; Constans et al., 1999; Stopa and Clark, 2000; Amir et al., 2012), studies conducted in children and adolescents have yielded more mixed results with some studies finding that biases are not linked to social anxiety (In-Albon et al., 2009; Creswell et al., 2014).

One possibility as to why robust associations between interpretation bias and anxiety are not consistently found in youth studies is that age may moderate this association (Haller et al., 2013). With the growing importance of peers and sociocultural norms increasingly guiding behaviour, it is likely that social cue interpretation fine-tunes during puberty and across adolescence. With increasing age, youths have a greater quantity of social experiences to inform their thinking styles, and cognitive styles may also become more stable and global (e.g. Nolen-Hoeksema et al., 1992). Interpretational style may only become stable and function as a maintenance factor in adolescence, not earlier in development (Nolen- Hoeksema et al., 1992; Nolen-Hoeksema, 1996). However, it should be noted that there are alternative explanations; for instance, the assessment tools commonly used to identify interpretation biases may also not work as well for developing populations and there are far fewer youth samples in general.

Social concerns are typical in adolescence. In many ways, SAD represents a more exaggerated version of the typical developmental phenomenon of increased salience and reactivity to social cues and sensitivity to social exclusion or rejection. Understanding whether changes in sensitivity to, and interpretation of, social information are adolescent non-specific, emergent, or idiosyncratic trends, and whether these cognitions consistently link with SAD will help understand the cognitive aetiology of SAD and identify possibly changing SAD correlates. How negative and positive peer experiences shape trajectories will provide further clues about periods at which these processes may be specifically malleable and external influences may have particular impact on trajectories. Hence, mapping typical trajectories and social anxiety-linked variability will put us in a better position to determine how these biases should be targeted and when. It is possible that interpretational style is more malleable to interventions before adolescence. Attentional control may have a more prolonged maturational trajectory as networks underpinning attentional control networks are still maturing throughout adolescence (Henderson et al., 2014), but these remain empirical questions. Mapping these cognitive correlates of social anxiety onto key functions investigated in neuroimaging studies (i.e. understanding the role of attention and (re) interpretation in emotion generation and regulation), will allow us to address these questions at different levels of analyses.

Structural brain development and (social) anxiety

There is only very limited literature on structural brain development and (social) anxiety—significantly more research has focused on structural indices and depression. Morphometric studies with group comparisons in clinical paediatric anxiety have yielded relatively inconsistent results in both limbic (amygdala) and cortical areas (e.g. De Bellis et al., 2000; Milham et al., 2005; Monk, 2008). This is likely due to samples varying in anxiety conditions and comorbid depression. Additionally, anxiety-related structural differences in youths have to be examined against a backdrop of significant and protracted age- and puberty-linked structural changes in social-affective networks (Goddings et al., 2014; Mills et al., 2014). Hence, varying age range and pubertal status across studies is likely contributing to inconsistencies across findings, too. Recent consortium efforts, which bring together data from different imaging studies, hold promise in providing solid estimates of effect sizes in any differences found between healthy and clinical groups. These large-scale efforts are powered to assess age-related differences as linked to anxiety cross-sectionally. However, in order to understand when differences arise and what they represent (i.e. a maturational difference or a true trait difference or a combination of both), longitudinal designs are key.

Functional brain responses

Increased sensitivity to ambiguous and threatening social cues have been shown to manifest in functional responses in specific brain networks that are involved in the expression or regulation of emotion (Bar-Haim et al. 2007, Haller et al., 2015). Most of this work has been conducted with adult clinical populations, but there is now a growing body of work on youths with different anxiety diagnoses and a few studies that have selected for high social anxiety or SAD. Increased affective responses to negative social cues (e.g. angry or fearful faces) have been linked to increased amygdala sensitivity as well as differential responses in several frontal regions such as the anterior cingulate cortex, medial and lateral PFC, and anterior insula in adolescents with SAD or adolescents selected for increased social worries (Killgore and Yurgelun-Todd, 2005; McClure et al., 2007; Battaglia et al., 2012). These data have been replicated and extended with tasks that present more dynamic social exchanges online (Guyer et al., 2008; Lau et al., 2011; Jarcho et al., 2013).

Interestingly, networks implicated in perturbed processing in SAD are those documented to undergo prolonged functional restructuring across adolescence. Cross-sectional data on typically developing youths suggest peak sensitivities in the neural responses of subcortical affect- and reward-processing regions such as the amygdala and striatum to simple threatening or rewarding stimuli around adolescence (Ernst et al., 2005; Hare et al., 2008; Passarotti et al., 2009; Van Leijenhorst et al., 2010;

Somerville et al., 2011; Chein et al., 2012). There is some contention as to whether these peak sensitivities occur before, at the start, or in mid-adolescence (Hare et al., 2008; Somerville et al., 2011, 2013; Gee et al., 2013).

Functional developmental trajectories of frontal areas in response to socio-affective stimuli are equally complex, with reports of adolescent-emerged or adolescent-idiosyncratic trends in tasks that require automatic or effortful emotion regulation (e.g. McRae et al., 2012; Somerville et al., 2013). Inconsistencies in the directionality of developmental differences in child/adolescent/adult groups across studies have made it difficult to draw firm conclusions about developmental change (Crone and Dahl, 2012). Speculatively, inconsistencies may stem from the use of different tasks tapping slightly different processes. Alternatively, variations may also arise from differences in the salience and relevance of the task context (Crone and Dahl, 2012; Braams et al., 2014). More systematic, longitudinal investigations are clearly needed to map out critical maturational changes and individual trajectories more comprehensively and to understand individual differences and variability in peak sensitivities and how these relate to social anxiety and important social experiences. This also highlights the difficulty with group comparisons of paediatric samples of wide age ranges: it is plausible that age and/or pubertal status may significantly affect how social stimuli are processed, possibly obscuring more subtle SAD-related differences. Ideally, paediatric imaging studies should include pubertal status indices as puberty may be particularly relevant to neural development and SAD symptom onset—more so than age (Patton and Viner, 2007). Overall, it is clear that we need to integrate findings on SAD-linked functional responses of key emotion generation and regulation regions with the emerging corpus of work on typical developmental trajectories of peak sensitivities of regions in these networks to understand when and how neural trajectories diverge.

As well as studying differences in individual regions, recent studies have also explored SAD-linked and typical developmental changes in functional connectivity between regions of the networks implicated in social and emotional processing. Task-related functional connectivity is an indicator of co-activation between different areas during engagement in conditions of an in-scanner task designed to probe a relevant process (e.g. anticipation, reward processing, emotion regulation). Different functional connectivity patterns and age-related changes of these patterns in response to emotionally evocative stimuli in youths with increased levels of social concerns/SAD (as well as with other anxiety disorders) have now been reported in a handful of studies. Studies seem to suggest differences in associations between amygdala and prefrontal engagement, although the directionality is not always consistent (e.g. Hare et al., 2008; Monk et al., 2008; Roy et al., 2013). Two studies, which investigated age-related change in addition to examining relationships with anxiety, both found developmental effects in the link between task-based functional connectivity and anxiety (Gold et al., 2016; Kujawa et al., 2016).

These results are particularly interesting in the context of cross-sectional work on typical developmental changes in functional connectivity (Gee et al., 2013; Wu et al., 2016). Both studies found a normative developmental 'switch' from positive to negative connectivity in the amygdala-medial PFC network during the viewing of emotional faces.

In order to move developmental imaging work on SAD forward, it is crucial to understand whether the transition to adolescence represents an inflection point or a central point of divergence of functional connectivity between these key regions. Are anxiety-related differences in functional connectivity already present before puberty? If so, do differences become more pronounced? Is a delay in valence change of coupling related to a rise of social anxiety and linked to poorer emotion regulation skills? How much 'normative' variability is there at the juncture to adolescence and how does this relate to indices of pubertal status and significant social experiences (e.g. parenting, positive and negative peer interactions)? Only when we go beyond cross-sectional approaches to chart individual trajectories and links with social anxiety, can we answer these questions comprehensively. Once we have determined when critical maturational time courses occur, we can move to determine whether these changes in coupling also represent windows at which external influences (i.e. interventive efforts) have increased impact, whether training abilities pre-emptively can shape trajectories towards more adaptive outcomes, or whether these functions remain plastic and malleable into adulthood.

Interim summary: what can a developmental angle contribute to this social anxiety research?

This review has highlighted that it is important to go beyond extrapolating predictions from adult models to understand (1) developmental changes in cognitive profiles and (2) timing of symptom onset by assessing how potentially unique cognitive and emotional trajectories in normative development may shape and bring out risks at certain developmental periods. It is plausible that typical developmental processes exaggerate social fears and increase functional impairment during the adolescent developmental period (via adolescent-idiosyncratic or adolescent-emergent developmental trends in affect, reward, and social–cognitive processing), accentuating individual differences and pushing individuals towards the more extreme ends of the distribution (Haller et al., 2013). It is only when we chart developmental trajectories more continuously, that we can test these hypotheses directly.

Where do we go from here?

Longitudinal studies are a significant investment of time and resources. There has been a move towards longitudinal cohort designs in developmental cognitive neuroscience, including large-scale projects such as the ABCD study, which follows thousands of youths through the second decade of life. There are also numerous smaller longitudinal imaging studies examining social–emotional brain function across adolescence (see Crone and Elzinga (2014) for an overview). It is time to join forces with clinical neuroscience and paediatric psychiatry to harness knowledge on individual differences and disorder-related trajectories in parallel to examining typical change over time. Analytical tools that allow the modelling of several dynamic factors across time will be crucial. Ultimately, this will be a significant step towards deriving comprehensive, integrative models of psychiatric conditions. Developmental ideas of timing of environmental events, cascading effects, and (mal)adaptations of the developing brain should make up key components of these models.

Conclusion

A developmental framework is crucial to understand how common and impairing psychopathologies and their subclinical manifestations emerge and are maintained. As such, this approach emphasizes both normal and abnormal developmental trajectories and both risk and protective factors involved in the development of psychopathology and mental health. It is only within the context of dynamically developing abilities that we can fully understand the pathways and mechanisms by which risk factors are expressed. We need to trace the causal structure from the early decades of life to adulthood as the complexities of interactions between genetic and environmental factors increase along the developmental time line. Lastly, a better understanding of the relationship between cognitive and brain development across the first decades of life would also play a large role in making recommendations for the early intervention or treatment approaches.

References

Amin, N., Foa, E.B., and Coles, M.E. (1998). Negative interpretation bias in social phobia. *Behaviour Research and Therapy*, **36**(10), 945–957.

Amir, N., Prouvost, C., and Kuckertz, J.M. (2012). Lack of a benign interpretation bias in social anxiety disorder. *Cognitive Behaviour Therapy*, **41**(2), 119–129.

Alexander-Bloch, A.F., Reiss, P.T., Rapoport, J., McAdams, H., Giedd, J.N., Bullmore, E.T., and Gogtay, N. (2014). Abnormal cortical growth in schizophrenia targets normative modules of synchronized development. *Biological Psychiatry*, **76**(6), 438–446.

Anticevic, A., Cole, M.W., Murray, J.D., Corlett, P.R., Wang, X.J., and Krystal, J.H. (2012). The role of default network deactivation in cognition and disease. *Trends in Cognitive Sciences*, **16**(12), 584–592.

Bacanu, S.A. and Kendler, K.S. (2013). Extracting actionable information from genome scans. *Genetic Epidemiology*, **37**(1), 48–59.

Barnett, J.H., McDougall, F., Xu, M.K., Croudace, T.J., Richards, M., and Jones, P.B. (2012). Childhood cognitive function and adult psychopathology: associations with psychotic and non-psychotic symptoms in the general population. *British Journal of Psychiatry*, **201**, 124–130.

Bar-Haim, Y., Lamy, D., Pergamin, L., Bakermans-Kranenburg, M.J., and Van Ijzen-doorn, M.H. (2007). Threat-related attentional bias in anxious and nonanxious individuals: a meta analytic study. *Psychological Bulletin*, **133**(1), 1–24.

Battaglia, M., Zanoni, A., Taddei, M., Giorda, R., Bertoletti, E., Lampis, V., and Tettamanti, M. (2012). Cerebral responses to emotional expressions and the development of social anxiety disorder: a preliminary longitudinal study. *Depression and Anxiety*, **29**(1), 54–61.

Beddington, J., Cooper, C.L., Field, J., Goswami, U., Huppert, F.A., Jenkins, R., Jones, H.S., Kirkwood, T.B.L., Sahakian, B.J., and Thomas, S.M. (2008). The mental wealth of nations. *Nature*, **455**, 1057–1060.

Blakemore, S.J. (2008). The social brain in adolescence. *Nature Reviews Neuroscience*, **9**(4), 267–277.

Burnett, S., Sebastian, C., Cohen Kadosh, K., and Blakemore, S.-J. (2011). The social brain in adolescence: evidence from functional magnetic resonance imaging and behavioural studies. *Neuroscience and Biobehavioral Reviews*, **35**(8), 1654–1664.

Braams, B.R., Peters, S., Peper, J.S., Güroğlu, B., and Crone, E.A. (2014). Gambling for self, friends, and antagonists: differential contributions of affective and social brain regions on adolescent reward processing. *Neuroimage*, **100**, 281–289.

Callicott, J.H., Mattay, V.S., Verchinski, B.A., Marenco, S., Egan, M.F., and Weinberger, D.R. (2003). Complexity of prefrontal cortical dysfunction in schizophrenia: more than up or down. *American Journal of Psychiatry*, **160**(12), 2209–2215.

Casey, B.J. (2013). The teenage brain: an overview. *Current Directions in Psychological Science*, **22**(2), 80–81.

Casey, B.J., Tottenham, N., Liston, C., and Durston, S. (2005). Imaging the developing brain: what have we learned about cognitive development? *Trends in Cognitive Sciences*, **9**(3), 104–110.

Chein, J., Albert, D., Brien, L.O., Uckert, K., and Steinberg, L. (2012). Peers increase adolescent risk taking by enhancing activity in the brain's reward circuitry. *Developmental Science*, **14**(2), 1–16.

Clark, D.M. and Wells, A. (1995). A cognitive model of social phobia. In: R.G. Heimberg, M.R. Liebowitz, D.A. Hope, and F.R. Schneier (Eds.), *Social Phobia: Diagnosis, Assessment, and Treatment* (pp. 69–93). New York: The Guilford Press.

Cohen Kadosh, K., Cohen Kadosh, R., Dick, F., and Johnson, M.H. (2011). Developmental changes in effective connectivity in the emerging core face network. *Cerebral Cortex*, **21**(6), 1389–1394.

Cohen Kadosh, K. and Johnson, M.H. (2007). Developing a cortex specialized for face perception. *Trends in Cognitive Sciences*, **11**(9), 267–269.

Cohen Kadosh, K., Johnson, M.H., Dick, F., Cohen Kadosh, R., and Blakemore, S.J. (2013a). Effects of age, task performance, and structural brain development on face processing. *Cerebral Cortex*, **23**(7), 1630–1642.

Cohen Kadosh, K., Linden, D.E.J., and Lau, J.Y. (2013b). Plasticity during childhood and adolescence: innovative approaches to investigating neurocognitive development. *Developmental Science*, **16**(4), 574–583.

Conklin, H.M., Luciana, M., Hooper, C.J., and Yarger, R.S. (2007). Working memory performance in typically developing children and adolescents: behavioral evidence of protracted frontal lobe development. *Developmental Neuropsychology*, **31**(1), 103–128.

Constans, J.I., Penn, D.L., Ihen, G.H., and Hope, D.A. (1999). Interpretive biases for ambiguous stimuli in social anxiety. *Behaviour Research and Therapy*, **37**(7), 643–651.

Corlett, P.R. and Fletcher, P.C. (2012). The neurobiology of schizotypy: fronto-striatal prediction error signal correlates with delusion-like beliefs in healthy people. *Neuropsychologia*, **50**(14), 3612–3620.

Cougnard, A., Marcelis, M., Myin-Germeys, I., De Graaf, R., Vollebergh, W., Krabbendam, L., Lieb, R., Wittchen, H.U., Henquet, C., Spauwen, J., and Van Os, J. (2007). Does normal developmental expression of psychosis combine with environmental risk to cause persistence of psychosis? A psychosis proneness-persistence model. *Psychological Medicine*, **37**(4), 513–527.

Creswell, C., Murray, L., and Cooper, P. (2014). Interpretation and expectation in childhood anxiety disorders: age effects and social specificity. *Journal of Abnormal Child Psychology*, **42**(3), 453–465.

Crone, E.A. and Dahl, R.E. (2012). Understanding adolescence as a period of social- affective engagement and goal flexibility. *Nature Reviews Neuroscience*, **13**(9), 636–650.

Crone, E.A. and Elzinga, B.M. (2015). Changing brains: how longitudinal functional magnetic resonance imaging studies can inform us about cognitive and social-affective growth trajectories. *Wiley Interdisciplinary Reviews: Cognitive Science*, **6**(1), 53–63.

De Bellis, M.D., Casey, B.J., Dahl, R.E., Birmaher, B., Williamson, D.E., Thomas, K.M., Axelson, D.A., Frustaci, K., Boring, A.M., Hall, J., and Ryan, N.D. (2000). A pilot study of amygdala volumes in pediatric generalized anxiety disorder. *Biological Psychiatry*, **48**(1), 51–57.

De Herdt, A., Wampers, M., Vancampfort, D., De Hert, M., Vanhees, L., Demunter, H., Van Bouwel, L., Brunner, E., and Probst, M. (2013). Neurocognition in clinical high risk young adults who did or did not convert to a first schizophrenic psychosis: a meta-analysis. *Schizophrenia Research*, **149**(1–3), 48–55.

Dickson, H., Cullen, A.E., Reichenberg, A., Hodgins, S., Campbell, D.D., Morris, R.G., and Laurens, K.R. (2014). Cognitive impairment among children at-risk for schizophrenia. *Journal of Psychiatric Research*, **50**, 92–99.

Dima, D., Jogia, J., and Frangou, S. (2014). Dynamic causal modeling of load-dependent modulation of effective connectivity within the verbal working memory network. *Human Brain Mapping*, **35**(7), 3025–3035.

Downs, J.M., Cullen, A.E., Barragan, M., and Laurens, K.R. (2013). Persisting psychotic-like experiences are associated with both externalising and internalising psychopathology in a longitudinal general population child cohort. *Schizophrenia Research*, **144**(1–3), 99–104.

Drakesmith, M., Caeyenberghs, K., Dutt, A., Zammit, S., Evans, C.J., Reichenberg, A., Lewis, G., David, A.S., and Jones, D.K. (2015). Schizophrenia-like topological changes in the structural connectome of individuals with subclinical psychotic experiences. *Human Brain Mapping*, **36**(7), 2629–2643.

Dumontheil, I., Burgess, P.W., and Blakemore, S.J. (2008). Development of rostral prefrontal cortex and cognitive and behavioural disorders. *Developmental Medicine and Child Neurology*, **50**(3), 168–181.

Dumontheil, I. and Klingberg, T. (2012). Brain activity during a visuospatial working memory task predicts arithmetical performance 2 years later. *Cerebral Cortex*, **22**(5), 1078–1085.

Dutt, A., Tseng, H.-H., Fonville, L., Drakesmith, M., Su, L., Evans, J., Zammit, S., Jones, D., Lewis, G., and David, A.S. (2015). Exploring neural dysfunction in 'clinical high risk' for psychosis: a quantitative review of fMRI studies. *Journal of Psychiatric Research*, **6**, 122–134.

Ernst, M., Nelson, E.E., Jazbec, S., McClure, E.B., Monk, C.S., Leibenluft, E., and Pine, D.S. (2005). Amygdala and nucleus accumbens in responses to receipt and omission of gains in adults and adolescents. *Neuroimage*, **25**(4), 1279–1291.

Fair, D.A., Cohen, A.L., Dosenbach, N.U.F., Church, J.A., Miezin, F.M., Barch, D.M., Raichle, M.E., Petersen, S.E., and Schlaggar, B.L. (2008). The maturing architecture of the brain's default network. *Proceedings of the National Academy of Sciences*, **105**(10), 4028–4032.

Fair, D.A., Dosenbach, N.U.F., Church, J.A., Cohen, A.L., Brahmbhatt, S., Miezin, F.M., Barch, D.M., Raichle, M.E., Petersen, S.E., and Schlaggar, B.L. (2007). Development of distinct control networks through segregation and integration. *Proceedings of the National Academy of Sciences*, **104**(33), 13507–13512.

Fonville, L., Cohen Kadosh, K., Drakesmith, M., Zammit, S., Lewis, G., Jones, D., and David, A. (2015). Psychotic experiences, working memory and the developing brain: a multimodal neuroimaging study. *Cerebral Cortex*, **25**(12), 4828–4838.

Friston, K.J., Harrison, L., and Penny, W. (2003). Dynamic causal modelling. *Neuroimage*, **19**(4), 1273–1302.

Fusar-Poli, P. (2012). Voxel-wise meta-analysis of fMRI studies in patients at clinical high risk for psychosis. *Journal of Psychiatry & Neuroscience*, **37**(2), 106–112.

Fusar-Poli, P., Deste, G., Smieskova, R., Barlati, S., Yung, A.R., Howes, O., Stieglitz, R.D., Vita, A., McGuire, P., and Borgwardt, S. (2012). Cognitive functioning in prodromal psychosis: a meta-analysis. *Archives of General Psychiatry*, **69**(6), 562–571.

Fusar-Poli, P., Perez, J., Broome, M., Borgwardt, S., Placentino, A., Caverzasi, E., Cortesi, M., Veggiotti, P., Politi, P., Barale, F., and McGuire, P. (2007). Neurofunctional correlates of vulnerability to psychosis: a systematic review and meta-analysis. *Neuroscience & Biobehavioral Reviews*, **31**(4), 465–484.

Gamble, A.L. and Rapee, R.M. (2009). The time-course of attentional bias in anxious children and adolescents. *Journal of Anxiety Disorders*, **23**(7), 841–847.

Gee, D.G., Humphreys, K.L., Flannery, J., Goff, B., Telzer, E.H., Shapiro, M., Hare, T.A., Bookheimer, S.Y., and Tottenham, N. (2013). A developmental shift from positive to negative connectivity in human amygdala–prefrontal circuitry. *The Journal of Neuroscience*, **33**(10), 4584–4593.

Giedd, J.N., Blumenthal, J., Jeffries, N.O., Castellanos, F.X., Liu, H., Zijdenbos, A., Paus, T., Evans, A.C., and Rapoport, J.L. (1999). Brain development during childhood and adolescence: a longitudinal MRI study. *Nature Neuroscience*, **2**(10), 861–863.

Goddings, A.L., Mills, K.L., Clasen, L.S., Giedd, J.N., Viner, R.M., and Blakemore, S.J. (2014). The influence of puberty on subcortical brain development. *Neuroimage*, **88**, 242–251.

Gold, A.L., Shechner, T., Farber, M.J., Spiro, C.N., Leibenluft, E., Pine, D.S., and Britton, J.C. (2016). Amygdala–cortical connectivity: associations with anxiety, development, and threat. *Depression and Anxiety*, **33**(10), 917–926.

Guyer, A.E., Lau, J.Y., McClure-Tone, E.B., Parrish, J., Shiffrin, N.D., Reynolds, R.C., Chen, G., Blair, R.J., Leibenluft, E., Fox, N.A., Ernst, M., Pine, D.S., and Nelson, E.E. (2008). Amygdala and ventrolateral prefrontal cortex function during anticipated peer evaluation in pediatric social anxiety. *Archives of General Psychiatry*, **65**(11), 1303–1312.

Gregory, A.M., Caspi, A., Moffitt, T.E., Koenen, K., Eley, T.C., and Poulton, R. (2007). Juvenile mental health histories of adults with anxiety disorders. *American Journal of Psychiatry*, **164**(2), 301–308.

Haller, S.P.W, Cohen Kadosh, K., and Lau, J.Y.F. (2014). A developmental angle to understanding the mechanisms of biased cognition in social anxiety. *Frontiers in Human Neuroscience*, **7**, 846.

Haller, S.P.W., Cohen Kadosh, K., Scerif, G., and Lau, J.Y.F. (2015). Social anxiety disorder: a new developmental cognitive neuroscience approach to uncover risk factors during adolescence. *Developmental Cognitive Neuroscience*, **13**, 11–20.

Hare, T.A., Tottenham, N., Galvan, A., Voss, H.U., Glover, G.H., and Casey, B.J. (2008). Biological substrates of emotional reactivity and regulation in adolescence during an emotional go-nogo task. *Biological Psychiatry*, **63**(10), 927–934.

Harris, J.J., Reynell, C., and Attwell, D. (2011). The physiology of developmental changes in BOLD functional imaging signals. *Developmental Cognitive Neuroscience*, **1**(3), 199–216.

Henderson, H.A., Pine, D.S., and Fox, N.A. (2014). Behavioral inhibition and developmental risk: a dual-processing perspective. *Neuropsychopharmacology*, **40**(1), 207–224.

In-Albon, T., Dubi, K., Rapee, R.M., and Schneider, S. (2009). Forced choice reaction time paradigm in children with separation anxiety disorder, social phobia, and non-anxious controls. *Behaviour Research and Therapy*, **47**(12), 1058–1065.

Ingvar, D.H. and Franzen, G. (1974). Abnormalities of cerebral blood flow distribution in patients with chronic schizophrenia. *Acta Psychiatrica Scandinavica*, **50**(4), 425–462.

Jarcho, J.M., Leibenluft, E., Walker, O.L., Fox, N.A., Pine, D.S., and Nelson, E.E. (2013). Neuroimaging studies of pediatric social anxiety: paradigms, pitfalls and a new direction for investigating the neural mechanisms. *Biology of Mood and Anxiety Disorders*, **12**, 3–14.

Johnson, M.H., Grossmann, T., and Cohen Kadosh, K. (2009). Mapping functional brain development: building a social brain through interactive specialization. *Developmental Psychology*, **45**, 151–159.

Johnson, M.H., Jones, E.J., and Gliga, T. (2015). Brain adaptation and alternative developmental trajectories. *Developmental Psychopathology*, **27**(2), 425–442.

Kaymaz, N., Drukker, M., Lieb, R., Wittchen, H.U., Werbeloff, N., Weiser, M., Lataster, T., and van Os, J. (2012a). Do subthreshold psychotic experiences predict clinical outcomes in unselected non-help-seeking population-based samples? A systematic review and meta-analysis, enriched with new results. *Psychological Medicine*, **42**(11), 2239–2253.

Kaymaz, N., Drukker, M., Lieb, R., Wittchen, H.U., Werbeloff, N., Weiser, M., Lataster, T., and van Os, J. (2012b). Do subthreshold psychotic experiences predict clinical outcomes in unselected non-help-seeking population-based samples? A systematic review and meta-analysis, enriched with new results. *Psychological Medicine*, **42**(11), 2239–2253.

Kelleher, I., Connor, D., Clarke, M.C., Devlin, N., Harley, M., and Cannon, M. (2012). Prevalence of psychotic symptoms in childhood and adolescence: a systematic review and meta-analysis of population-based studies. *Psychological Medicine*, **42**(9), 1857–1863.

Keshavan, M.S., Giedd, J., Lau, J.Y.F., Lewis, D.A., and Paus, T. (2014). Changes in the adolescent brain and the pathophysiology of psychotic disorders. *The Lancet Psychiatry*, **1**(7), 549–558.

Kessler, R.C., Angermeyer, M., Anthony, J.C., De Graaf, R., Demyttenaere, K., Gasquet, I., De Girolamo, G., Gluzman, S., Gureje, O., Haro, J.M., Kawakami, N., Karam, A., Levinson, D., Medina Mora, M.E., Oakley Browne, M.A., Posada-Villa, J., Stein, D.J., Adley Tsang, C.H., Aguilar-Gaxiola, S., Alonso, J., Lee, S., Heeringa, S., Pennell, B.E., Berglund, P., Gruber, M.J., Petukhova, M., Chatterji, S., and Ustun, T.B. (2007). Lifetime prevalence and age-of-onset distributions of mental disorders in the World Health Organization's World Mental Health Survey Initiative. *World Psychiatry*, **6**(3), 168–176.

Kessler, R.C., Berglund, P., Demler, O., Jin, R., Merikangas, K.R., and Walters, E.E. (2005). Lifetime prevalence and age-of-onset distributions of DSM-IV disorders in the National Comorbidity Survey Replication. *Archives of General Psychiatry*, **62**(6), 593–602.

Killgore, W.D. and Yurgelun-Todd, D.A. (2005). Social anxiety predicts amygdala activation in adolescents viewing fearful faces. *Neuroreport*, **16**(15), 1671–1675.

Kirchner, W.K. (1958). Age differences in short-term retention of rapidly changing information. *Journal of Experimental Psychology*, **55**(4), 352–358.

Klingberg, T. (2006). Development of a superior frontal-intraparietal network for visuo-spatial working memory. *Neuropsychologia*, **44**(11), 2171–2177.

Kloep, M. (1999). Love is all you need? Focusing on adolescents' life concerns from an ecological point of view. *Journal of Adolescence*, **22**(1), 49–63.

Kujawa, A., Wu, M., Klumpp, H., Pine, D.S., Swain, J.E., Fitzgerald, K.D., Monk, C.S., and Phan, K.L. (2016). Altered development of amygdala-anterior cingulate cortex connectivity in anxious youth and young adults. *Biological Psychiatry: Cognitive Neuroscience and Neuroimaging*, **1**(4), 345–352.

Lau, J.Y., Gregory, A.M., Goldwin, M.A., Pine, D.S., and Eley, T.C. (2007a). Assessing gene–environment interactions on anxiety symptom subtypes across child- hood and adolescence. *Development and Psychopathology*, **19**(4), 1129–1146.

Lau, J.Y., Rijsdijk, F., Gregory, A.M., McGun, P., and Eley, T.C. (2007b). Pathways to childhood depressive symptoms: the role of social, cognitive, and genetic risk factors. *Developmental Psychology*, **43**(6),1402.

Lau, J.Y.F., Guyer, A.E., Tone, E.B., Jenness, J., Parrish, J.M., Pine, D.S., and Nelson, E.E. (2011). Neural responses to peer rejection in anxious adolescents: contributions from the amygdala-hippocampal complex. *International Journal of Behavioral Development*, **36**(1), 36–44.

Lebel, C. and Beaulieu, C. (2011). Longitudinal development of human brain wiring continues from childhood to adulthood. *Journal of Neuroscience*, **31**(30), 10937–10947.

Lerner, R.M. and Steinberg, L. (2004). *Handbook of Adolescent Psychology*. Hoboken, NJ: John Wiley & Sons.

Linscott, R.J. and van Os, J. (2013). An updated and conservative systematic review and meta-analysis of epidemiological evidence on psychotic experiences in children and adults: on the pathway from proneness to persistence to dimensional expression across mental disorders. *Psychological Medicine*, **43**(6), 1133–1149.

Ma, L., Steinberg, J.L., Hasan, K.M., Narayana, P.A., Kramer, L.A., and Moeller, F.G. (2012). Working memory load modulation of parieto-frontal connections: evidence from dynamic causal modeling. *Human Brain Mapping*, **33**(8), 1850–1867.

McClure, E.B., Monk, C.S., Nelson, E.E., Parrish, J.M., Adler, A., Blair, R.J.R., and Pine, D.S. (2007). Abnormal attention modulation of fear circuit function in pediatric generalized anxiety disorder. *Archives of General Psychiatry*, **64**(1), 97–106.

McGorry, P.D., Purcell, R., Goldstone, S., and Amminger, G.P. (2011). Age of onset and timing of treatment for mental and substance use disorders: implications for preventive intervention strategies and models of care. *Current Opinion in Psychiatry*, **24**(4), 301–306.

McIntosh, A.M., Owens, D.C., Moorhead, W.J., Whalley, H.C., Stanfield, A.C., Hall, J., Johnstone, E.C., and Lawrie, S.M. (2011). Longitudinal volume reductions in people at high genetic risk of schizophrenia as they develop psychosis. *Biological Psychiatry*, **69**(10), 953–958.

McRae, K., Gross, J.J., Weber, J., Robertson, E.R., Sokol-Hessner, P., Ray, R.D., Gabrieli, J.D., and Ochsner, K.N. (2012). The development of emotion regulation: an fMRI study of cognitive reappraisal in children, adolescents and young adults. *Social Cognitive and Affective Neuroscience*, **7**(1), 11–22.

Meier, M.H., Caspi, A., Reichenberg, A., Keefe, R.S.E., Fisher, H.L., Harrington, N., Houts, R., Poulton, R., and Moffitt, T.E. (2014). Neuropsychological decline in schizophrenia from the premorbid to the postonset period: evidence from a population-representative longitudinal study. *American Journal of Psychiatry*, **171**(1), 91–101.

Miers, A.C., Blöte, A.W., Heyne, D.A., and Westenberg, P.M. (2014). Developmental pathways of social avoidance across adolescence: The role of social anxiety and negative cognition. *Journal of Anxiety Disorders*, **28**(8), 787–794.

Milham, M.P., Nugent, A.C., Drevets, W.C., Dickstein, D.P., Leibenluft, E., Ernst, M., Charney, D., and Pine, D.S. (2005). Selective reduction in amygdala volume in pediatric anxiety disorders: a voxel-based morphometry investigation. *Biological Psychiatry*, **57**(9), 961–966.

Mills, K.L., Lalonde, F., Clasen, L.S., Giedd, J.N., and Blakemore, S.J. (2014). Developmental changes in the structure of the social brain in late childhood and adolescence. *Social Cognitive and Affective Neuroscience*, **9**(1), 123–131.

Monk, C.S. (2008). The development of emotion-related neural circuitry in health and psychopathology. *Development and Psychopathology*, **20**(4), 1231.

Monk, C.S., Telzer, E.H., Mogg, K., Bradley, B.P., Mai, X., Louro, H.M., Chen, G., McClure-Tone, E.B., Ernst, M., and Pine, D.S. (2008). Amygdala and ventrolateral prefrontal cortex activation to masked angry faces in children and adolescents with generalized anxiety disorder. *Archives of General Psychiatry*, **65**(5), 568–576.

Nishida, A., Sasaki, T., Nishimura, Y., Tanii, H., Hara, N., Inoue, K., Yamada, T., Takami, T., Shimodera, S., Itokawa, M., Asukai, N., and Okazaki, Y. (2010). Psychotic-like experiences are associated with suicidal feelings and deliberate self-harm behaviors in adolescents aged 12–15 years. *Acta Psychiatrica Scandinavica*, **121**(4), 301–307.

Nolen-Hoeksema, S. (1996). Chewing the cud and other ruminations. In: R.S. Wyer, Jr. (Ed.), *Advances in Social Cognition, Vol. 9. Ruminative Thoughts* (pp. 135–144). Hillsdale, NJ: Lawrence Erlbaum Associates, Inc.

Nolen-Hoeksema, S., Girgus, J.S., and Seligman, M.E. (1992). Predictors and con- sequences of childhood depressive symptoms: a 5-year longitudinal study. *Journal of Abnormal Psychology*, **101**(3), 405–422.

Passarotti, A.M., Sweeney, J.A., and Pavuluri, M.N. (2009). Neural correlates of incidental and directed facial emotion processing in adolescents and adults. *Social Cognitive and Affective Neuroscience*, **4**(4), 387–398.

Patton, G.C. and Viner, R. (2007). Pubertal transitions in health. *The Lancet*, **369**(9567), 1130–1139.

Pauly, K., Seiferth, N.Y., Kellermann, T., Ruhrmann, S., Daumann, B., Backes, V., Klosterkotter, J., Shah, N.J., Schneider, F., Kircher, T.T., and Habel, U. (2010). The interaction of working memory and emotion in persons clinically at risk for psychosis: an fMRI pilot study. *Schizophrenia Research*, **120**(1–3), 167–176.

Paus, T., Keshavan, M., and Giedd, J.N. (2008). Why do many psychiatric disorders emerge during adolescence? *Nature Reviews Neuroscience*, **9**(12), 947–957.

Petanjek, Z., Judas, M., Simic, G., Rasin, M.R., Uylings, H.B.M., and Rakic, P. (2011). Extraordinary neoteny of synaptic spines in the human prefrontal cortex. *Proceedings of the National Academy of Sciences*, **108**(32), 13281–13286.

Pine, D.S., Cohen, P., and Brook, J. (1996). Emotional problems during youth as predictors of stature during early adulthood: results from a prospective epidemiologic study. *Pediatrics*, **97**(6 Pt 1), 856–863.

Pine, D.S., Cohen, E., Cohen, P., and Brook, J. (1999). Adolescent depressive symptoms as predictors of adult depression: moodiness or mood disorder? *American Journal of Psychiatry*, **156**(1), 133–135.

Polanczyk, G., Moffitt, T.E., Arseneault, L., Cannon, M., Ambler, A., Keefe, R.S.E., Houts, R., Odgers, C.L., and Caspi, A. (2010). Etiological and clinical features of childhood psychotic symptoms results from a birth cohort. *Archives of General Psychiatry*, **67**(4), 328–338.

Reichenberg, A., Caspi, A., Harrington, H., Houts, R., Keefe, R.S., Murray, R.M., Poulton, R., and Moffitt, T.E. (2010). Static and dynamic cognitive deficits in childhood preceding adult schizophrenia: a 30-year study. *American Journal of Psychiatry*, **167**(2), 160–169.

Rose, A.J. and Rudolph, K.D. (2006). A review of sex differences in peer relationship processes: potential trade-offs for the emotional and behavioral development of girls and boys. *Psychological Bulletin*, **132**(1), 98–131.

Roy, A.K., Fudge, J.L., Kelly, C., Perry, J.S., Daniele, T., Carlisi, C., Benson, B., Castellanos, F.X., Milham, M.P., Pine, D.S., and Ernst, M. (2013). Intrinsic functional connectivity of amygdala-based networks in adolescent generalized anxiety disorder. *Journal of the American Academy of Child & Adolescent Psychiatry*, **52**(3), 290–299.

Roy, A.K., Vasa, R.A., Bruck, M., Mogg, K., Bradley, B.P., Sweeney, M., Bergman, R.L., McClure-Tone, E.B., Pine, D.S., CAMS Team. (2008). Attention bias toward threat in pediatric anxiety disorders. *Journal of the American Academy of Child & Adolescent Psychiatry*, **47**(10), 1189–1196.

Seidman, L.J., Giuliano, A.J., Smith, C.W., Stone, W.S., Glatt, S.J., Meyer, E., Faraone, S.V., Tsuang, M.T., and Cornblatt, B. (2006). Neuropsychological functioning in adolescents and young adults at genetic risk for schizophrenia and affective psychoses: results from the Harvard and Hillside Adolescent High Risk Studies. *Schizophrenia Bulletin*, **32**(3), 507–524.

Sekar, A., Bialas, A.R., de Rivera, H., Davis, A., Hammond, T.R., Kamitaki, N., Tooley, K., Presumey, J., Baum, M., Van Doren, V., Genovese, G., Rose, S.A., Handsaker, R.E., Schizophrenia Working Group of the Psychiatric Genomics Consortium, Daly, M.J., Carroll, M.C., Stevens, B., and McCarroll, S.A. (2016). Schizophrenia risk from complex variation of complement component 4. *Nature*, **530**(7589), 177–183.

Simon, A.E., Cattapan-Ludewig, K., Zmilacher, S., Arbach, D., Gruber, K., Dvorsky, D.N., Roth, B., Isler, E., Zimmer, A., and Umbricht, D. (2007). Cognitive functioning in the schizophrenia prodrome. *Schizophrenia Bulletin*, **33**(3), 761–771.

Steinberg, L., and Silverberg, S.B. (1986). The vicissitudes of autonomy in early adolescence. *Child Development*, **57**(4), 841–851.

Stirling, L.J., Eley, T.C., and Clark, D.M. (2006). Preliminary evidence for an association between social anxiety symptoms and avoidance of negative faces in school- age children. *Journal of Clinical Child and Adolescent Psychology*, **35**(3), 431–439.

Stopa, L. and Clark, D.M. (2000). Social phobia and interpretation of social events. *Behaviour Research and Therapy*, **38**(3), 273–283.

Somerville, L.H., Hare, T.A., and Casey, B.J. (2011). Fronto striatal maturation predicts behavioral regulation failures to appetitive cues in adolescence. *Journal of Cognitive Neuroscience*, **23**(9), 2123–2134.

Somerville, L.H., Jones, R.M., Ruberry, E.J., Dyke, J.P., Glover, G., and Casey, B.J. (2013). The medial prefrontal cortex and the emergence of self-conscious emotion in adolescence. *Psychological Science*, **24**(8), 1554–1562.

Tamnes, C.K., Walhovd, K.B., Dale, A.M., Østby, Y., Grydeland, H., Richardson, G., Westlye, L.T., Roddey, J.C., Hagler, D.J., Jr., Due-Tønnessen, P., Holland, D., Fjell, A.M., and Alzheimer's Disease Neuroimaging Initiative. (2013). Brain development and aging: overlapping and unique patterns of change. *Neuroimage*, **68**, 63–74.

Thermenos, H.W., Keshavan, M.S., Juelich, R.J., Molokotos, E., Whitfield-Gabrieli, S., Brent, B.K., Makris, N., and Seidman, L.J. (2013). A review of neuroimaging studies of young relatives of individuals with schizophrenia: a developmental perspective from schizotaxia to schizophrenia. *American Journal of Medical Genetics Part B: Neuropsychiatric Genetics*, **162B**(7), 604–635.

Valli, I., Tognin, S., Fusar-Poli, P., and Mechelli, A. (2012). Episodic memory dysfunction in individuals at high-risk of psychosis: a systematic review of neuropsychological and neurofunctional studies. *Current Pharmaceutical Design*, **18**(4), 443–458.

Van Leijenhorst, L., Zanolie, K., Van Meel, C.S., Westenberg, P.M., Rombouts, S.A.R.B., and Crone, E.A. (2010). What motivates the adolescent? Brain regions mediating reward sensitivity across adolescence. *Cerebral Cortex*, **20**(1), 61–69.

van Os, J., Linscott, R.J., Myin-Germeys, I., Delespaul, P., and Krabbendam, L. (2009). A systematic review and meta-analysis of the psychosis continuum: evidence for a psychosis proneness-persistence-impairment model of psychotic disorder. *Psychological Medicine*, **39**(2), 179–195.

Whitfield-Gabrieli, S. and Ford, J.M. (2012). Default mode network activity and connectivity in psychopathology. *Annual Review of Clinical Psychology*, **8**, 49–76.

Wittchen, H.U., Stein, M.B., and Kessler, R.C. (1999). Social fears and social phobia in a community sample of adolescents and young adults: prevalence, risk factors and co-morbidity. *Psychological Medicine*, **29**(2), 309–323.

Wolf, D.H., Satterthwaite, T.D., Calkins, M.E., Ruparel, K., Elliott, M.A., Hopson, R.D., Jackson, C.T., Prabhakaran, K., Bilker, W.B., Hakonarson, H., Gur, R.C., and Gur, R.E. (2015). Functional neuroimaging abnormalities in youth with psychosis spectrum symptoms. *JAMA Psychiatry*, **72**(5), 456–465.

Wu, M., Kujawa, A., Lu, L.H., Fitzgerald, D.A., Klumpp, H., Fitzgerald, K.D., Monk, C.S., and Phan, K.L. (2016). Age-related changes in amygdala–frontal connectivity during emotional face processing from childhood into young adulthood. *Human Brain Mapping*, **37**(5), 1684–1695.

Zalesky, A., Fornito, A., Seal, M.L., Cocchi, L., Westin, C.-F., Bullmore, E.T., Egan, G.F., and Pantelis, C. (2011). Disrupted axonal fiber connectivity in schizophrenia. *Biological Psychiatry*, **69**(7), 80–89.

Zammit, S., Kounali, D., Cannon, M., David, A.S., Gunnell, D., Heron, J., Jones, P.B., Lewis, S., Sullivan, S., Wolke, D., and Lewis, G. (2013). Psychotic experiences and psychotic disorders at age 18 in relation to psychotic experiences at age 12 in a longitudinal population-based cohort study. *American Journal of Psychiatry*, **170**(7), 742–750.

Chapter 6

Which biopsychosocial view of mental illness?

Walter Sinnott-Armstrong
and Jesse S. Summers

Introduction

This chapter will clarify the biopsychosocial (BPS) view of mental illness and then apply it to scrupulosity and other particular mental illnesses. These applications will clarify and raise challenging questions for the BPS view of mental illness. One overarching issue is whether there is any interpretation of the BPS view that steers between the Scylla of being empty and the Charybdis of being wrong. We will argue that the BPS view is wrong when used to *define* mental illnesses but is still important and useful as a theory of the *causes* and *treatments* of mental illnesses.

Disjunction

One interpretation of the BPS theory of mental illness makes it so obvious that nobody would deny it. This interpretation is suggested by the definition of mental illness in the fifth edition of the American Psychiatric Association's *Diagnostic and Statistical Manual of Mental Disorders* (DSM-5):

> A mental disorder is a syndrome characterized by clinically significant disturbance in an individual's cognition, emotion regulation, or behavior that reflects a dysfunction in the psychological, biological, or developmental processes underlying mental functioning. (American Psychiatric Association, 2013, p. 20)

What makes this view so uncontroversial is the repeated 'or', which is clearly inclusive. In order to reach consensus, the American Psychiatric Association did not want to restrict mental disorders to psychological dysfunctions or to biological dysfunctions or to developmental dysfunctions. That is why its definition deploys a disjunction of dysfunctions (rhyme intended). Of course, what is developmental is not necessarily social, but the BPS theory of mental illness could use the same logic to include biological, psychological, and social into its account of mental illness by claiming this:

> *Disjunction BPS*: mental illnesses must be understood in terms of either psychological, biological, or social processes, dysfunctions, or causes.

All this says is that we cannot understand any mental illness except by viewing it at one or more of these levels. That disjunctive claim could and should be accepted by theorists who think that the only way to understand any mental illness is in terms of biology, and it could and should also be accepted by theorists who think that the only way to understand any mental illness is in terms of psychology or in terms of social relations. If any one or more of the disjuncts is true, then the whole disjunction is true.

The problem, of course, is that the very feature of this view that makes it uncontroversial also makes it uninteresting. The lack of controversy stems from its lack of content. A bare disjunction tells us neither which of the disjoined levels matters nor how they are related nor whether one disjunct is true of one case and another disjunct is true of other cases. Inquiring minds want to know more.

Causation

So, what is the relation among the biological, psychological, and social levels? One obvious candidate is causation, and it seems plausible that every mental illness somehow involves some causal relations among biological, psychological, and social factors. After all, it is biological organisms that have mental illnesses, and some aspects of their biological processes are bound to affect their psychological states somehow. Brain activity affects how we feel and think. The biological organisms also live in societies that affect their thoughts and feelings in various ways. Nobody denies these causal relations unless they deny the reality or causal efficacy of psychological states, societies, or organisms. Even such eliminativist views often allow our ordinary way of *speaking* about such causal relations, despite their claim that causal relations really occur only at the physical level.

We will ignore those eliminativist views, and everybody else accepts:

> *Causation BPS*: mental illnesses are caused or affected by biological, psychological, and social processes.

The reason why this view is uncontroversial is that it claims only causal relations among the biological, psychological, and social levels. There are many important questions about how such causal relations work, but nobody, except extreme eliminativists, denies or should deny those causal relations.

The central thesis of the BPS theory is not simply that such causal relations exist. After all, most of the living things we interact with—our friends, food, and flowers—also have biological, psychological, and social causes: the thoughts and social conventions of people who grow apples and cultivate orchids affect how apples and orchids turn out. The crucial question is not just what caused the organism to be what it is but also how we should understand its essential features and, relatedly, how we should help it flourish. The same goes for mental illnesses. The BPS theory of mental illness intends to say more than that biological, psychological, and social processes caused mental illnesses to be the way they are.

Explanation

What more does the BPS view claim? At least in part, the BPS theory is about how we should explain mental illnesses, so it might seem to claim this:

> *Explanation BPS* (EBPS): in order to explain a mental illness fully, we need to look at its psychological, biological, and social causes and aspects.

Notice that this view conjoins ('and') different levels of explanation. This conjunction makes the view controversial, because it implies that psychology by itself is not enough for complete explanation of a mental illness.

In contrast, many mental disorders in the *DSM-5* include only psychological and behavioural symptoms without listing anything about the underlying biology or about the social circumstances that lead to the disorder. For example, the *DSM-5* criteria for substance dependence include only patterns of use, impairment or distress, tolerance, withdrawal, desires, activities, and knowledge. None of these criteria requires any biological or social factor (but see later). True, tolerance and withdrawal are often understood to be the manifestation of some underlying biological changes, but the criteria themselves only cite these as psychological symptoms, not as biological factors. Thus, the *DSM-5* fails to provide a full understanding of substance dependence, according to the EBPS view. Of course, defenders of the *DSM-5* can reply that they never intended to provide a full explanation in their list of criteria, but that reply in effect admits that these criteria alone do not provide a full explanation, just as the EBPS view says.

As a result, it is hard to see why anyone would or should question the EBPS view. To see this, apply it to substance dependence. If we want to fully understand a person's dependence on cocaine, for example, we need to know something about how cocaine affects the person's brain, which is a biological organ. We also need to know something about the person's social circumstances, because those affect why the person was motivated to take cocaine as well as how the person obtained cocaine. These social factors shape the person's use of cocaine, such as whether he used crack or powdered cocaine, whether he hid or used publicly, with whom, and so on. Details of an individual's pattern and style of use are bound to be affected by social circumstances. That is why the EBPS view is right to say that we cannot fully explain—or understand all aspects of—this mental disorder without considering its biological and social causes and aspects in addition to its psychological causes and aspects.

Treatment

The BPS theory is not always only about how we should explain or understand mental illnesses. Most advocates of the BPS view are also interested in treatment. If a mental illness has biological and social causes in addition to its psychological causes, and if doctors do and should treat illnesses by removing their causes, then a mental illness must be treated by removing not only its psychological causes but also its biological and social causes. If doctors target only the psychological aspects without changing the biological substrate and the social circumstances, then the treatment is unlikely to succeed in the long run. Perhaps this is why addicts so often relapse after merely psychological treatment. At least, that is what many BPS theorists suggest, so they seem to claim something like this:

> *Treatment BPS* (TBPS): in order to treat a mental illness fully, we need to treat not only its psychological causes and aspects but also its biological and social causes and aspects.

Notice that the TBPS view does not claim that an incomplete treatment is no good at all. What it claims is only that a treatment is not full or complete unless it treats all three levels together.

This thesis might seem controversial. Many psychiatrists prescribe medications without talk therapy or cognitive behavioural treatment for the psychological aspects of the condition and also without family therapy and occupational therapy for the social aspects of the condition. On the other hand, many therapists give cognitive behavioural treatment or talk therapy for the psychological aspects of the condition without medications for the biological aspects of the condition or family and occupational therapy for the social aspects of the condition. They would (and should) not act in this way if they accepted the TBPS view, unless they assume that the cognitive behavioural or talk therapies somehow will cure occupational and family problems and will cause biological effects similar to those of medications. In contrast, the TBPS view suggests that neither kind of treatment will work (at least fully or optimally) without the others.

Still, we doubt that most therapists would deny the TBPS view. After all, there is strong evidence that treatments work better when they target all three levels together. There is less relapse to opioid use when a patient is not only on naltrexone but also moves to a neighbourhood with fewer drug cues, engages in regular talk therapy sessions, and has job training plus help in finding and keeping a job (cf. Ahmed et al., 2013). Nobody should deny that. But then why do therapists not treat all levels in accordance with the TBPS view? Because they cannot do everything. Sure, their patients would be better off if they received treatments at all levels (biological, psychological, and social), but one practitioner cannot provide equally competent treatments at all of these levels at once, and certainly not while also helping other clients, so they do as much as they can at the level at which they specialize. If this is why they engage in incomplete treatment, then they do not really deny the TBPS view after all. They merely provide a partial treatment because they cannot provide a full treatment of the kind that they and the TBPS view would prefer.

Constitution

All of these interpretations of the BPS view—disjunction, causation, explanation, and treatment—seem unquestionable. So, where's the beef? What specific claim is made by advocates of the BPS view that opponents deny?

One possibility is a claim about what constitutes or defines a particular mental illness:

> *Constitutive BPS* (CBPS): each mental illness is constituted by features at all three levels—psychological, biological, and social.

This claim is about what is essential to the mental illness rather than about what causes, explains, or treats it. It identifies the illness with a complex of traits at all three levels.

A claim about what partly constitutes (or defines or is essential to) a mental illness tells us what is necessary for that condition to be the particular mental illness it is rather than some other mental illness or no mental illness. When a condition is constituted or defined by a complex set or a conjunction of traits, nothing can possibly be an instance of that condition if any of those traits is missing.

The difference between constitution and causation can be illustrated by piano tuning. What *constitutes* a piano being in tune is a certain relation among sounds produced by striking its keys. It is out of tune when it produces sounds that are not related in the right way (but not when it is so badly broken that it produces no sounds at all). What *causes* it to be out of tune might be the temperature producing too much or too little tension in its strings, so we can *treat* the problem by adjusting these tensions. However, these tensions do not constitute or define what it is to be in or out of tune, because different strings could be in tune with different tensions. What is essential to being in tune is only the relations among the sounds produced. If any of the requisite relations is missing, then the piano is not in tune.

Analogously, the CBPS view implies that a condition is not the mental illness in question if any of the traits is missing—that is, if it lacks the defining psychological features or if it lacks the defining biological features or if it lacks the defining social features. For example, suppose that substance dependence is constituted not only by certain psychological traits but also by certain neurological traits, including, perhaps, abnormal activity in the ventral striatum in response to drug cues. Then, if an individual patient has all of the psychological traits of people with substance dependence but lacks that abnormal brain activity, that patient does not really have any substance dependence. And if all mental illnesses have to be constituted or defined by features at all levels, as the CBPS view claims, and if this patient has no biological abnormality, then this patient does not really have any mental illness, regardless of the abnormal behaviour.

It is not clear whether advocates of the BPS view really embrace the CBPS view. Many of them probably do not go that far. Nonetheless, it is still instructive to ask whether the CBPS view is true. We will argue that it is not. Although the other interpretations of the BPS view are obvious or at least defensible, the CBPS view is not plausible when taken literally as applied to all mental illnesses. If we are correct, the plausibility and attractiveness of the BPS approach must lie not in the CBPS view but rather in the weaker interpretations or, perhaps, in some exceptional examples in which the CBPS view holds.

In addition to this negative claim, we will also argue for a positive claim about what is essential to a certain mental illness—or at least most mental illnesses. Our alternative view is that biological and social forces cause mental illnesses but do not constitute or define those mental illnesses except in unusual cases. In most cases, their psychological aspects or features are what make them the illnesses that they are. In short, its mental features constitute a mental illness.

To see why, first consider an analogy: a person's height is caused by her or his biology (including genes) and environment (including nutrition). It can be measured in many different units, depending on which units a society uses. Still, height is height. It is not defined, constituted, or identified with genes or nutrition, nor does the height itself change when it is measured using different units. That is shown by the fact that a person who measures 5 feet tall when his or her genes and environment would have predicted a height of 6 feet is still really only 5 feet—or 1.52 metres—tall. The causes of height and the socially determined ways in which we measure it do not constitute height.

Our question, then, is whether a mental illness is defined or constituted by its biological or social features or only by its psychological features. To answer this question, we first need to test our intuitions in imaginary cases. In particular, we need to think about cases where an individual lacks the biological and social aspects of a condition but has its psychological aspects, and vice versa.

For example, suppose we established that 99% of people with a certain biomarker (such as a pattern of neural activity) had depressed feelings (such as sadness) and thoughts (such as that life is meaningless) that lead to depressed activity (lethargy or suicide attempts). Furthermore, 99% of people with depressed feelings, thoughts, and actions have that biomarker. This is fiction, of course, because no current biomarker of depression is anywhere near that accurate; but imagine it in the year 2525. Still, a person who genuinely has the same strong and persistent feelings, thoughts, and actions of depression but who lacks that biomarker would, we contend, have the mental illness of depression. Conversely, a person who has that biomarker but who lacks any depressed feelings, thoughts, or actions would *not* have the mental illness of depression. Just imagine someone with the biomarker who smiles and laughs, is energetic and sociable, and says, 'Life is great. I am so happy'. We might not understand what is going on in this case, but we would not suspect the mental illness of depression. These intuitions suggest that the psychological aspects of depression—the depressed feelings, thoughts, and actions—are what constitute or define the mental illness of depression. In contrast, the biological aspects or correlates of those psychological aspects are not constitutive or definitive of depression, even if they are causal or explanatory.

This is not to deny that some people could prefer to use a biomarker instead of current clinical criteria of depression. Some might even declare that a person who lacks the biomarker isn't 'really' depressed while a person who has the biomarker without the psychological symptoms 'really' is depressed. People can stipulate whatever idiolect they prefer and even insist that the rest of us change what we mean by 'depression'. Moreover, if enough people come to share their view, 'depression' might even come to refer to all and only people with this biomarker, regardless of their psychological symptoms. Our project is neither prescriptive nor in opposition to such potential changes. Our only conclusion is that this is not the way we would define or diagnose depression now, so there are no grounds now to claim that such a biomarker would be a discovery about 'real' depression.

The same point applies to social causes of mental illness. Take a challenging example: if someone uses cocaine and has tolerance, withdrawal, lack of control, related harms, and all of the other criteria of substance dependence in the *DSM-5*, then that person is dependent on cocaine. But not so if the person has similar problems with caffeine, since we socially value people using caffeine. Doesn't this show that dependence is socially constituted, since there is no caffeine dependence? Continuing this line of thought, perhaps there's an even deeper reason that we socially define dependence or addiction the way we do: such as because we have other social goals promoted by these definitions, like stigmatizing certain groups as addicts while not stigmatizing others (cf. Hart, 2013).

There is some evidence for such a view in the *DSM* itself. In the *DSM-5*, three of seven criteria must be met for a diagnosis of substance dependence. One of those criteria explicitly mentions a social condition: 'Important social, occupational, or recreational activities are given up or reduced because of [substance] use' (American Psychiatric Association, 2013, p. 491; cf. pp. 509, 520, 523, 534, 541, 550, 561, 571, 577). Since only three of seven criteria must be met, this single criterion is neither necessary nor sufficient for substance dependence, but this social factor is still partially diagnostic of substance dependence in the *DSM-5*.

It would be a mistake, however, to think that this diagnostic information is constitutive or definitive of addiction (Summers, 2015). Note first that what matters is that the person gives up important activities in order to use the drug, not whether these important activities are 'social, occupational, or recreational'. If the person gave up important activities that were neither social nor occupational nor recreational, and if giving up those activities caused significant harm to the person, then that person's substance dependence could still be a mental disorder deserving treatment.

While it is true that the criterion includes the word 'important', which seems to suggest some social constitution—our society thinks jobs and families are important, playing video games is not—this is a slender reed on which to build the case for the social constitution of addiction. The point of the word 'important' is to acknowledge that everything I do will cause me to give up some activities, but most of what I give up is less important than what I give it up for, so I shouldn't be diagnosed simply because I gave up *something*. How particular clinicians interpret 'important' is an empirical question to which we don't have an answer, but they no doubt often defer to the patient's own evaluation of what 'important' means, not substituting what the clinician believes 'society' would value.

Crucially, though, this diagnostic criterion isn't necessary to any particular case of substance dependence: some addicts might be dependent without any such harm at all. Consider George, who gambles a lot, keeps gambling longer than intended, would suffer withdrawal if he stopped, and spends a lot of time going to different casinos as well as reading books about how to gamble better. His job was important to him, but he gives it up to gamble more. This sounds like a behavioural addiction to gambling, except that George is a good gambler: he wins much more than he loses, makes new friends through gambling, and becomes rich by gambling. As his gambling activities became prominent in his life, George gave up and reduced 'social, occupational, or recreational activities' that were important to his life before he became a gambler. However, his new gambling activities are fruitful financially and personally. He might even be happier and more satisfied with his life than before. Despite these benefits, George could still be addicted to gambling.

If our view is correct, then these common social consequences are not really essential to addiction or substance dependence. Instead, a patient would have the same substance dependence if he had the psychological aspects of substance dependence without those social consequences or harms. And, of course, he would not have any substance dependence if he had those social consequences without the psychological features. These intuitions, then, suggest that, if any aspects of substance dependence are constitutive or definitive, it is the psychological and not the social.

Similarly, whether someone is *diagnosed* as addicted to cocaine or to coffee does depend in part on what drugs our society cares about. Psychiatry does not generally worry about addiction to caffeine, and this may reflect the personal judgements of clinicians or of society at large. But this is not to say that the disorders psychiatry focuses on are the only possible disorders. Psychiatrists may not care about caffeine addiction, perhaps because society doesn't care about caffeine addiction, but that does not mean that caffeine dependence is not really dependence unless it is socially recognized as such. In fact, all the elements of a potential diagnosis are present in the *DSM-5* (tolerance, withdrawal, lack of control, harm, and the various other problems common to all dependences), ready to be applied to caffeine or to any new or unrecognized drug. If our evidence that cocaine dependence is socially constituted is only that caffeine dependence is not recognized, this only points out that some disorders are of concern for clinicians and researchers while others are not. But whether or not they are of concern, those disorders are, we maintain, psychologically constituted.

Tricky cases

We haven't proven that there are no social aspects to any mental illness, nor do we intend to. We also have not proven—nor do we believe—that there is no biological aspect to any mental illness. We agree with many proponents of BPS models that mental illnesses are best understood in and by their biological and social contexts. Nonetheless, we have still resisted the stronger conclusion that mental illnesses are all constituted by biological, psychological, and social elements.

Perhaps a more modest conclusion is defensible, however, and the CBPS view is meant to apply only to *some* mental illnesses. The social or biological causes might be essential to some mental illnesses even if they are not essential to other mental illnesses (cf. Davies, 2016). We will consider a few cases that make a strong claim to being understood as disorders only biopsychosocially.

Consider post-traumatic stress disorder (PTSD). The *DSM-5* (American Psychiatric Association, 2013, pp. 271–274) defines PTSD in terms of a complex set of psychological features that originate in a traumatic event. That traumatic event can be biological (such as a severe injury) or social (such as rape or abuse). The biological and social features are therefore essential to this mental illness on this definition, right? That conclusion would confuse the cause of the disorder with the essential features of the disorder itself. Imagine two cases that have exactly the same current psychological symptoms, but these symptoms derive from trauma in one case but arise without trauma in the other case. It is trivially true that only one of these two stress disorders is literally 'post-traumatic', but insisting on that would beg the question: the CBPS view shouldn't depend on the name we have given to any particular disorder. (If I call a particular substance dependence 'illegal cocaine dependence', that doesn't change the underlying disorder. It remains the same disorder in places where cocaine is illegal as in places where cocaine is legal.) The treatment might be different in these two cases, and perhaps there are very good practical reasons that we want to distinguish the traumatically induced stress disorders from stress disorders with other aetiologies. But that alone will not show that they are different mental illnesses.

Similarly, disinhibited social engagement disorder (DSED) is defined in the *DSM-5* by psychological symptoms (such as children's 'reduced or absent reticence in approaching and interacting with unfamiliar adults') caused by past neglect ('a pattern of extremes of insufficient care') (American Psychiatric Association, 2013, pp. 268–269; cf. Singh and Sinnott-Armstrong, 2015). As with PTSD, this cause is or can be social or biological in nature, but it is a mistake to include this cause in the definition of DSED. Imagine cases with parallel psychological symptoms, but neglect causes those symptoms in one case and not in the other. It seems to us that these cases exemplify the same mental illness with different causes and perhaps also different treatments.

If we are right, then these mental illnesses should be defined by their psychological symptoms rather than by their social or biological causes. Of course, one reason that we care about the biological and social aetiologies of various disorders is that their causes correlate with current symptoms and often help us to determine which treatments will be effective. It would be very unusual and unexpected for two people to have the same current symptoms when their pasts were relevantly so different, for example, that someone has PTSD-like symptoms without any past trauma. Indeed, if we did run into such a patient, then we might look again more closely at the patient's history to find anything that the patient might have interpreted as traumatic. Nonetheless, the possibility that we might not find any such trauma yet still be faced with a patient who otherwise shows the symptoms of PTSD shows that past trauma (or neglect, for DSED) is not really essential to the mental illness.

If the social isn't essential even in cases in which it appears in the name of the disorder, is that because there was an underlying biological disorder that unifies the cases? Perhaps. The two patients who both share PTSD-like symptoms while only one of them has a history of trauma might nevertheless share the same neurological substrate. Does our objection to a constitutive social element therefore show that there is a constitutive biological element?

To answer this, consider a different case of two different neural substrates of similar symptoms. Imagine two patients who exhibit extremely impulsive behaviour where one patient has neural abnormalities only in one brain area associated with strong emotions or desires (such as the limbic system) and the other patient has abnormalities only in another brain area associated with lack of executive control (such as the prefrontal cortex). Don't these different neural substrates suggest that these patients have different mental illnesses? If so, then the neural substrate seems to be part of what constitutes or at least individuates the particular mental illness.

However, why do these mental illnesses seem distinct at all? It is not because the neurological substrates are different but only because the relevant neural substrates are themselves related to different psychological processes: strong emotions and desires in the one case and weak executive control in the other case. To see this, remember that areas of the brain are not all clearly demarcated biologically by neuron types, neurotransmitters, and such. Anatomical divisions are sometimes used to identify various nuclei, but what will matter to mental illness are functional demarcations and their psychological correspondences. We contend that it is this psychological difference that suggests distinct mental illnesses rather than the mere difference in neural substrate.

This reply is supported by considering how we would classify the cases if the neural differences were not related at all to any psychological difference. Imagine cases with similar impulsivity where one has abnormalities in one brain area (such as the claustrum) and the other has abnormalities in another (such as the frontal eye fields) where neither area is associated with any psychological symptom related to impulsivity. Then we are not inclined to count these patients as having distinct mental illnesses. That suggests that neural differences count in classifying mental illnesses only when those neural differences matter to psychology.

Overall, then, we conclude that psychological aspects rather than biological or social aspects are what constitute or define a particular mental illness—except maybe in unusual cases. Biological and social factors are still very important for diagnosis, treatment, and prevention, because it is sometimes easier to manipulate social and biological factors. However, the issue is *not* what is important or useful but what is essential to mental illness in most cases. What is essential is at least usually the psychological level.

Scrupulosity

We have not argued that it is impossible for the biological and social to constitute any mental illness even partially. What we have argued is only that the biological and social should not generally be viewed as constitutive of a mental illness. One potential objection to this view is that we have selected only examples of mental illnesses that are conducive to our position. If we had instead considered a mental illness that can only be understood as such in terms of its biological and social aspects in addition to its psychological aspects, then we would have to admit that the CBPS view is plausible for least some mental illnesses. The question would then be which mental disorders are best defined biopsychosocially and which are essentially only psychological.

This response is quite plausible, and no argument can prove that no mental disorders at all are best characterized biopsychosocially. This would require moving disorder by disorder through a complete list. Moreover, this claim would apply not only today but in the future. We cannot rule out the possibility that future neuroscience will change the way we look at mental illnesses so that we will start individuating them by biology instead of psychology. That is why we do not claim to prove anything universal or timeless. We hope only to place the burden of proof on anyone who would argue that mental illnesses are constituted biopsychosocially, rather than psychologically, as they have typically been understood.

It will be worth our effort, though, to look more closely at a disorder that makes a good case for being characterized biopsychosocially. This example will make clearer how we are likely to respond to any proposed counterexample, and why we believe that a counterexample must meet a high burden of proof before we revise our understanding of mental illness as essentially mental.

The disorder we examine is scrupulosity. Scrupulosity is a form of obsessive-compulsive disorder (OCD) in which the person has religious or moral obsessions or compulsions. In most ways, it resembles OCD, with fears of contamination and feelings of extreme personal responsibility. Characteristically, its patients have a high degree of perfectionism, doubt, and distress directed at morality. They also often do not distinguish the badness of having a bad thought from the badness of performing a bad action, being (nearly) as critical of their own bad thoughts as they would be if they had performed equivalently bad actions (moral thought–action fusion) (Summers and Sinnott-Armstrong, 2019).

No biological marker of OCD has yet been discovered. Abramowitz and colleagues (2009, p. 491) report, 'Biological models of obsessive-compulsive disorder propose anomalies in the serotonin pathway and dysfunctional circuits in the orbito-striatal area and dorsolateral prefrontal cortex'. However, they immediately add, 'Support for these models is mixed and they do not account for the symptomatic heterogeneity of the disorder'. Still, it is not hard to imagine that future research might pin down a precise biological marker of OCD in general or even of scrupulosity in particular. After all, the effectiveness of some medications for OCD might seem to suggest that there must be some biological cause of OCD. Of course, we could repeat some of the above-mentioned reasoning to evaluate any proposed biomarker. If the biomarker does not perfectly predict every case of scrupulosity, then we must wonder whether we have only found *a* biomarker of *some* cases of scrupulosity or whether we have found *the* biomarker of *all* real cases of scrupulosity and we were wrong in how we classified the cases that do not fit the discovered biomarker. No biological discovery alone will settle for us whether what we currently call scrupulosity should be reconceptualized as separate disorders—one to correspond to each biomarker—or if instead it remains a single disorder with multiple biomarkers. It is unclear how we can make progress in this debate without taking seriously the psychological category with which we began, which defined scrupulosity in terms of religious or moral obsessions or compulsions rather than in terms of any biomarker.

Despite these problems, let's assume for the sake of argument that there is a single (though probably complex) biomarker, and that scrupulosity is unified biologically in the same way that it is unified psychologically. In other words, let's assume that all and only cases of scrupulosity identified psychologically also have this particular biomarker. This assumption, even if implausible today, should allow us to set aside the biological question so that we can focus on a distinct and perhaps more challenging issue with scrupulosity: can it be characterized only psychologically or must it be characterized socially as well?

To put this broad question more precisely, consider how scrupulosity manifests in actual cases. A scrupulous Catholic often will attend confession much more than a non-scrupulous Catholic, and she will feel afterwards that she may not have succeeded in confessing all of her sins, and, as a result, she may not have succeeded in receiving the absolution she desires. In contrast, a scrupulous orthodox Jew will not, of course, engage in the Catholic ritual of confession. Instead, a scrupulous Jew might doubt that he correctly said his obligatory prayers, therefore causing him either to move extremely slowly through the prayers or to repeat them. Yet another kind of case is a patient with secular scrupulosity who worries constantly about the suffering of others, so he gives away almost all of his money, and he and his family are then forced to live on only a very small percentage of what he earns—even though these donations still do not relieve his anxiety and guilt feelings. (Examples of these sorts are described in Summers and Sinnott-Armstrong (2019).)

Despite these differences in manifestation, all three cases could be diagnosed as scrupulosity. Crucially for our question here, social circumstances seem to play several roles in understanding these cases.

First, social factors clearly shape the particular practices of people with scrupulosity. In religious cases, the disorder is differently expressed depending on the religion of the person with the disorder. A Catholic does not worry about keeping kosher or fasting during Ramadan, nor does a Jew or Muslim worry about confessing or going to mass on Sundays.

However, the fact that a mental disorder is *shaped* by social elements does not imply or support the CBPS view's claim that the disorder is socially *constituted*. One cannot be a scrupulous Catholic without being a Catholic, and one cannot be a scrupulous Jew without being a Jew. Scrupulous Catholics will act differently from scrupulous Jews. Nonetheless, what is socially shaped is the manifestation or expression of the illness rather than the illness itself. Scrupulous Catholics, Jews, Muslims, Hindus, Buddhists, and even atheists can have the same basic mental illness even if they manifest that illness in different actions (much as allergies can have various manifestations in various environments).

Second, and more profoundly, comparisons with the patient's society might seem to be part of what justifies calling these conditions a mental illness. After all, Catholics see confession as admirable or even required, Jews see prayers as obligatory, and most people admire helping others in need. So, why do these same practices manifest a disorder in our cases? The answer might seem to lie in the extent to which these patients engage in these acts. Confession is healthy, but not five times a day. Prayers can support one's other religious beliefs and practices, but an hour each time is too much. Charity is encouraged, but enough is enough. Of course, how much is seen as enough or too much varies historically as well as between societies. What looks to us here and now as a disorder might be (or might be seen as) a relatively tame religious practice in other places and times. Conversely, what looks to us here and now as a tame religious practice might someday appear to be disordered religious extremism. If a comparison to what other people in society normally do and to what they see as appropriate is what turns our three cases into cases of disorders, then society seems to play an essential role in determining which people have the mental illness of scrupulosity.

We think this suggestion is inaccurate because it misses what really distinguishes patients with scrupulosity from other people who practise extreme religion or charity. What really makes scrupulosity a disorder is its source in anxiety. Monks who give up worldly pleasures, live in a monastery, and pray long hours each day do not necessarily have scrupulosity. If they choose this lifestyle out of their love for God, then this is not a psychological disorder (even if their beliefs are false). In contrast, if they become monks only in order to escape constant and intense anxiety that is too much for them to bear, this could suggest a disorder. This underlying anxiety leads to abnormal focus on some moral or religious issues to the exclusion of others, especially others that are more important, and reinforces the person's own inflated sense of personal responsibility. Although anxiety itself is not a disorder, and it is not disordered to act to eliminate one's own anxiety, what makes cases of scrupulosity a mental illness is that the underlying anxiety leads to disordered practices. The practices are not disordered because society deems them so. Even if a society included lots of monks, so that their practices were not out of the norm—statistically or normatively—for that society, the monks who were more strongly motivated to eliminate their anxiety would likely have these other psychological problems, which would manifest in disordered actions. Thus, what makes scrupulosity a mental illness is not a social comparison but rather a collection of psychological problems due to underlying anxiety. Accordingly, this mental illness, like others, is essentially psychological rather than social.

Details complicate but support this basic picture. In the earlier examples, the practices of the scrupulous person are of a piece with religious or ethical practices. The scrupulous Catholic goes to confession to find absolution from sins, real or imagined, but so does the non-scrupulous Catholic. The differences aren't in the practices alone, and the disorder isn't just that the scrupulous Catholics go more often, since there are many reasons that a person may go more often that have nothing to do with mental disorder. Likewise, someone with secular scrupulosity—though this is an understudied area—gives much more to charity than most people, but we are not going to diagnose someone as having any kind of a disorder simply on the basis of giving more than others since, again, there are many reasons that a person may give much more than others.

We can't diagnose scrupulosity on the basis of someone acting more religiously or morally than others, but we also can't easily diagnose it based solely on some other part of their behaviour, since the behaviour might not match the relevant religion or system of morality. Although we began with examples in which the person's actions are an extreme version of more ordinary actions, scrupulosity also leads to actions that are so different from ordinary religious or moral actions that the connection between the supposed beliefs and the person's actions is tenuous at best. The scrupulous Catholic who goes to confession multiple times a day, however extreme this is, is comprehensible to the ordinary Catholic; but the Catholic who must confess in order to keep her children from dying is much less so; and the Catholic who confesses daily to imaginary 'sins' so minor that the priest feels no need to give absolution is no longer the devout version of a Catholic but someone with a mental disorder that expresses itself in Catholic ritual. Similarly, the orthodox Jew who won't draw a religious picture in order not to make an image of god is understandable even to less orthodox believers, but one who refuses even to look at a photo or painting, looking only at the frame, looks like something else entirely (Traig, 2006).

What could explain both extreme religious practices and also the practices that are only nominally related to a religious tradition? Despite the initial suggestion, it cannot be simply that the scrupulous are more extreme than the ordinarily religious or moral. No, when we look more closely at the cases, what we see in these extremes are the manifestation of the person's narrow focus on certain issues that the person sincerely believes or merely rationalizes as being religious or moral. This focus is to the exclusion of other moral or religious issues, including issues that are more important, and focusing primarily on issues where the patient feels—with or without justification—an exaggerated sense of personal responsibility. What underlies this focus on only a few issues to the exclusion of more important issues is the patient's desire to soothe her own anxiety, which she may feel most acutely in evaluating her own moral worth.

This suggests that we are not diagnosing a disorder defined as one extreme end of a religious or moral practice. Instead, we are looking at a psychological disorder constituted by an underlying anxiety, which is then characteristically expressed as an extreme of moral or religious practice. The underlying disorder is characterized in purely psychological terms, and, while it often finds its expression in such extreme practices, it needn't. It is not a disorder because of these extreme manifestations. Instead, it is extreme because it expresses a psychological disorder.

Conclusion

For these reasons, scrupulosity is constituted by psychological rather than biological or social factors. Of course, that does not prove that no other mental illness is constituted by biological and social factors in addition to psychological factors. Critics can respond to our arguments by proposing other apparent counterexamples. We hope, however, that the example of scrupulosity clarifies what is needed in order to claim that any particular mental illness is not just shaped or explained by biological and social factors but also at least partly constituted by them.

A claim about what partly constitutes (or defines or is essential to) a mental illness is a claim about what is needed to make that condition the mental illness it is rather than another mental illness or no mental illness. In order to show that a biological factor partly constitutes a certain mental illness, one would need to show that any case of that particular mental illness has that biological condition. Similarly, to show that a social factor partly constitutes a certain mental illness, one would need to show that the social factor must be present in any case of that mental illness. Both claims deny that the psychological elements that had previously been used to define or diagnose the mental illness are sufficient by themselves—without biological or social accompaniments—to constitute a case of that particular mental illness.

Of course, when we refer to 'any case' of a mental illness, we are not referring to mere logical possibility. What matters are cases that are realistic psychologically, biologically, and socially (as well as physically). Still, we are not limited to cases that have actually arisen or been observed. We need to imagine societies and organisms somewhat different from our own in order to test claims about what partially constitutes a certain mental illness.

Thus, in order to respond to a proposal that some mental illness is partly constituted by some biological or social factor, we need to imagine cases where the psychological elements are all present but the biological and social elements are absent. Then we need to ask whether it is best (accurate, precise, informative, or useful) to classify that imagined case as a case of the mental illness. If not, then the biological and social elements might be essential to that mental illness. But if the case with the psychological but not the biological and social elements is still a case of that mental illness, then the biological and social elements are not really essential or constitutive of that mental illness.

When we apply this test to the mental illnesses that we are familiar with, we do not find any mental illness that meets the requirements of the CBPS view. Admittedly, that might just show the limits of our knowledge or imagination. However, it at least shifts the burden of proof onto proponents of the CBPS view. If they can come up with a counterexample of a mental illness that is constituted even partly by its biological or social elements, then we will have learned something.

Overall, then, the problem for the BPS view of mental illness is that it wavers between the obvious and the implausible. There is a lot of truth in some interpretations of the BPS view, including disjunction, causation, explanation, and treatment BPS views. However, there is not much controversy about those claims. They seem obvious, though it can sometimes be useful to remind ourselves of obvious truths. What is perhaps less obvious but also worth a reminder is another lesson of the BPS model of mental illness, namely that we need to keep an open mind before we decide that any difference is a disorder. That lesson is also worth remembering even if the CBPS view should be rejected as too strong as a general claim. There still might be some exceptional mental illnesses that fit the CBPS model, but that remains to be seen.

References

Abramowitz, J.S., Taylor, S., and McKay, D. (2009). Obsessive-compulsive disorder. *The Lancet*, **374**(9688), 491–499.

Ahmed, S.H., Lenoir, M., and Guillem, K. (2013). Neurobiology of addiction versus drug use driven by lack of choice. *Current Opinion in Neurobiology*, **23**(4), 581–587.

American Psychiatric Association (2013). *Diagnostic and Statistical Manual of Mental Disorders* (5th ed.). Washington, DC: American Psychiatric Association.

Davies, W. (2016). Externalist psychiatry. *Analysis*, **76**(3), 290–296.

Hart, C. (2013). *High Price: A Neuroscientist's Journey of Self-Discovery That Challenges Everything You Know About Drugs and Society*. New York: HarperCollins.

Singh, D. and Sinnott-Armstrong, W. (2015). The DSM-5 definition of mental disorder. *Public Affairs Quarterly*, **29**(1), 5–31.

Summers, J. (2015). What is wrong with addiction. *Philosophy, Psychiatry and Psychology*, **22**(1), 25–40.

Summers, J., and Sinnott-Armstrong, W. (2019). *Clean Hands? Philosophical Lessons from Scrupulosity*. New York: Oxford University Press.

Traig, J. (2006). *Devil in the Details: Scenes from an Obsessive Girlhood*. Boston, MA: Back Bay Books.

Chapter 7

The truth in social construction

Neil Levy

Introduction

Psychiatry has long been a contested site. It has been one of the central places where a battle for our souls—or perhaps over whether we *have* souls—has been conducted. On one side, we have arrayed the forces of science with its momentous, data-driven, achievements. On the other we have humanists, who acknowledge the great power and insights of science but who argue that it has limits: that social and psychological explanations cannot be replaced by mechanist explanations. This kind of conflict might be seen as a successor to a centuries-long cultural battle between poetry and science, between Romanticism and Enlightenment, and between the irreducibly human and (perhaps proudly) soulless mechanism.

In psychiatry, the battle pits advocates of the biopsychosocial model against advocates of the medical model. The first camp acknowledges that explanations couched in terms of brain chemistry (say) can be illuminating, but claim that they can never be the whole story, while the second identifies psychiatric diseases with a lesion or a dysfunction in a brain mechanism (or even in gene expression). This battle maps well, though not perfectly, onto another: between those who think that treatment should emphasize psychotherapy and psychopharmaceuticals used sparingly, and those who see no special reason to prefer talk therapy. It is in this form that the conflict has had widest cultural relevance, with many people beyond the domain of psychiatry worried about the possible over-prescription of antidepressants and (perhaps especially due to the fact that most patients are children) pharmaceutical treatments for attention deficit hyperactivity disorder. Both in the philosophical literature and in the popular press, there are many advocates of psychotherapy over psychopharmaceuticals, often arguing that the latter risk mechanizing us and thereby failing to treat us as rational agents (see Hari (2018) for a recent example).

The latest front in this battle is the announcement by Thomas Insel (2013), the then director of the US National Institute of Mental Health (NIMH), that the NIMH will direct funding away from research using categories from the *Diagnostic and Statistical Manual of Mental Disorders*, fifth edition (*DSM-5*) (American Psychiatric Association, 2013). Insel wants to replace the lists of symptoms and behavioural disturbances by which the *DSM-5* and its predecessors classify patients with more biological categories. Mental disorders, he writes, 'are biological disorders involving brain circuits that implicate specific domains of cognition, emotion, or behavior'. They are not mere lists of symptoms. Insel points out that with somatic disease, diagnosis cuts across symptomatology: 'chest pain' is not a disorder; rather it is a symptom of any number of problems, some trivial and some life-threatening. Insel argues that psychiatry needs to follow the other branches of medicine and understand illness as physical in nature.

Under Insel's leadership, the NIMH has launched its *Research Domain Criteria* (RDoC) project, which aims to lay the foundations for a new classification scheme by utilizing biological information drawn from genetics, neuroimaging, molecular biology, and other parts of cognitive science. It is tempting to see RDoC as representing the extreme wing of the mechanistic forces. Their less extreme allies may concede some role for social factors to modulate the experience of mental illness, while nevertheless insisting that it is an essentially biological phenomenon (Guze, 1992). On the humanist side, we might see proponents of the biopsychosocial model, which acknowledges the importance of biological approaches to understanding mental illness, as representing the moderate wing while a more extreme current—the complement of RDoC—is represented by those who claim that mental illness is a social construction. In this chapter, however, I shall argue that social construction and the RDoC are in fact natural allies. RDoC *requires* social construction to make good on its promise to illuminate mental illness.

The RDoC project is motivated by several different things. One important driver is frustration at the failure of psychiatry to follow the path that other areas of medicine laid down, often decades earlier. All branches of medicine began with a descriptive taxonomy of the kind that psychiatry still utilizes. But over time, this taxonomy was revised as the biological basis for illness and disease was uncovered. Similar symptoms were discovered to be caused by quite different pathologies. Kapur and colleagues (2012) give the example of breast lumps; it took histopathological differentiation and molecular markers to move beyond symptomatology to distinguish pathologies. That initial breakthrough laid the grounds for others, with subtypes of breast cancer identified and treatments specifically targeted at these subtypes developed. An understanding of the specific biology of the subtypes led to treatments not only for these ailments but also for other cancers sharing molecular pathways with them. Understanding the underlying biology therefore can lead to better understanding and better treatments.

The example of breast lumps—and others, Kapur and colleagues also mention arthritides—suggests that some of the mental illnesses we currently identify by descriptive taxonomies may turn out to be distinct pathologies. Conversely, some of those we currently distinguish on the basis of symptomatology may actually be manifestations of the same underlying dysfunction. The failure of current diagnostic categories to predict treatment responses is some evidence that they do not cut nature at its joints (Insel et al., 2010). More direct evidence comes from genetics, neuroscience, and epidemiological findings. Extensive comorbidity of apparently distinct conditions suggests that they may not be all that distinct (Kapur et al., 2012). Nearly all genetic risk factors for schizophrenia convey comparable risks for bipolar disorder, and for even more—intuitively—distant disorders such as depression, substance abuse, and epilepsy (Insel and Cuthbert, 2010). All of this suggests that the underlying pathologies do not line up at all well with *DSM* categories.

A central aim of the RDoC is to reclassify disorders by identifying their molecular, genetic, and neurological basis. It conceives of mental illnesses as brain disorders arising not from lesions but from disorders of brain circuits. The project calls for the tools of neuroscience to be used for identifying which brain circuits are dysfunctional, thereby providing a target for molecular and genetic work which will uncover the cellular mechanisms causally involved in the disorder. Neuroscience will be guided in its investigations by symptomatology (not by diagnostic categories: the target population will not be sufferers from schizophrenia, say, but disorders of attention or declarative memory) and also by existing work on the genetics of mental illness.

All of this may sound like the triumph of mechanism. It seems to promise—or threaten—to replace the lived experience of mental illness, whether that of the sufferer or of the clinician, with brain circuits, genes, and molecules. But its proponents recognize, however imperfectly, that this can't be the end of the story. Though it is surely correct that uncovering the underlying molecular causes of dysfunctional brain circuitry is essential to developing new treatments, understanding mental illness—and treating it too—requires much more. I will argue that it requires attention to the kind of forces that social constructionists insist on.

The building blocks of social construction

The phrase 'social construction', and its derivatives, is used across a wide variety of debates and with a correspondingly broad range of meanings. In its very weakest sense, to say that something is socially constructed is to say that social forces (institutions, cultural norms, cultural practices) play a role in determining that it exists or the actual form it takes. In this form, the claim is trivial: human beings are social animals, dependent for their survival on socially transmitted skills and almost always also dependent on the labour of others. If to say that something is socially constructed is just to say that it is causally dependent on social institutions and practices, then every aspect of the human phenotype is socially constructed. Advocates of claims like 'mental illness is socially constructed' have a stronger claim in mind.

Typically, they have a deflationary and debunking aim. When someone claims that something is socially constructed with these aims in mind, they commit themselves to three claims, in addition to the claim that the target is causally dependent for its existence or its actual form on social forces (Hacking, 1999):

1. The social forces in question are, in a sense to be explained, *contingent*.

2. The social forces are disguised.

3. The final form of whatever it is that is socially constructed is very undesirable.

The sense of contingency that is referred to in claim (1) is not the standard philosopher's sense, in which 'contingency' is contrasted with metaphysical or nomological necessity. Rather, the contrast is with *social* necessity. The claim is not that there are possible worlds in which the laws might have been different, say, but that realistic changes in the actual history of our society would have resulted in significant differences in the target. The claim is not merely historical, in most cases; rather, the contingency is ongoing: it remains realistic for us to eliminate or alter the social forces in question, compatible with our having flourishing lives (so in this sense food production or childcare is not contingent—we can't eliminate either and continue to have flourishing lives—though the precise form which each takes *is* contingent). Claiming that mental illness is socially constructed is claiming that it is practically possible to shape social forces so that mental illness is significantly altered (or even eliminated), compatible with us continuing to have good lives.

Claim (1) is obviously true with regard to certain targets. It will surprise no one that newsstands are socially constructed in this kind of way (we could easily alter their layout or even eliminate them without seriously impacting the quality of our lives). Social constructionists assert the first claim only when claim (2) is also true. Social constructionists aim to *unmask* the fact that something that is taken to be natural, or at least inevitable, is in fact the product of contingent social forces. It is claim (2) that makes social constructionism a debunking project. In the case of mental illness, social constructionists might see in the RDoC the latest attempt to pass off mental illness as biological—and therefore natural or inevitable—when it is in fact socially constructed. Someone taking this line might see the attempt to identify genetic pathways and neural correlates of disorders as ideological; as attempts to hide the fact that people are classified as mentally ill when (say) they violate social norms.

Claim (3) is tightly connected to claim (1), at least when social constructionism is a debunking project. The social forces are contingent because we can eliminate them without (undue) cost; since eliminating mental illness is surely a benefit, we have good reason to do so. The status quo is, all things considered, undesirable, and maintained because it serves the interests of powerful actors (note that those who benefit from the maintenance of the status quo need not be aware of this fact).

Few people would regard a *global* debunking social constructionism with regard to mental illness as plausible. It is implausible that we could alter social forces so that no one, or almost no one, suffered from a (significant) mental illness. A *local* debunking project is much more plausible: it is plausible that some mental illnesses are socially constructed and that they, or much of the suffering associated with them, could be eliminated by altering social conditions. Consider—to take Murphy's (2006) example—bulimia. There is evidence that bulimia is socially constructed. Bulimia seems to be higher in groups that are more exposed to particular conceptions of female beauty (Wilson et al., 1996), which are more prevalent in Western societies. So, for instance, there is a correlation between use of English at home and body dissatisfaction among Chinese girls in Singapore (Ung, 2003), and rates of bulimia among girls from Indian and Pakistani immigrant families in the UK seem to be orders of magnitude higher than rates among girls in Pakistan (Mumford et al., 1991, 1992). These facts suggest that bulimia may be the product of social forces which are socially contingent and which we could eliminate without cost. Bulimia may therefore satisfy conditions (1) and (3). If it is also true that the role of these social forces is widely denied or dissimulated, then bulimia may also satisfy condition (2). This, too, is a plausible, though hardly uncontroversial, contention; think here of debates over whether standards of female beauty are evolutionarily innate—such that they can be altered only at great cost, in terms of resources or consequences—or are historically contingent. In light of the importance of debates like this, we can better understand why some social constructionists see pop versions of evolutionary psychology, which often advance the innateness claim, as ideological propaganda (see Buss (1994) for a defence of the claim that standards of beauty are innate and Pinker (2002) for an explicit defence of the claim that our political institutions must respect our evolved dispositions).

Explanatory or debunking?

The claim that bulimia is socially constructed can come in two forms, one stronger and one weaker. The stronger claim, of the kind more optimistic debunkers seem to have in mind, is that if the contingent social norms that are causally responsible for bulimia were altered in the right kind of way, bulimia *and* all the suffering associated with it would also disappear. The weaker claim is agnostic on whether all the suffering associated with bulimia would disappear. The best-known philosophical defender of social construction, Ian Hacking, often seems to have a version of the weaker claim in mind when discussing actual cases. On his view, sufferers from the transient mental illnesses on which he focuses, like dissociative fugues, were people whose suffering was shaped and moulded by social forces in distinctive ways for a relatively short stretch of time. Dissociative fugue provided a way for them to *express* their suffering, rather than *causing* their suffering. Indeed, Hacking actually suggests something even weaker than the weak claim. He identifies a number of 'vectors' that are necessary for a particular socially constructed mental illness to exist, among them what he calls 're-lease' (Hacking, 1999). 'Release' refers to the ways in which a possible mental illness actually *alleviates* distress, at least in the short term. Hacking's apparent commitment to the claim that particular socially constructed mental illnesses may reduce distress rather than increase it makes his entitlement to the mantle of debunker somewhat suspect, so far as the social construction of mental illness is concerned. In any case, it is an empirical question whether we ought to advocate a strong or weak form of the claim: the answer depends on whether it is possible (sufficiently cheaply) to elim-inate the social conditions responsible for the existence of the suffering or only its dis-tinctive manifestation. The answer is likely to vary from condition to condition, and very often the right answer may be 'both', to differing degrees. It is plausible to think, for instance, that if our social expectations with regard to body weight were more re-laxed, some bulimia sufferers would not have developed any significant mental illness at all, whereas others would have manifested distress in some other way.

If social construction can reveal that social vectors shape the form that suffering takes, rather than its very existence, then it need not take a debunking form. It might instead take an *explanatory* form. An explanatory social constructionism is not com-mitted to claims (1) or (3). Rather, it aims to show only that mental illness, or par-ticular illnesses, take the form they do due to social forces. It need not hold that these social forces are eliminable (though it may). It need not hold that the social forces are undesirable (though again it may). It is committed only to some version of claim (2): that the role of social forces has gone unrecognized. We are not faced with a choice between debunking and explanatory forms of social constructionism: different kinds of socially constructed phenomena, including different mental disorders, may aptly be explained by one or the other. Some mental illnesses may be apt for debunking.

Others may be the product of socially contingent forces, though altering those forces would eliminate only the form the suffering takes, and not its very existence, and the suffering arising from some may depend, in an interesting and unrecognized way, on social forces we can't eliminate sufficiently cheaply to make the enterprise worthwhile.

RDoC and social construction

Attention to the evidence cited by proponents of the RDoC itself indicates the need to supplement its preferred explanatory tools with social forces. The RDoC *begins* from the gap between symptomatology and neural circuits. Given that the categories distinguished by the descriptive taxonomies of the *DSM* fail to match up with the neuroscience and genetics of mental illness, we require some other explanation of the behaviour and the phenomenology. Now, that explanation cannot be independent of the cellular and the neural correlates of mental disorder: the brain is the primary proximate cause of behaviour and feeling and it responds to information only in so far as that information is translated into a format to which it is sensitive. Thoughts are neural processes and affect behaviour only because they are physically realized. But if our best science has not been able to find systematic correlations between specific neurological pathologies and schizophrenia alone (as opposed to, say, schizophrenia and bipolar disorder), that is good evidence that the features of disorders on which the descriptive taxonomy turn are not systematic at the neural level. There must be differences at the level of the brain, but the inability to find them using the techniques of neuroscience and molecular biology suggests that the proximate (neural) causes of the properties the *DSM* focuses on do not constitute a neural or a genetic kind. If brain circuits, regions, and genetics cross-cut *DSM* categories, then the proximate (neural) causes of the phenotypic properties must themselves be explained by distal causes that do not fall within the province of the RDoC.

Why does systematicity matter? For two related reasons. In developing a taxonomy, we seek to identify the *kind* to which something belongs. Kinds are things the members of which share something important in common; something without which they fail to belong to the kind. The kind 'democracies' consists (roughly) in the set of nations which elect governments through mechanisms designed to reflect the preferences of citizens; the kind 'mammals' consists (again, roughly) in the set of animals that lactate to feed their young, and so on. Differences between kinds are systematic: that is, kinds have something in common (an essence, a history, a decision procedure, and so on) which things which do not belong to the kind lack (of course, the systematicity may be much less neat than this; it may consist in satisfying a sufficient number of disjunctive conditions, for example). If mental illnesses are appropriately grouped into kinds, then we must find systematic differences between members of one kind (say, schizophrenia) and another (say, depression).

Second, and closely related to this taxonomic concern, knowing the kind to which something belongs provides useful information about it because members of a kind have certain properties in common. The more precise the kind, the more information we have. Knowing that an animal is a mammal tells us a little bit about it, but knowing that it is a giraffe tells us a lot more: we know what kind of habitat it needs, what kind of food it requires, the extent to which it is a social animal, and so on. When it comes to disease, knowing the kind to which something belongs provides targets for intervention. If a disease is genetic—that is, if members of the kind to which it belongs share properties at the genetic level, and these properties distinguish those who have the disease from those who lack it—then we can develop therapies for the disease that target that gene. We can also use this information to discover who is at risk for the disease, and take steps to prevent it. We can make predictions and inferences about vulnerability to the disease given that we know that a person has the relevant gene or genes, and we can make predictions and inferences about genes given that we know the person has the disease.

If the differences between phenotypes that differ (symptomatologically) are not systematic at the neural or the genetic level, the symptomatological differences must have causes at some other level. If the brain differences that are proximate causes of behaviour and symptoms are heterogeneous—not apt to feature in a natural kind—then to the extent to which the observed phenotypic properties are themselves systematic, they are not fully explained by these brain differences (though, again, neural events are the proximate causes of symptomology). For this reason, it is overwhelmingly likely that the differences in symptomatology which the *DSM* taxonomy captures reflect the contribution of the neural, neurochemical, and genetic differences that the RDoC focuses on, *plus* differences in higher-level factors: broadly, social and cultural factors. These include (but are not limited to) the ways in which different mental illnesses are conceptualized in a society, the ways in which social roles are assigned and understood, and perhaps idiosyncratic facts about the individual and her history which result in her having beliefs that modulate the form that her illness takes.

Thus, explaining mental illness requires both biological psychiatry and attention to social and historical facts about the individual, about mental illness, and about social roles. Social constructionists like Hacking are correct—perhaps more correct than some of them realize. Social factors may play a decisive role in how an underlying pathology is expressed; that is, in systematic phenotypic differences between patients. In so far as social constructionists restrict their claims to transient mental illnesses, they are not ambitious enough. Given that there is no systematic difference between genes or brain circuits that correlates with the difference between (say) schizophrenia and bipolar disorder, it may be that social and cultural factors play a role in explaining the difference between them, and not just the difference between, say, depression and hysterical fugue. Further, social and cultural factors may play a causal role not only in how a mental illness is expressed, but also in whether a particular individual develops a mental illness in the first place. Some sufferers from bulimia may have an underlying vulnerability to mental illness, but though some of them may have developed a *different* pathology were cultural norms different, some of them probably would not have developed a mental illness at all. Sufferers from culture-bound delusions might have developed another delusion in a different context, or another serious mental illness, but they may not have developed a mental illness at all. That will depend on the causal mechanisms involved, and how they interact with environmental conditions.

To see how social construction might work, even in cases for which an identifiable brain lesion is causally necessary for the pathology, consider a standard two-factor account of a delusion (Stone and Young, 1997; Davies et al., 2001). Factor one is typically held to be an abnormal experience, consequent on brain insult or disease. For instance, factor one in the formation of Capgras delusion—the delusion that familiar people (typically spouses, children, and other relatives) and occasionally even animals have been replaced with impostors—might be a brain abnormality that strips away the normal feeling of familiarity accompanying perception of a loved one. The deficit is presumed to be the result of a dysfunction in the dorsal perceptual stream, which is (largely) unconscious. Capgras delusion is therefore sometimes held to be the mirror image of prosopagnosia, in which patients have difficulty in recognizing faces; in prosopagnosia, the ventral processing stream is hypoactive, but the dorsal stream may be normal; hence prosopognosics may exhibit normal signs of autonomic arousal in response to familiar faces (Ellis and Lewis, 2001). However, two-factor theorists argue that the first, experiential, factor is insufficient to account for the delusion. They have two main reasons for thinking that there must be a second factor. First, it seems implausible that an anomalous experience could be sufficient to explain a bizarre belief, at least in a person who is globally rational (and delusional patients may seem quite rational in other spheres). After all, the person may be entirely capable of understanding the fact that they have had a stroke (say), and even of understanding how a stroke might fully account for their unusual experience. Since they know that their belief is bizarre, and they may know that a brain lesion explains their abnormal experience of familiar faces, it seems that mere anomalous experience is not sufficient to explain why they nevertheless go on to form the delusional belief. Second, some patients who apparently have the kind of anomalous experiences hypothesized to be partial causes of delusions do not go on to form delusional beliefs. It is the second factor, two-factor theorists maintain, that distinguishes these patients from those who suffer from delusions.

The second factor is typically held to be some kind of bias in reasoning: perhaps a disposition to accept hypotheses on the basis of flimsy evidence. There is some evidence for reasoning biases in delusional patients. For instance, schizophrenics seem to have a tendency to form beliefs on the basis of evidence that normal controls judge to be insufficient (Bentall et al., 1991). Further, once they have formed a belief, deluded patients apparently require significantly more disconfirming evidence to change their minds (Woodward et al., 2008). Now it is certainly possible that this reasoning bias, on the assumption that it is necessary for the delusion, is also best explained at the level of the brain or genes. But it is also very possible that a brain or genetic explanation—even if it is part of the story regarding the second factor—is insufficient, and that we need to explain the reasoning bias by reference to social and cultural factors. A delusional patient might, for instance, have a genetic disposition toward such a bias, but it might not have developed in a culture that encouraged more reflection (or if they had had a family environment that emphasized reflection). If that were the case, then explaining the delusion requires attention to the cultural and the individual, and not just the biological, level.

A biological essence?

Proponents of the RDoC might insist that though cultural and social factors may play the kind of role just mentioned, nevertheless the pathology itself is a neural pathology: a brain disease. Suppose it is true that a particular person would not have developed bulimia, dissociative fugue, or a delusion had it not been for social and cultural factors that disposed them toward developing that illness, or some mental illness or other. Nevertheless, they will insist, the effects will be seen in the brain and central nervous system, whether in gene expression or functional connectivity. That shows that the biological level is of special significance in understanding mental illness. More centrally still, it shows that mental illnesses *are* brain diseases: they are identical to patterns of pathology in the brain.

There is an important grain of truth to this claim. The brain does play a special role in behaviour and emotions, and cultural forces that produce or shape mental illness will always be mediated by the brain. Languages, institutions, rituals, and so on all affect behaviour, in very important part (but not exclusively: they also shape the physical environment and thereby also affect behaviour) by being represented in the brain (Murphy, 2006). These mental representations are, or supervene on, brain events; it is true that the social and cultural forces on which social constructionists insist play their role by causing brain changes.[1] To that extent, the social constructionist claim should not be seen as a rival to the claim that mental illnesses work through the brain: rather, it is a claim about *how* these brain changes come about.

Understanding social constructionism as a claim about how brain changes come about is not the same thing as understanding it as a mere terminological variant of the RDoC. The claim is rather that important systematic causal factors of symptomology are (also) to be found at the level of culture and the social. The fact that a patient presents with a disorder with such and such symptoms, or even with a disorder at all, may be counterfactually sensitive to contingent cultural and social facts. Thus, we might be able say something like this: schizophrenia is a disease that is caused by a genetic vulnerability (of a specific sort) and certain social factors; both are causally necessary for its development. The systematic factors are found at both levels. That gives us two different kinds of targets for intervention. We may be able to prevent the development of the illness by targeting either or both. In so far as they are systematic, we can identify these risk factors prior to the development of the illness. We can test for the gene and can target people who occupy certain social conditions (e.g. low socioeconomic status or familial history of immigration to an urban area; see Cooper (2005) for interventions). If the person develops the illness, we may be able to intervene at either the neurobiological level or the social level. It may be that social support or cognitive behavioural therapy is as, or more, effective than drug treatment, say. Sites of intervention will vary from illness to illness: in some cases, psychopharmaceuticals may be preferable (cheaper or more efficacious); in others, we may have good reason to prefer

---

[1] Haslanger (2003) points out that one need not understand an institution or a ritual, or even a sentence, for it to make a causal difference to one. However, in all cases in which the social factor plays a causal role *as* a social factor, that role is mediated by mental representations (it is certainly possible for a social institution to play a brute causal role that is not mediated by mental representations. When I read a book, its causal influence on me is mediated by my representing its contents; when a book falls on my head, its causal role is brute, rather than mediated by mental representations).

a social intervention. In some cases, social factors might be crucial to the aetiology of a disorder but not present an effective site for interventions once it has developed; in other cases, the reverse may be true.[2]

But if it is true that systematic properties of the phenotype are caused—even if not proximally caused—by social factors as well as neurobiological factors, and if it is true that social factors are sometimes the best targets for intervention, then we have good reason to think that the kinds into which we appropriately group these phenotypes (recall that it is systematic properties with which we are concerned) are not simply neurobiological kinds. They are partially social or cultural kinds: in learning that someone has such a condition, we may learn as much about their society or their circumstances as we do about their genes or their neurobiology. How much we learn about one or the other depends on their relative contribution to the phenotype, in so far as it is possible to apportion causal contributions.[3]

Conclusion

The RDoC aims to replace *DSM* taxonomy with another that better carves mental illness at its joints. As we have seen, taxonomy matters; the stakes are not merely a better description of mental illness or a neater classification. A better taxonomy has implications for understanding the causes of mental illness, and therefore for prevention and treatment. However, if the RDoC project is to capture the phenotypic differences between mental illnesses, it can't explain these differences in terms of neurobiology or genes alone: it must also advert to the social and cultural factors that are (also) causes of mental illnesses. It must make peace with social construction.

This raises an intriguing possibility: the resulting taxonomy may actually look much more like the current *DSM* than RDoC proponents think. There is nothing special

---

[2] Murphy argues that the most basic biological level, the molecular level, is special because of the amount of precision that molecular targets for intervention provide. 'It is possible, by contrasting wild types and experimental types, to keep everything except the effect of one gene constant and trace the effects of that change, or to manipulate elements of the system while holding others constant', while the psychological level does not offer this kind of precision: it is extremely difficult to change a person's beliefs 'without any psychological ramifications' (Murphy, 2006, pp. 130–131). I don't think this is correct: manipulating either will have far-reaching ramifications. Consider the range and the breadth of functions in which serotonin is causally involved: social affiliative behavior, cardiovascular regulation, respiration, sleep–wake cycles, appetite, pain sensitivity, and reward learning (Churchland, 2011, p. 98).

[3] There are well-known difficulties with calculating the degree to which genetic and environmental properties are responsible for the final phenotype. Estimates of the degree of variance in the phenotype which one or the other explains are not projectible: though it may be true that in one environment, genes explain (say) 70% of the variance, in another environment they might explain much less or much more. We can, however, relativize the degree to which each is responsible for the phenotype to those environments which are typical. Exactly the same set of issues and the same solution seems to apply when we broaden the range of causally relevant factors, to include (on the one hand) those which proponents of the RDoC emphasize and (on the other) social and cultural factors.

about the neural and genetic causes of mental illness that entails that our classifications should respect them and ignore or downplay social causes.[4] That is not to say that the *DSM*, as it stands, is likely to be vindicated: the disorders the *DSM* recognizes are symptomatically heterogeneous, suggesting that it does not capture distinctions into genuine kinds. A better taxonomy will attend to all the systematic causes of mental illness, distal and proximate, neurobiological and social. It is in that direction that hope for a truly scientific psychology lies.

Acknowledgements

I am grateful to Will Davies and Steve Clarke for extremely helpful comments on this paper.

References

American Psychiatric Association (2013). *Diagnostic and Statistical Manual of Mental Disorders* (5th ed.). Washington, DC: American Psychiatric Publishing.

Bentall, R.P., Kaney, S., and **Dewey, M.E.** (1991). Paranoia and social reasoning: an attribution theory analysis. *British Journal of Clinical Psychology*, **30**(1), 13–23.

Buss, D.M. (1994). *The Evolution of Desire: Strategies of Human Mating*. New York: Basic Books.

Churchland, P.S. (2011). *Braintrust: What Neuroscience Tells Us About Morality*. Princeton, NJ: Princeton University Press.

Cooper, B. (2005). Immigration and schizophrenia: the social causation hypothesis revisited. *British Journal of Psychiatry*, **186**, 361–363.

Cuthbert, B.N. and **Insel, T.R.** (2010). Toward new approaches to psychotic disorders: the NIMH Research Domain Criteria project. *Schizophrenia Bulletin*, **36**(6), 1061–1062.

Davies, M., Coltheart, M., Langdon, R., and **Breen, N.** (2001). Monothematic delusions: towards a two-factor account. *Philosophy, Psychiatry, and Psychology*, **8**(2–3), 133–158.

Ellis, H.D. and **Lewis, M.B.** (2001). Capgras delusion: a window on the face of recognition. *Trends in Cognitive Sciences*, **5**(4), 149–156.

Guze, S.B. (1992). *Why Psychiatry is a Branch of Medicine*. New York: Oxford University Press.

Hacking, I. (1999). *The Social Construction of What?* Cambridge, MA: Harvard University Press.

Hari, J. (2018). *Lost Connections*. London: Bloomsbury.

Haslanger, S. (2003). Social construction: the 'Debunking' Project. In: F.F. Schmitt (Ed.), *Socializing Metaphysics: The Nature of Social Reality* (pp. 301–325). Lanham, MD: Rowman and Littlefield.

Insel, T. (2013). Post by former NIMH director Thomas Insel: transforming diagnosis. http://www.nimh.nih.gov/about/director/2013/transforming-diagnosis.shtml

---

[4] Perhaps there is some reason for a taxonomy to give greater weight to proximate causes than to distal causes. I don't find the suggestion compelling, but in any case, a taxonomy that rejected distal causes would not vindicate the RDoC as a taxonomic approach either: genetic causes are (typically) distal causes of disease, as much as are social causes.

Insel, T., Cuthbert, B., Garvey, M., Heinssen, R., Pine, D.S., Quinn, K., Sanislow, C., and Wang, P. (2010). Research Domain Criteria (RDoC): toward a new classification framework for research on mental disorders. *American Journal of Psychiatry*, **167**(7), 748–751.

Kapur, S., Phillips, A.G., and Insel, T.R. (2012). Why has it taken so long for biological psychiatry to develop clinical tests and what to do about it? *Molecular Psychiatry*, **17**(12), 1174–1179.

Mumford, D.B., Whitehouse, A.M., and Choudry, I.Y. (1992). Survey of eating disorders in English-medium schools in Lahore, Pakistan. *International Journal of Eating Disorders*, **11**(2), 173–184.

Mumford, D.B., Whitehouse, A.M., and Platts, M. (1991). Sociocultural correlates of eating disorders among Asian schoolgirls in Bradford. *British Journal of Psychiatry*, **158**, 222–228

Murphy, D. (2006). *Psychiatry in the Scientific Image*. Cambridge, MA: MIT Press.

Pinker, S. (2002). *The Blank Slate: The Modern Denial of Human Nature*. New York: Penguin.

Stone, T. and Young, A. (1997). Delusions and brain injury: the philosophy and psychology of belief. *Mind and Language*, **12**(3/4) 327–364.

Ung, E. (2003). Eating disorders in Singapore: a review. *Annals of the Academy of Medicine, Singapore*, **32**(1), 19–24.

Wilson, G.T., Nathan, P.E., O'Leary, K.D., and Clark, L.A. (1996). *Abnormal Psychology: Integrating Perspectives*. Boston, MD: Allyn & Bacon.

Woodward, T.S., Moritz, S., Menon, M., and Klinge, R. (2008). Belief inflexibility in schizophrenia. *Cognitive Neuropsychiatry*, **13**(3), 267–277.

Chapter 8

Minority report: Values, teamwork, and implementing biopsychosocial psychiatry

K.W.M. (Bill) Fulford

Introduction

From its inception, the biopsychosocial model has been understood primarily in scientific terms. Engel's original formulation (Engel, 1977), building on antecedent theories (Ghaemi, 2009), and followed by most subsequent commentators (Roache, Chapter 2, this volume), represents the biopsychosocial model as combining biological, psychological, and social aspects of the presentation, aetiology, and treatment of mental disorders. The dominant perspective, then, the majority report if you will, is empirical. Yet right from the start there has been recognition that when it comes to implementation something more than the dominant empirical perspective will be required. Expressing this minority perspective, Engel himself urged combining the humanities with science for better patient care (Engel, 1978). Ghaemi (2010) takes a similar line, arguing that his proposed replacement of biopsychosocial thinking with 'methodological consciousness' reconciles the art and science of psychiatry.

It is with the minority—humanities-led—perspective on the biopsychosocial model that this chapter is concerned. The argument of the chapter is that while scientific understanding of the biopsychosocial model is important for technical aspects of psychiatry (concerned with the diagnosis, aetiology, and treatment of mental disorders), values are key to implementing the model in practice in the context of contemporary person-centred clinical care. The first section describes the underpinnings of this approach in an empirical study of biopsychosocial thinking in multidisciplinary mental health teams and their patients called the Models Project. The second section gives a brief introduction to values-based practice as a resource for implementing the findings of the Models Project in practice. The third section gives examples of values-based practice in mental health. The fourth section notes some of the new resources for values-based implementation of biopsychosocial psychiatry to be found in contemporary developments in person-centred clinical care.

The chapter finishes with a note on what the philosopher Isaiah Berlin called the challenge of pluralism (Berlin, 1958). Biopsychosocial thinking is nothing if not pluralistic. Small wonder then, if Berlin is right, that it has proved challenging to deliver in practice. It may be, though, the chapter concludes, that as in Steven Spielberg's cult sci-fi film of the same name, it is the minority report that will be crucial to implementation.

The Models Project: team values and person-centred care

The Models Project (Colombo et al., 2003) combined philosophical and social science methods (Fulford and Colombo, 2004) in a study of implicit models of disorder in multidisciplinary teams involved in the community care of people with long-term mental disorders. This section briefly describes the Project and indicates the wider significance of its findings for understanding the importance of values in implementing the biopsychosocial model.

The Models Project

In earlier work, the lead researcher in the Models Project, the British social scientist Anthony Colombo (1997), had shown that models of mental disorder could be analysed and compared according to how they conceived the diagnosis, aetiology, and treatment of mental disorders. This approach had proved particularly helpful in comparing explicit models (the models people claimed they held) with implicit models (the models reflected in the way they understood and managed mental disorders in practice).

The distinction between explicit and implicit models underpinned the Models Project. Asked directly, psychiatrists, social workers, nurses, and other team members all said they worked with a broadly biopsychosocial model. This was their shared *explicit model*. Team members' responses, however, to a standardized case vignette (reflecting the kind of patient with whom they were concerned in day-to-day practice), showed that their *implicit models*, the models actually guiding their practice, were very different. Psychiatrists gave predominantly biological responses, while the responses of social workers were mainly psychological and social. Nurses were split: they were 'bio' on diagnosis but 'psychosocial' on aetiology and treatment. The contrast between the implicit models respectively of psychiatrists and social workers is shown diagrammatically in Figure 8.1.

In subsequent feedback sessions, team members were initially sceptical about their implicit models as suggested by these findings. 'Surely', they protested, 'that's not us!' But on further reflection they came to see that their different implicit models, precisely *because* they were unaware of them, lay behind what were otherwise inexplicable disagreements over case management. One practical outcome of the study was thus improved communication and decision-making among team members through raised awareness of their differences in implicit models.

The more significant outcome, though, for understanding the importance of values in the implementation of the biopsychosocial model, came in a second phase of the Models Project when the same methods were used to assess the implicit models of patients. Patients in the study were recruited not from teams but through a local branch of a mental health advocacy non-governmental organization called MIND. The expectation was that patients so recruited would include a significant number of people

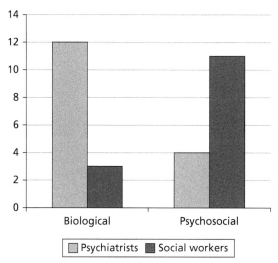

Figure 8.1 Diagrammatic representation of the contrasting implicit models of mental disorder exhibited respectively by psychiatrists (blue columns) and social workers (red columns) in the Models Project. They (and other team members) all believed they were working with much the same biopsychosocial model of mental disorder. This was their shared explicit model. The figure, however, shows that their implicit models were quite different: psychiatrists exhibited a predominantly biological implicit model; social workers exhibited a predominantly psychosocial implicit model.

who rejected psychiatric 'labels'—whether biological or psychosocial—altogether, construing their difficulties rather in sociopolitical terms.

As it turned out, however, patients' implicit models closely reflected those of team members. Patients' implicit models are shown diagrammatically in Figure 8.2. Comparing Figure 8.2 with Figure 8.1 indicates the extent of the match between patients' implicit models and those respectively of psychiatrists (biological) and social workers (psychosocial). The conclusion, then, from this second phase of the Models Project, was that team members brought a range of implicit models to understanding and managing mental disorders that corresponded closely with the implicit models of their patients. Just how this conclusion plays out in practice depends on how the implicit models in question are understood. The next section looks at the implications of a values-based understanding of implicit models for implementing biopsychosocial thinking in practice.

Values and implementing the biopsychosocial model in clinical care

In an exclusively science-based understanding of the biopsychosocial model, it is natural to ask which of the implicit models exhibited by team members in the Models Project is 'right'. This was how team members initially reacted in the feedback described previously. Having accepted the findings—that notwithstanding their shared

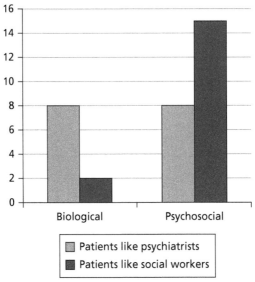

Figure 8.2 Diagrammatic representation of the implicit models of mental disorder exhibited by patients in the Models Project. Patients in the study exhibited implicit models similar to those found for psychiatrists and social workers. Comparing Figure 8.2 with Figure 8.1 indicates that while some patients (blue columns) exhibited broadly biological implicit models (corresponding with psychiatrists in the study), other patients (red columns) exhibited broadly psychosocial implicit models (corresponding with social workers in the study).

explicit biopsychosocial model they exhibited very different implicit models—team members fell into discussion about which aspect of the biopsychosocial model was 'really' most important. Similar discussions are familiar in academic contexts. In discussions of gene–environment interactions, for example, 'biological' psychiatrists generally acknowledge the influence of psychological and social factors while reserving pole position for the biological, while psychologists and social scientists offer counterpart arguments for the primacy of psychological and social factors.

Such discussions, anchored in robust empirical evidence derived for well-defined groups, are clearly appropriate in academic contexts. The clinical context is, however, different. In clinical contexts, what is important means (in part) *what is important from the perspective of the particular patient concerned*. The patient's perspective is central to the shared decision-making that, as will be described more fully later, underpins contemporary person-centred clinical care. But 'what is important' from this or that person's perspective is just another way of referring to that person's *values*. Hence, shared clinical decision-making means decision-making that is based (in part) on the values of the patient concerned. In values-based practice, this is called person-*values*-centred care (see Table 8.1, element 5, in the next section).

Examples of the clinical significance of person-*values*-centred care are given in the next section and in 'Values-based practice in mental health'. But the point for now is that if this values-based understanding is right, the range of implicit models exhibited by team members becomes a resource for shared clinical decision-making. This is clear from the match in implicit models shown by comparing Figure 8.1 (team members) with Figure 8.2 (patients). Figure 8.2 shows that for some patients the more appropriate approach ('appropriate' because it reflects what matters to the patient concerned) will be biological, while for others it will be psychosocial. Figure 8.1 shows that different team members will be well placed to offer these different approaches in virtue of their different implicit models.

This finding is the basis of the 'extended multidisciplinary team' of values-based practice (see element 6 in Table 8.1 in the next section). The Models Project extended the importance of the multidisciplinary team from the range of knowledge and skills it offers to include also a range of implicit models. In values-based practice, this range of implicit models implies a range of values (a range of what matters or is important from the perspectives of different team members). So understood, the extended multidisciplinary team becomes a resource for delivering person-values-centred care.

Notice, however, the parenthetical 'in part' appearing in the earlier statement about what is important. This reflects the significance of the *shared* clinical decision-making underpinning person-centred care. For what is important in shared clinical decision-making includes not only what is important from the perspective of the patient (the patient's values) but also what is important from the perspective of the clinician (the clinician's values). This is what makes a clinical decision a *shared* clinical decision: it is a decision that is shared between the patient and the clinician, or, in multidisciplinary teamwork, between the patient and the clinical team. Shared clinical decision-making thus necessarily involves a complex range of values. These values moreover will sometimes come into conflict: what is important may appear different from the perspectives of different team members (reflecting their different implicit models); and what is important may appear different from the perspective of the clinician or clinical team and that of the patient. This is where the resources of values-based practice for working with complex and conflicting values in clinical care come into play.

An introduction to values-based practice

Values-based practice is a skills-based approach to working with complex and conflicting values in clinical care (Fulford et al., 2012). As such, it offers a process—no more and no less—for working with values. Derived analytically, from work on the meanings of value terms (Fulford, 1989; Fulford and van Staden, 2013), values-based practice is not a branch of substantive ethics. It supplies no answers, no prescriptions, no preset values guiding decision-making. It aims instead to support decision-makers in finding answers for themselves. This is one of the many respects in which values-based practice is a partner to evidence-based practice. Both are decision support tools. Evidence-based practice offers a process that supports balanced decision-making where complex and conflicting *evidence* is in play. Values-based practice offers a process that supports balanced decision-making where complex and conflicting *values* are in play.

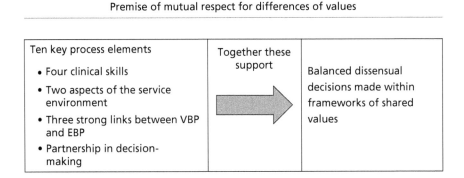

Figure 8.3 Diagram of values-based practice. Starting from a premise of mutual respect for differences of values, values-based practice uses clinical skills and other key process elements to support balanced dissensual decisions on individual cases. EBP, evidence-based practice; VBP, values-based practice.

This section gives a brief outline of values-based practice. The next section, 'Values-based practice in mental health', gives examples of how values-based practice supports implementation of biopsychosocial thinking in mental health. The following section, 'New resources for implementing biopsychosocial psychiatry', indicates how values-based practice works alongside other resources for working with values in mental health and in other areas of healthcare.

The main elements of values-based practice are shown diagrammatically in Figure 8.3 and defined briefly in Table 8.1. As these indicate, values-based practice builds on a premise of mutual respect for differences of values. Supported by this broadly 'democratic' first principle, the process of values-based practice includes learnable clinical skills, a particular service environment, close links with evidence-based practice, and partnership in decision-making. This process in turn supports the outputs of values-based practice in balanced dissensual decisions on individual cases made within frameworks of shared values.

On first inspection it may seem that it is the service environment of values-based practice that is key to implementing the biopsychosocial model. Certainly, the 'extended multidisciplinary team' (element 6) and 'person-values-centred care' (element 5) of values-based practice, derived as they are from the Models Project, are essential. Yet as indicated at the end of the previous section, the shared decision-making through which the extended multidisciplinary team contributes to person-values-centred care depends on resolving complex and conflicting values. This makes the skills for values-based practice (elements 1–4) integral to shared decision-making. But shared decision-making is evidence based as well as values based: as described further later, shared decision-making depends on bringing together the clinician's or clinical team's knowledge of the evidence base for the options available with the values of (with what is important or matters to) the individual patient concerned. Understanding therefore how evidence and values come together in clinical decision-making (elements 7–9) is also crucial. The process as a whole moreover depends on partnership between

Table 8.1 Brief definitions of the elements of values-based practice. Among other process elements of values-based practice, two aspects of its model of service delivery are central to its role in supporting biopsychosocial approaches in mental health: the 'extended multidisciplinary team' (element 6) is crucial to the delivery of 'person-values-centred care' (element 5). The effective operation of these elements in turn depends on other elements of the model: training in key clinical skills, attention to evidence as well as values, and a particular (dissensual) model of partnership in decision-making. The process as a whole is underpinned by the premise of mutual respect.

Values-based practice	Brief definition
Premise of mutual respect	Mutual respect for differences of values
1. **Skills—awareness**	Awareness of values and of differences of values
2. **Skills—knowledge**	Knowledge retrieval and its limitations
3. **Skills—reasoning**	Used to explore the values in play rather than to 'solve' dilemmas
4. **Skills—communication**	Especially for eliciting values and for conflict resolution
5. **Person-values-centred care**	Care centred on the actual rather than assumed values of the patient
6. **Extended MDT**	MDT role extended to include a range of value perspectives as well as of knowledge and skills
7. **'Two feet' principle**	All decisions are based on the 'two feet' of values and evidence
8. **Squeaky wheel principle**	We notice values when they cause difficulties (like the squeaky wheel) but (like the wheel that doesn't squeak) they are always there and operative
9. **Science-driven principle**	Advances in medical science drive the need for VBP (as well as EBP) because they open up choices and with choices go values
10. **Partnership**	Decisions in VBP (although informed by clinical guidelines and other sources) are made by those directly concerned working together in partnership
Frameworks of shared values	Values shared by those in a given decision-making context (e.g. the Guiding Principles for the Mental Health Act 2007—see Figure 8.5) and within which balanced decisions can be made on individual cases
Balanced dissensual decision	Decisions in which the values in question remain in play to be balanced sometimes one way and sometimes in other ways according to the circumstances of a given case

EBP, evidence-based practice; MDT, multidisciplinary team; VBP, values-based practice.

clinician/clinical team and patient (element 10) in coming to balanced dissensual decisions within a framework of shared values (the output of values-based practice). Such partnership is, however, possible only where there is mutual respect: this is why the premise of values-based practice underpins the process as a whole.

The examples given in the next two sections illustrate how the elements of values-based practice support implementation of the biopsychosocial model in clinical care respectively in mental health and (supported by other resources) in other areas of healthcare.

Values-based practice in mental health

The examples given in this section are derived mainly from a programme run under the auspices initially of the National Institute for Mental Health England (NIMHE) and then of its successor, the Care Services Improvement Partnership (CSIP), within the UK's Department of Health. The programme reflected input from a wide range of stakeholders including not only various professions involved in mental health but also leads representing service user (Laurie Bryant) and carer (Lu Duhig) perspectives. It was this co-production (equality of voices between stakeholders) that was key to the programme just as it is key to values-based practice in general and hence to the role of values-based practice in implementing the biopsychosocial model.

As indicated in the previous section, the elements of values-based practice work together as a whole. The NIMHE/CSIP programme correspondingly included initiatives in each of the key areas of values-based practice from premise through process to outputs.

The premise of values-based practice: the NIMHE Values Framework

Mutual respect for differences of values (the premise of values-based practice) is clearly one of the keys to implementing biopsychosocial thinking through effective multidisciplinary teamwork. Without mutual respect between clinical team members, no amount of awareness of each other's perspectives will lead to effective communication and team decision-making. Without mutual respect between team members and their patients, differences of values operate as a barrier to rather than a resource for shared clinical decision-making. Yet a concern is that 'mutual respect' might open the door to anything-goes relativism in mental health.

This concern led in the early days of the NIMHE programme to the development of a Values Framework by a project group—comprising representative multidisciplinary team members, patients, and carers—convened by the Department of Health to support service development (Fulford et al., 2015a). The NIMHE Values Framework (National Institute for Mental Health England, 2004) recognized that 'mutual respect for differences of values' in and of itself sets limits to the values that can be included in the balanced decisions of values-based practice. Thus *mutual* respect precludes, by definition, racism or any other form of discrimination since these are by their very nature not mutually respectful. The key passage though of particular relevance to values-based implementation of the biopsychosocial model comes in the Framework's definition of patient-centred care. A common misunderstanding about person-centred care is that it equates to a consumer model of 'the patient is always right'. The definition of 'respect' in the NIMHE Values Framework was carefully drafted to avoid this. It reads:

> NIMHE respects diversity of values and will support ways of working with such diversity that makes the principle of service-user centrality a unifying focus for practice. This means that the values of each individual service user/client and their communities must be the starting point and key determinant for all actions by professionals. (National Institute for Mental Health England, 2004)

The 'service-user centrality' of this statement is thus the 'person-*values*-centred care' of values-based practice (it makes central the 'values of each individual service user/ client and their communities', consistently with element 5 in Table 8.1). But the exact wording is crucial: person-values-centred care, as defined in the NIMHE Values Framework, means making the values of the individual service user/client the *starting* point (but not therefore the *only* point) of actions by professionals; and it means making the values of the service user/client the *key* determinant (but not therefore the *sole* determinant) of actions by professionals. Implementing the NIMHE Values Framework in individual cases will thus require balancing the values of those concerned. This is one key area where the diverse values of the 'extended multidisciplinary team' of values-based practice (element 6 in Table 8.1) have a key role to play. Multidisciplinary teamwork, correspondingly, is included later in the Framework in its own right as a service development priority for NIMHE (it subsequently became the focus of the 'Ten Essential Shared Capabilities' ('10 ESCs') and related training and service development initiatives outlined later in this chapter).

The NIMHE Values Framework, then, in the precise way it defines respect for diversity of values, provides a robust foundation for values-based implementation of the biopsychosocial model. It provides a basis for person-values-centred care supported by the extended multidisciplinary team.[1] It was on this foundation that the training and service development initiatives of the NIMHE/CSIP programme were developed.

The process of values-based practice: training and service development initiatives

The NIMHE/CSIP programme included an ambitious series of training and service development initiatives aimed at supporting multidisciplinary teamwork as the basis of person-centred care in mental health. These initiatives will be described briefly focusing on the resources they represent for implementing biopsychosocial thinking in mental health.

The first stage of the NIMHE/CSIP training and service development initiatives was an extensive consultation among service users and service providers. Based on pilot

---

[1] The NIMHE Values Framework provides an example of the importance of co-production of values-based practice. We owe the careful drafting of the definition of respect underpinning the Framework as a whole, not to any of the various professionals in the development group, but to Simon Allard, an ex-service user with several years at the sharp end of service experience (Fulford et al., 2015a).

Box 8.1 The 'Ten Essential Shared Capabilities' ('10 ESCs')

1. Working in partnership.
2. Respecting diversity.
3. Practising ethically.
4. Challenging inequality.
5. Promoting recovery.
6. Identifying people's needs and strengths.
7. Providing service user-centred care.
8. Making a difference.
9. Promoting safety and positive risk taking.
10. Personal development and learning.

The 10 ESCs summarize the capabilities that all staff working in mental health services require as the basis of best practice. They were developed co-productively between clinicians, patients. and carers, and thus reflect their shared priorities.

---

work by Peter Lindley and others at the Sainsbury Centre for Mental Health (a Mental Health non-governmental organization), the aim of the consultation was to identify the generic capabilities with which anyone working in or concerned with mental health should be equipped, whatever their particular professional background or training.

The '10 ESCs' derived from the consultation are shown in Box 8.1. As this indicates, the required capabilities cover a range of attitudes, behaviours, and values that, being shared by all stakeholders, provide a robust agenda for training. Training materials implementing the 10 ESCs were developed and have since been widely distributed (Department of Health, 2004a; see also McGonagle et al., 2015). In developing these materials, the NIMHE/CSIP programme again drew on earlier development work by the Sainsbury Centre for Mental Health published as *Whose Values?: A Workbook for Values-Based Practice in Mental Health Care* (Woodbridge and Fulford, 2004).[2] The training materials in turn supported a series of policy and service development initiatives aimed at extending and strengthening multidisciplinary teamwork in mental health as the basis of more effective person-centred care (see, e.g. Department of Health, 2005, 2007[3]). Underpinning the programme as a whole was a combined

---

[2] *Whose Values?* has subsequently become the foundation also for recent training initiatives in values-based practice in other areas of healthcare such as surgery (see 'New resources for implementing biopsychosocial psychiatry').

[3] Further initiatives included the development of the National Occupational Standards (NOS) for training in mental health. The NOS have since been further revised to make explicit the importance of co-production and values-based practice as the basis of recovery oriented service

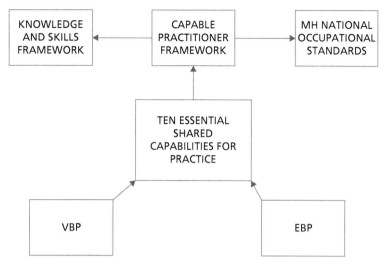

Figure 8.4 The values-based and evidence-based roots of the '10 ESCs'. The NIMHE/CSIP programme 'New ways of working' aimed to achieve more effective multidisciplinary mental health teamwork through training in the required generic capabilities, the 10 ESCs. This diagram (which is from the 10 ESCs policy document) shows how the programme as a whole built on values-based and evidence-based sources. EBP, evidence-based practice; MH, mental health; VBP, values-based practice.
Source: Adapted from 'The Ten Essential Shared Capabilities: A Framework for the Whole of the Mental Health Workforce'. Department of Health (2004). © Crown copyright 2004. Available from http://www.dualdiagnosis.co.uk/uploads/documents/originals/ten%20shared%20care%20 capabilities.pdf

values-based and evidence-based approach consistent with elements 7–9 of values-based practice. This is shown diagrammatically in Figure 8.4 (taken from the original 10 ESCs publication).

The NIMHE/CSIP programme, like other service development initiatives at the time, reflected the importance of recovery practice in mental health. It went beyond other initiatives, however, in developing a programme on the diagnostic as well as the more familiar treatment aspects of recovery. The '3 Keys',[4] as this programme came to be called, will be worth looking at in a little more detail as an example of how the various process elements of values-based practice come together to support implementation of biopsychosocial thinking in mental health.

---

provision (see Skills for Health, 2013). There were also a number of more specific policy initiatives such as the introduction of *community development workers* (Department of Health, 2004b), promotion of *recovery* (Department of Health, 2004c; Care Services Improvement Partnership, 2006), and a *review of the care programme approach* (Department of Health, 2008).

[4] *The 3 Keys to a Shared Approach to Assessment in Mental Health*, NIMHE and CSIP (2008).

Table 8.2 The '3 Keys' to a shared approach to assessment in mental health. In a wide-ranging consultation, all stakeholders (clinicians of various kinds, patients and carers) agreed on the importance of these three aspects of mental health assessment

Assessment in mental health should be	
1 **Person centred**	Based on *active partnership* with the service user concerned and their carers, where appropriate
2 **Multidisciplinary**	Drawing together *different provider perspectives*
3 **Strengths based**	Focusing on *individual strengths, resiliencies, and aspirations* as well as needs and difficulties

'Recovery' in the context of mental health means recovering a good quality of life as defined by the values of (by what is important from the perspective of) the person concerned (Slade, 2009). So defined, 'recovery practice' is the mental health equivalent of the 'person-values-centred practice' of values-based clinical care (see element 5, Table 8.1). As just noted, recovery practice has focused largely on treatment. But treatment (broadly construed as how a problem is managed) depends critically on diagnostic assessment (how a problem is understood). Hence, the traditional focus on treatment has been on the face of it overly restrictive. Applying the 'two feet' principle of values-based practice (that values as well as evidence come into all areas of mental health[5]) thus led naturally to the idea that recovery practice should be broadened to include looking at the role of values in mental health assessment.

The '3 Keys' arising from the resulting programme are summarized in Table 8.2. They represent three assessment values (three things that matter about assessment) identified through a wide consultation shared across all stakeholders—including patients and carers as well as clinicians of various kinds. The relevance of the 3 Keys to biopsychosocial thinking is evident from Keys 1 and 2. Key 1 is about person-centred care (element 5 of values-based practice, Table 8.1). Key 2 is about the importance of the multidisciplinary team (element 6 of values-based practice, Table 8.1). Combining Keys 1 and 2 with the findings from the Models Project thus leads directly to the importance of biopsychosocial thinking in recovery-oriented mental health assessment.

The third Key, 'Strengths-based assessment', illustrates two further points about values-based practice as a resource supporting implementation. First, it shows the importance of looking at positives as well as negatives. Thus, a familiar acronym in communication skills training is ICE: this reminds us to explore Ideas, Concerns, and Expectations (Fulford et al., 2012, chapter 7). But ICE is generally understood as being

---

[5] See element 7, Table 8.1. The NIMHE Values Framework (see 'The premise of values-based practice: the NIMHE Values Framework') adopted the 'two feet' principle in a headline statement that read: '*Recognition*—NIMHE recognizes the role of values alongside evidence in all areas of mental health policy and practice.'

concerned with the patient's presenting needs and difficulties. Key 3 reminds us that, important as needs and difficulties may be, we should also explore positive aspects of the patient's presentation, specifically their strengths, aspirations, and resiliencies. The corresponding mnemonic for values-based communications skills training has thus become ICE StAR: with a slight tweak to Key 3, this reminds us to explore the patient's Strengths, Aspirations, and Resources.[6]

The second point about values-based practice and implementation illustrated by Key 3 is the importance of co-production. Key 3 was initially a potential barrier to a shared approach in that many clinicians feared (not unreasonably) that they would be expected to deliver on too wide a range (perhaps even an impossible range) of individual aspirations from service users. It was, however, the service user lead for the programme, Laurie Bryant, who was able to allay these clinicians' concerns (Fulford et al., 2015b). He pointed to the evidence showing that individual aspirations are not only essential to recovery but that in practice such aspirations tend to be modest (e.g. 'to go for a walk in the park'). The result was that 'Aspirations' stayed in. Not only that, but aspirations proved to be a particularly rich aspect of the good practice examples collected in a second stage of the programme.[7]

The outputs of values-based practice: the Guiding Principles for the Mental Health Act 2007

The outputs of values-based practice are balanced dissensual decisions within frameworks of shared values (Figure 8.3 and Table 8.1). Dissensus is best understood by contrast with the more familiar consensus. Consensual decision-making involves some of those concerned in a given decision ceding their position to an agreed right answer. Consensus on the evidence is the output of evidence-based practice. The process of evidence-based practice (its meta-analyses, etc.) produces an answer that until further evidence comes in, claims priority as the right answer against competing views. Consensus is also important in values-based practice in establishing its shared frameworks of values.[8]

Dissensus by contrast comes into play when a shared framework of values is applied in practice. Applying a shared framework involves balancing its constituent values according to the particular concrete circumstances presented by a given situation. In this 'particularist' approach, the balance may come out one way in one situation and quite differently in another. This is 'dissensus', then, in that instead of a given value claiming priority against competing values, the values making up the framework as a whole *remain in play* to be balanced sometimes one way and sometimes in quite different ways in different cases.

The interplay between consensual and dissensual elements of values-based practice is illustrated by a set of training materials produced by the NIMHE/CSIP programme to support implementation of the UK's 2007 Mental Health Act (CSIP and

---

[6] A detailed case example illustrating the importance of moving from ICE to ICE StAR is given in Fulford et al. (2012, chapter 7).

[7] A selection of these examples is given in the 3 Keys report (NIMHE and CSIP, 2008, pp. 9–31).

[8] For a worked example of developing a framework of shared values, see Fulford et al. (2012, chapter 14).

NIMHE, 2008; Fulford et al., 2015a). Thus, consensus was important in the origins of the training materials. The Act in question updated the law in England and Wales on involuntary psychiatric treatment. As such it was deeply contentious, resulting in a public consultation extending over 5 years. One important outcome of this consultation, however, was the identification of a number of shared values, that is, aspects of involuntary treatment that were regarded as important by those on all sides of the debate about how the law should be updated. These shared values were incorporated into the wording of the Act and spelled out in the accompanying Code of Practice as a set of Guiding Principles. The Guiding Principles in turn became the basis for the values-based training materials produced by the NIMHE/CSIP programme.

But if the Guiding Principles were derived by consensus, the way they were used required dissensus. This is indicated diagrammatically in Figure 8.5 that is reproduced from the training materials. The 'round table' layout indicates that each of the Guiding

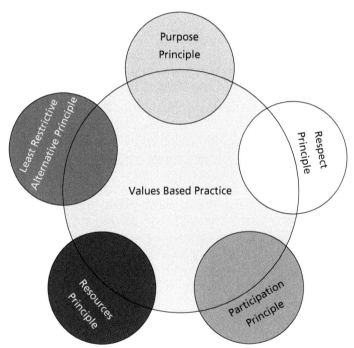

Figure 8.5 The Guiding Principles for the Mental Health Act 2007 as a framework of shared values. This diagram is from the Foundation Module of the training materials produced by the NIMHE/CSIP programme to support implementation of the UK's Mental Health Act 2007. It illustrates how the skills and other process elements of values-based practice are used to balance the shared values represented by the Guiding Principles for the use of the Act. This illustrates the outputs of values-based practice in balanced dissensual decision-making within frameworks of shared values (Table 8.1).
Source: Reproduced from 'Brief Workbook to Support Implementation of the Mental Health act 2007'. National Institute of Mental Health (NIMH) 2007. Available from: https://www.pennine-gp-training.co.uk/res/Mental%20Health%20Act%20updated%202009.pdf

Principles carries in principle equal weight. In practice, though, the principles will be balanced sometimes in one way and sometimes in other ways according to the circumstances of the particular case. This dissensual process requires (as the 'Values Based Practice' at the centre of the diagram indicates) the skills and other process elements of values-based practice.[9]

New resources for implementing biopsychosocial psychiatry

Recent developments in values-based practice have extended the approach to other areas of healthcare. Work has continued in mental health: a Commission for Values-based Child and Adolescent Mental Health Services, for example, building on a strongly co-productive methodology, identified, consistently with the NIMHE/CSIP programme, the importance of multidisciplinary teamwork as the basis of person-centred care (Royal College of Psychiatrists, 2016). But there have also been completely new programmes in values-based practice, for example, in surgery (Handa et al., 2016) and in radiography (Fulford et al., 2018).

In developing these new programmes, values-based practice has been able to draw on the resources of other tools in what has been called the 'values tool kit' (Fulford et al., 2012, chapter 3). Other tools in the tool kit include medical law and regulation, and, perhaps more surprisingly, evidence-based practice. Medical law and regulation indeed came together in a recent UK Supreme Court ruling on consent, the *Montgomery* judgement (*Montgomery* v *Lanarkshire Health Board*, 2015). Drawing on established guidance from the UK medical regulator, the General Medical Council (2008), the *Montgomery* judges' decision made shared decision-making based on evidence and values the legal basis of consent to treatment in all areas of health and social care (Herring et al., 2017).[10] As to evidence-based practice as a resource for working with values, the shared decision-making required by *Montgomery* is reflected in the preface to every evidence-based guideline produced by the National Institute for Health and Care Excellence (NICE).[11] The preface to all such guidelines specifies

---

[9] Dissensus requires the skills and other process elements of values-based practice because the shared values expressed in the Guiding Principles are individually complex and jointly conflicting. The principle of 'Respect' for example is a complex value in the sense that 'respect' means different things to different people of different ages and from different backgrounds. The principle of 'Respect' moreover may come into conflict with other Guiding Principles. It may conflict for example with the 'Purpose' principle (which is about the purpose of the Act being to treat people without consent and hence without respect to their wishes). Balanced decision-making within the framework of Guiding Principles, then, depends, in any given case, first on interpreting the meaning of the Principles as they apply in that case, and then balancing them one against another to the extent that they conflict. This is where as described earlier in 'An introduction to values-based practice' the resources of values-based practice for working with complex and conflicting values comes into play.

[10] Cases cited in *Montgomery* from international law have similar implications for consent in other administrations such as the European Union and Australia.

[11] NICE produces evidence-based guidelines for use in the UK's National Health Service.

that 'When exercising their judgement, professionals are expected to take this guideline fully into account, alongside the *individual needs, preferences and values* of their patients or service users' (see, e.g. National Institute for Health and Care Excellence, 2015, emphasis added).

Such resources, therefore, to the extent that they support the implementation of values-based practice in healthcare generally, by the same token support values-based implementation of biopsychosocial psychiatry.

Conclusion—the challenge of pluralism

This chapter has explored the implications of values-based practice for implementing biopsychosocial psychiatry. The chapter opened by characterizing the values-based perspective on biopsychosocial thinking as a minority report in contrast to the more familiar majority scientific perspective. The two perspectives as was made clear are complementary. The scientific perspective works well for the technical aspects of psychiatry. But a values-based perspective, the chapter has argued, is needed for implementation. This as was indicated was foreshadowed by Engel. The argument of the chapter as a whole has been that a values-based perspective is the key to implementing biopsychosocial psychiatry in the context of the shared decision-making that underpins contemporary person-centred clinical care.

The first section described the origins of this approach in the Models Project, an empirical study of biopsychosocial thinking in multidisciplinary mental health teams and their patients. Combining empirical with philosophical methods, the Models Project showed the importance of values (alongside evidence) in the way biopsychosocial thinking among team members could help to deliver person-centred care. The second section gave a brief introduction to values-based practice. As a partner to evidence-based practice, values-based practice supports multidisciplinary teams in delivering biopsychosocial approaches to person-centred care. The third section gave examples of values-based practice (working in partnership with evidence-based practice) in mental health. The fourth section noted the new resources for implementation provided by contemporary developments in the values tool kit: the tool kit included, besides values-based practice, medical law and regulation, and, importantly, evidence-based guidelines.

Values-based practice is not for everyone. It is indeed much debated (Loughlin, 2014). Key challenges have been made to all aspects of values-based practice from its premise (Thornton, 2014) through to its outputs (Venkatapuram, 2014). Perhaps the biggest challenge, though, when it comes to implementation, is what the political philosopher, Isaiah Berlin, writing over 50 years ago in the shadow of National Socialism, identified as the challenge of pluralism (Berlin, 1958). Biopsychosocial thinking as was indicated in the introduction to this chapter is pluralistic. So too is values-based practice. Values-based practice is indeed top-to-toe pluralistic from its premise of mutual respect to its outputs in dissensual decision-making. Our default position though, as Berlin pointed out, is not pluralism but monism. Berlin's default to monism has been evident in the developments outlined in the third section, 'Values-based practice in mental health', in this chapter. Psychiatrists opted for their own workstream separate from other mental health professionals in the 'New Ways of Working' and '10 ESC' programmes. Diagnosis in mental health remains, despite a number of '3 Keys' initiatives, predominantly medical and needs based rather than multidisciplinary and strengths based. The balanced decision-making required by the Guiding Principles has been largely sidestepped in the way the Mental Health Act 2007 has been used in practice.

This is not to say that we should give up. To the contrary, many of the worst abuses of psychiatry can be traced to the default to monism (Fulford et al., 2015b). Correspondingly, therefore, the importance of biopsychosocial thinking in psychiatry is precisely that it holds out the promise of a pluralistic defence against the abuses of monism. Delivering on that promise by implementing biopsychosocial psychiatry is where the minority values-based perspective described in this chapter provides a new twist. John Anderton, the hero of Steven Spielberg's cult sci-fi film, *Minority Report*, outwits the PreCrime unit of his day by going up against his own predestination. When it comes to biopsychosocial pluralism there is a message there somewhere for implementation.

Acknowledgements

The work from the Department of Health NIMH/CSIP programme described in the third section of this paper was co-produced by an extended team representing a wide range of stakeholder perspectives including those of service users and carers. A similar co-productive approach underpins the new programmes being developed through the Collaborating Centre at St Catherine's College, Oxford (see 'Further reading and website'). I am grateful to all those involved in both programmes for our past and continued collaborations.

Further reading and website

Fulford, Peile, and Carroll's (2012) *Essential Values-Based Practice: Clinical Stories Linking Science with People* provides an introduction to values-based practice and illustrates the clinical impact of each of its main elements through a series of extended case histories from different areas of healthcare (dermatology, hypertension management, breast cancer, diabetes care, etc.).

The website for *The Collaborating Centre for Values-Based Practice* at St Catherine's College, Oxford, includes a detailed 'Reading guide' and a resource of teaching and other materials available as full-text downloads: see https://valuesbasedpractice.org/More-about-VBP/.

References

Berlin, I. (1958). *Two Concepts of Liberty*. Oxford: Clarendon Press.

Care Services Improvement Partnership (CSIP) (2006). *Pathways to Recovery Paper 1. Core Vision and Values for a Modern Health System*. London: Department of Health.

Care Services Improvement Partnership (CSIP) and the National Institute for Mental Health in England (NIMHE) (2008). *Workbook to Support Implementation of the Mental Health Act 1983 as amended by the Mental Health Act 2007*. London: Department of Health.

Colombo, A. (1997). *Understanding Mentally Disordered Offenders: A Multi-Agency Perspective.* Aldershot: Ashgate.

Colombo, A., Bendelow, G., Fulford, K.W.M., and Williams, S. (2003). Evaluating the influence of implicit models of mental disorder on processes of shared decision making within community-based multidisciplinary teams. *Social Science & Medicine,* **56**(7), 1557–1570.

Department of Health (2004a). *The Ten Essential Shared Capabilities: A Framework for the Whole of the Mental Health Workforce.* London: The Sainsbury Centre for Mental Health, the National Health Service University, and the National Institute for Mental Health England. [The 10 ESCs have been the basis of a number of ongoing training and service development initiatives—see, for example, from NHS Education for Scotland (2011) at: http://www.nes.scot.nhs.uk/media/351385/10_essential_shared_capabilities_2011.pdf.]

Department of Health (2004b). *Mental Health Policy Implementation Guide: Community Development Workers for Black and Minority Ethnic Communities.* London: Department of Health.

Department of Health (2004c). *NIMHE Guiding Statement on Recovery.* London: Department of Health.

Department of Health (2005). *New Ways of Working for Psychiatrists: Enhancing Effective, Person-Centred Services through New Ways of Working in Multidisciplinary and Multi-Agency Contexts.* London: Department of Health. [Final report 'but not the end of the story'.]

Department of Health (2007). *Mental Health: New Ways of Working for Everyone: Developing and Sustaining a Capable and Flexible Workforce.* London: Department of Health.

Department of Health (2008). *Refocusing the Care Programme Approach: Policy and Positive Practice Guidance.* London: Department of Health.

Engel, G. (1977). The need for a new medical model: a challenge for biomedicine. *Science,* **196**(4286), 129–136.

Engel, G. (1978). The biopsychosocial model and the education of health professionals. *Annals of the New York Academy of Sciences,* **310**, 169–181; reprinted in *General Hospital Psychiatry,* 1979, **1**(2), 156–165.

Fulford, K.W.M. (1989). *Moral Theory and Medical Practice.* Cambridge: Cambridge University Press. [Reprinted in paperback, 1995.]

Fulford, K.W.M. and Colombo, A. (2004). Six models of mental disorder: a study combining linguistic-analytic and empirical methods. *Philosophy, Psychiatry, & Psychology,* **11**(2), 129–144.

Fulford, K.W.M., Dewey, S., and King, M. (2015a). Values-based involuntary seclusion and treatment: value pluralism and the UK's Mental Health Act 2007. In: J.Z. Sadler, W. van Staden, and K.W.M. Fulford (Eds.), *The Oxford Handbook of Psychiatric Ethics* (Chapter 60). Oxford: Oxford University Press.

Fulford, K.W.M., Duhig, L., Hankin, J., Hicks, J., and Keeble, J. (2015b). Values-based assessment in mental health: The 3 keys to a shared approach between service users and service providers. In: J.Z. Sadler, W. van Staden, and K.W.M. Fulford (Eds.), *The Oxford Handbook of Psychiatric Ethics* (Chapter 73). Oxford: Oxford University Press.

Fulford, K.W.M., Newton-Hughes, A., Strudwick, R., and Handa, A. (2018). Values-based practice for imaging and radiotherapy professionals: an introduction. *Imaging and Oncology, 2018,* 26–33.

Fulford, K.W.M., Peile, E., and Carroll, H. (2012). *Essential Values-Based Practice: Clinical Stories Linking Science with People.* Cambridge: Cambridge University Press.

Fulford, K.W.M. and van Staden, W. (2013). Values-based practice: topsy-turvy take home messages from ordinary language philosophy (and a few next steps). In: K.W.M. Fulford, M. Davies, R. Gipps, G. Graham, J. Sadler, G. Stanghellini, and T. Thornton (Eds.), *The Oxford Handbook of Philosophy and Psychiatry* (pp. 385–412). Oxford: Oxford University Press.

General Medical Council (2008). *Consent: Patients and Doctors Making Decisions Together.* London: General Medical Council.

Ghaemi, S.N. (2009). The rise and fall of the biopsychosocial model. *British Journal of Psychiatry*, **195**, 3–4.

Ghaemi, S.N. (2010). *The Rise and Fall of the Biopsychosocial Model: Reconciling Art and Science in Psychiatry.* Baltimore, MD: Johns Hopkins University Press.

Handa, I.A., Fulford-Smith, L., Barber, Z.E., Dobbs, T.D., Fulford, K.W.M., and Peile, E. (2016). The importance of seeing things from someone else's point of view. *BMJ*, **354**, i1652. http://careers.bmj.com/careers/advice/The_importance_of_seeing_things_from_someone_else's_point_of_view

Herring, J., Fulford, K.W.M., Dunn, D., and Handa, A. (2017). Elbow room for best practice? Montgomery, patients' values, and balanced decision-making in person-centred care. *Medical Law Review*, **25**(4), 582–603.

Loughlin, M. (Ed.) (2014). *Debates in Values-Based Practice: Arguments For and Against.* Cambridge: Cambridge University Press.

McGonagle, I., Jackson, C.S., and Kane, R. (2015). The ten essential shared capabilities: reflections on education in values based practice: a qualitative study. *Nurse Education Today*, **35**(2), e24–e28.

Montgomery v *Lanarkshire Health Board* (judgment delivered March 11, 2015). https://www.supremecourt.uk/cases/uksc-2013-0136.html

National Institute for Health and Care Excellence (2015). Suspected cancer: recognition and referral. NICE guideline NG12 (last updated: July 2017). https://www.nice.org.uk/guidance/ng12 [Scroll down the page to the statement 'Your Responsibility'.]

National Institute for Mental Health England (2004). *The National Framework of Values for Mental Health.* [Originally published online on the NIMHE website. Available on the values-based practice website (see 'Further reading and website') or in hard copy in Woodbridge and Fulford (2004).]

National Institute for Mental Health in England (NIMHE) and the Care Services Improvement Partnership (2008). *3 Keys to a Shared Approach in Mental Health Assessment.* London: Department of Health. [Full text download available from the values-based practice website—see 'Further reading and website'.]

Royal College of Psychiatrists (2016). *What Really Matters in Children and Young People's Mental Health: Report of the Values-Based Child and Adolescent Mental Health System Commission.* London: The Royal College of Psychiatrists. [Available at: https://valuesbasedpractice.org/wp-content/uploads/2015/04/Values-based-full-report.pdf.]

Skills for Health (2013). *Revised National Occupational Standards for Mental Health.* Bristol: Skills for Health. [Available at: https://tools.skillsforhealth.org.uk/competence_search/.]

Slade, M. (2009). *Personal Recovery and Mental Illness: A Guide for Mental Health Professionals (Values-Based Medicine).* Cambridge: Cambridge University Press.

Thornton, T. (2014). Values-based practice and authoritarianism. In: M. Loughlin (Ed.), *Debates in Values-Based Practice: Arguments For and Against* (pp. 50–61). Cambridge: Cambridge University Press.

Venkatapuram, S. (2014). Values-based practice and global health. Chapter 11 In: M. Loughlin (Ed.), *Debates in Values-Based Practice: Arguments For and Against* (pp. 131–141). Cambridge: Cambridge University Press.

Woodbridge, K. and Fulford, K.W.M. (2004). *Whose Values?: A Workbook for Values-Based Practice in Mental Health Care.* London: The Sainsbury Centre for Mental Health. [Full text download available from the values-based practice website—see 'Further reading and website'.]

Chapter 9

Formulation in the face of complexity

Graeme C. Smith

Introduction

Health service professionals practise under the 'sword of Damocles' in trying to make sense of their clinical observations. The mission statements of their disciplines set up the expectation that they will use the integrated holistic,[1] humanist[2] biopsychosocial paradigm proposed by Engel (1977a) to address the abstraction[3] of twentieth-century medicine. However, this conflicts with another mantra, that of expecting clinicians to practise in a more 'evidence-based' way, the major model for which is an abstracted one that continues to privilege the biological (Gupta, 2003, 2011). In the mental health field, the issue is epitomized by the debate about whether in the process of clinical reasoning abstracted, operationalized diagnoses should be prioritized in making sense of the data or whether the process of patient-centred formulation, also known as case conceptualization, is more appropriate to the object of study, mental symptoms (Haslam, 2013; Smith, 2014a).

The definition of a formulation is itself a contentious matter, centred on the issue of abstraction. The person-centred definition of it is that it is the answer to the question, 'Why does this particular patient present with this diagnosis and these particular problems at this particular time?' (Perry et al., 1987). This is Engel's 'holistic diagnosis', a concept which underpins the biopsychosocial model (Engel, 1971). This definition

---

[1] In the holistic model, properties of individual elements are taken to be determined by relations they bear to other elements (Heil, 2005). Holism is the opposite of atomism and is not simply pluralism.

[2] Humanism, defined as the tendency to emphasize man and his status, importance, powers, achievements, interests, or authority (Lacey, 2005), eschews religious and magic explanations and prioritizes human experience, subjectivity, and meaning.

[3] The term abstraction is used here as being 'a concept or theory that, in order to focus on some features of things, ignores other features of those same things' (Schwartz and Wiggins, 1985). Abstraction constrains the process of gathering data as well as that of making sense of it. Abstraction may be deliberate, but is more likely to be tacit; the term 'spirit of abstraction' refers to the tendency for a person to become blind to the fact that they are using abstractions, and to then assume that their point of view represents the true being of reality (Schwartz and Wiggins, 1985). The parts are being taken as a whole.

provides a way of avoiding abstraction but is seen by some as being too subjective. The process-centred definition of a formulation, as 'a prescribed method for the orderly combination or arrangement of data … according to some rational principles' (Faulkner et al., 1985), on the other hand risks enshrining abstraction by leaving out integration and humanism. Both definitions are in use today. This chapter is based on the premise espoused in the biopsychosocial model that the 'rational principles' referred to in the process-centred definition must include those relating to holism (Smith, 2014a, 2014b). The need for a holistic and humanist formulation has been a recurring but contested proposition throughout the recorded history of medicine. Not only does the special nature of mental symptoms require such a formulation but so, too, does the increasingly frequent complex presentations of multimorbidity, which require integrated care (Smith, 2009). Thus all healthcare professionals need to be able to make such a formulation. The proposed greater patient/consumer participation (Tinetti et al., 2012) will require that they, too, will need to formulate rather than rely on diagnosis.

Plan of chapter

In keeping with the subject of this book, it is appropriate to first examine the place of formulation in Engel's biopsychosocial model. Rethinking this requires a review of the history of the concepts on which Engel drew, and of the history of formulation generally; these sections will follow. A review of the criticisms of the biopsychosocial model will lead to a discussion of the way in which developments in complexity theory have implications for formulation in a rethought biopsychosocial model. It sheds light on why holistic formulation is difficult, and about how this can be addressed in professional training and consumer participation.

Engel and formulation

Engel was a mid-twentieth-century physician with a strong interest in the developing field of psychosomatic medicine and its theoretical underpinning, psychoanalytic theory, in which he had some training (Ghaemi, 2011). He was not a psychiatrist, but he held an appointment in the Department of Psychiatry at the University of Rochester Medical School in the USA for many years. In the psychosomatic field, multiple models of illness and their theories had to be addressed, including biological ones; prioritization and integration of hypotheses was essential. In the 1950s, Engel 'formulated' (making a rare use by him of that term) a holistic and humanist model of ulcerative colitis based on prioritization of psychoanalytic and biological theories, after an extensive literature review and drawing on his own clinical experience (Engel, 1954a, 1954b, 1955, 1958).

In publications leading up to his formal proposal of the biopsychosocial model in 1977, Engel showed his familiarity with other emerging modernist ideas: the concept of totality, the limitations of the scientific method, the need to prioritize interaction in studying organismic systems, disease as a social construction, and the concept of the 'sick role' (Engel, 1960, 1965, 1973, 1977b). He was aware of the abstraction inherent in naming domains; nevertheless, he ultimately titled his model 'biopsychosocial' rather than 'total', 'compositionistic' or 'holistic', terms which he had considered. Grinker had made a similar error earlier when he argued most eloquently for the inclusion of biological, psychological, and social factors in a 'somatopsychosocial' model (Grinker, 1964).

In his articles on ulcerative colitis in the 1950s, Engel provided an example of what he called a 'holistic diagnosis' for one of his patients, based on his model of the disorder, with a discussion of how this impacted recommendations for a treatment plan.[4] In an article in which he described how he taught medical students an experiential approach to interviewing, Engel (1971) showed that he understood some of the epistemological issues of arriving at a 'holistic diagnosis', which others came to call a formulation. He helped students to explore subjectivity in their patients, and incorporate this in developing multiple hypotheses prioritized on the basis of evidence. The subjectivity of patients mattered to him, but having such procedures accepted as being scientific also mattered a great deal; much of his writing refers to the emerging systems theories and the need for ordering of data. He was thus combining person- and process-based models of formulation.

In the article in which Engel (1977a) proposed his biopsychosocial model of illness, he claimed that it was holistic and based on von Bertalanffy's general system theory (GST). This emphasized the limitations of the scientific method and the need to study the interrelationship of components of the hierarchical system in which organisms operate (von Bertalanffy, 1972).[5] Engel argued that by providing a hierarchical systems framework, GST allowed physicians to collect and order a wider range of data; this was 'scientific'. He paid scant attention to the main thrust of GST, which was to develop discipline-specific principles described mathematically where possible, to complement established common principles of organization across all systems. There was no elaboration of Engel's earlier proposition that multiple hypotheses could be developed from different theoretical viewpoints, thus no reference to prioritization of these by a process of abduction.[6] In subsequent publications, Engel provided a number of clinical examples of how he found 'focal points' in his interviews with patients that allowed him to develop hypotheses, based on psychoanalytic theory, about interactions of factors (Engel, 1977b, 1978, 1980, 1987, 1992). However, only rarely did he give an indication that he was thinking about the epistemological issues involved in formulation.

A clinical case reported by Engel exemplifies his application of his model (Engel, 1977b). A middle-aged woman with a history of intermittent drinking and fatty liver who had been abstemious for several years, was admitted with anorexia, fatiguability,

---

[4] Throughout his subsequent published works, Engel avoided using the term formulation, arguing that a 'holistic diagnosis' encompassed all pertinent factors. He used the terms 'clinical reasoning', 'clinical judgement', 'mechanisms', and 'explanatory principles' in describing the process of arriving at such a diagnosis.

[5] GST will be discussed in detail later in this chapter.

[6] Abduction—inference to the best explanation—is a model proposed by Peirce for prioritizing hypotheses (Hookway, 2005). Identifying that which is plausible and useful, is judged to have best fit in the circumstances, is fundamental to contemporary clinical reasoning and formulation (Sanford, 2005; Haig, 2005).

weakness, and loss of 'pep' and interest which had abruptly developed. She was extensively investigated, including having a liver biopsy. Following this, the treating physician reassured her and told her that he was glad that she could get home to her family. Engel interviewed her and elicited the fact that the symptoms had begun abruptly when she learned that her husband of 25 years was leaving her for another woman. In commenting that the physician had made decisions about her life without first investigating her current life situation and emotional status, he draws attention to a physical sign which the physician had overlooked: 'the hesitant response and the helplessness gesture'. Engel drew on the literature about such body-language signs and the concept of helplessness and conservation withdrawal that had been deduced from such studies to mount a 'scientifically plausible' hypothesis that the patient's symptoms were part of an emotional response to loss. He offered no other hypotheses such as behavioural or cognitive ones.

Engel acknowledged that 'the distinction between the observer and the observed, the subject and object, [can] become blurred, if indeed is does not at times disappear altogether' (Engel, 1987), an important contention of systems theories. He also acknowledged the importance of physicians' use of tacit knowledge[7] in comprehending patients and of the importance of finding ways of including data emerging from such practice 'scientifically' in 'holistic diagnosis':

> Each one of us is forever involved in exchanging information with others and interpreting its meaning, whether true, or valuable, or good, or bad, or useful, or whatever, and making decisions, or taking action thereupon. Hence it becomes difficult for most of us, especially scientists, to think of such ordinary everyday activities as having anything in common with scientific processes, much less as accessible to or requiring scientific study … They very much qualify as key elements of the human dimensions of medical practice and as such become proper areas for scientific enquiry. (Engel, 1987, p. 110)

Indeed, Engel argued that tacit knowledge was what physicians used in order to successfully engage with patients and make sense of the presentations, even if they did not know how they did this. Engel argued that the biopsychosocial model provided an opportunity for them to bring this to consciousness in a way that would be accepted as scientific, and that medical education should include training in how to do this. He recognized the importance of intuition, arguing that the first step in being scientific about psychosocial issues is to subject the intuition of them to the same sort of critical analysis as one would use with biological data (Engel, 1987). Engel argued for the importance of dialogue, the process of thinking about thinking, the necessary condition for the development of *nous*[8] (Engel, 1992).

Towards the end of his life, in the foreword for a book on the limits of scientific psychiatry and the role of uncertainty in mental health, Engel gives evidence of an awareness of emerging complexity theory in offering a justification for his use of 'focal points' in establishing hypotheses:

---

[7] The concept of tacit knowledge as developed by Polanyi (1966) is reviewed later in this chapter.

[8] The concept of *nous* is discussed in detail later in the chapter. It is something beyond intuition, and is captured in the term 'gut feeling'.

Primary causality will be forced to surrender its fundamental character in deference to complex circular networks of interdependent systems at multiple levels of complexity. Instead of seeking to correct one underlying root cause, we will search for ... focal points. (Engel, 1986, p. xviii)

In his final article, Engel focused on the abiding attention to 'humanness' that he claims has characterized medicine for thousands of years, and argues that 'That alone identifies biopsychosocial as a more complete and inclusive conceptual framework to guide clinicians in their everyday work with patients' (Engel, 1997, p. 57). This is an appeal to common sense. Engel then updates his previous comments on Heisenberg's dictum that 'What we observe is not nature itself but nature exposed to our method of questioning', now mentioning for the first time chaos and complexity theories, claiming that they are the conceptual developments that underlie this dictum.

Criticisms of the biopsychosocial model and development of new models of formulation

There have been substantial criticisms of the epistemological basis of the biopsychosocial model and of its apparent psychoanalytic bias (Smith and Strain, 2002; Ghaemi, 2011). Pertinent to the issue of formulation is the observation by Schwartz and Wiggins (1985) that the model is not humanist and integrative enough; they proposed an experiential model for integration, based on the concept of the 'lifeworld'. Some argued that the epistemological problem of integration had not been addressed (Beitman et al., 1989). Walsh and Peterson (1985) warned against premature attempts at synthesis, arguing instead that the most cognitively responsible yet comprehensive view available is the position of pluralism. Ghaemi (2011) emphasized this view, alluding to Jasper's work which advocated serial application of hypotheses. However, the main response has been that of trying to make the model more scientific in the positivist sense, using multidimensional models which, although claiming to be holistic, make little or no attempt at integration. Nor is there a place in them for the profundity captured by the term *nous*.

Although Engel included the word 'social' in his model, he did not develop that argument. He never followed up his reference to the concept of medicine's social construction of the meaning of disease with an exposition or critique of evolving systems-based sociological concepts such as that of 'the sick role' (Parsons,1977a, 1977b). Such a critique could have made Engel's argument for the inclusion of the social in his model more convincing.

Some have argued that formulation can have adverse effects when perceived by the patient as perpetuating the imbalance of power in the clinician–patient relationship (Eells, 1997, p. 13). The growing patient-centred medicine movement addresses this; it will require operationalization of the formulation process.

Developments in formulation

These criticisms of the biopsychosocial model were addressed to a varying extent as Engel's concept of 'holistic diagnosis' was taken up in the emerging concept of formulation. Two dedicated, peer-reviewed journals continue to address the issue, as have several reviews (Eells, 1997; Johnstone and Dallos, 2013). Although the major textbooks of Western psychiatry began using the term 'formulation' in the late twentieth century, their treatment of it remains cursory. Psychiatry and psychology training bodies introduced requirements for trainees to develop skills in formulation but give insufficient attention to the epistemological problems (Smith, 2014a, 2014b). Operational definitions were published. That of British psychiatrists Greenberg and colleagues ((1981) was process focused and described a grid, a tool which came to be used in a highly abstracted way that ignores holism. That of North American psychiatrists (Faulkner and colleagues (1985) was more pertinent; it attempted to capture the ambiguities of formulation. They argued that it should be integrated and pluralistic yet specific, fixed yet flexible, objective yet subjective, cross-sectional and descriptive yet longitudinal and developmental, historical yet futuristic, and comprehensive yet concise. In a landmark subsequent publication they discussed the problems of integrating factors in hierarchical levels and integrating explanatory models, indicating their familiarity with the epistemological tool of abduction, and of the need for judgement in employing the most effective and efficient combination of perspectives for patient evaluation and treatment (Sperry et al., 1992, p. 100). The British Psychological Society Division of Clinical Psychology (2011) produced a well-considered consensus about good practice guidelines on the use of formulation. Although their multidimensional definition of formulation is process based, the guidelines emphasize the need for reflective practice that embraces humanism to produce a plausible account which is 'a balanced synthesis of the intuitive and rational cognitive systems'.

History of concepts of formulation

Addressing in a humanist and holistic way the cosmic, unbounded question of why a person is presenting in a particular way asks a lot of clinicians; it is experienced as a very difficult task (Smith, 2014a). Engel's failure to address this problem comprehensively and subsequent incomplete attempts to rectify this leave clinicians insufficiently prepared to write formulations, even though, as Engel argued, they often do this in their head without realizing it. In training, placing the task in an historical context helps establish its validity and acknowledge its difficulty and contestation (Smith, 2014b).

Both the person- and process-based definitions of a formulation have evolved from the devices used in ancient medicine to make sense of data. During that evolution, medicine drew on long-standing ways and customs as well as emerging philosophical principles. There are two issues here; first, that of the impact of changing models of illness on the selection of data, and second, the impact of changing methods of clinical reasoning about such data.

Models and theories of health, illness, and disease

The type of formulation used reflects the model of illness within which it is produced. This in turn determines the focus of attention of both the clinician and the patient, and this may differ. The range of data available to the clinician and patient for the process of making sense of the symptoms and the presentation observed is thus constrained in a particular way. The history of medicine provides some striking examples of this.

In cultures which held highly abstracted models of illness, such as the ancient Mesopotamians who believed in divine cause and the practitioners of Hippocratic medicine who believed that illness was an imbalance of health associated with the bodily humours, there was little need to explore the contribution of natural factors. However, such models of illness required detailed study of the pattern of symptoms and signs, and of the lifestyle of the patient. For the Mesopotamians, it was necessary to discover in what way the patient had offended the spirit, and in what way the spirit was carrying out punishment, in order to select a treatment plan that would expiate the offence and bring about cure (Scurlock and Andersen, 2005, pp. 11–12, 549). Hippocratic practice required detailed pattern recognition including elicitation of lifestyle in order to infer the particular humoural disturbance at play, and then deduce the appropriate treatment (Porter, 1997, pp. 61; Nutton, 2013, pp. 90–92). Although the model was secular, physicians needed to be aware of the patient's spiritual beliefs, addressed by the Asclepian body of practice also used by patients and with which Hippocratic physicians needed to liaise (Nutton, 2013, pp. 104–115).

The resurgence of Greek fifth-century BCE humanism, as defined in footnote 2, at the beginning of the Renaissance, which now emphasized a move away from God in focusing on man and his status, importance, powers, achievements, interests, or authority (Lacey, 2005), brought a profound change in the way individuals viewed themselves and were viewed by others, including the physicians. Until then, 'Man was conscious of himself only as a member of a race, people, party, family, or corporation— only through some general category …[now] the subjective side asserted itself … Man became a spiritual individual and recognized himself as such' (Burckhard, J. (1860). *The Civilization of the Renaissance in Italy*, quoted by von Bertalanffy, 1975, p. 54). Data collection thus required attention to the patient's subjectivity (Porter, 1997, pp. 168–170). The metaphor of bodily humours was rejected and replaced by a model of illness based on natural rather than spiritual factors. Adoption of the positivist scientific method to explore such factors then met with such astounding success that by the end of the nineteenth century data collection encompassed a very wide range of physical factors. Data collection focused on these to the exclusion of subjective factors in this dualist, reductionist paradigm (Porter, 1997, pp. 306–308). This was the context in which psychiatry became a distinct discipline within medicine. As is the case today, psychiatrists were faced with the dilemma of how to be seen as scientific while needing somehow to be seen as humanist and capable of incorporating psychosocial determinants of behaviour, in the model of mental illness established by Pinel.[9] Psychiatry's data collection thus became somewhat broader than that of the medical model.

The modernist movement that began at the end of the nineteenth century led to a challenging of beliefs in all intellectual fields. In psychiatry, humanism again became

---

[9] Philippe Pinel, responsible for the mad at the Bicêtre and Salpêtrière in Paris during the French Revolution, showed that their behaviour was related to the way in which they were treated by observing what happened when he reduced mechanical restraints. He favoured a humanist therapy, *'traitement moral'*, aimed at instilling hope (Porter, 1997, pp. 495–497).

part of the model of illness, emerging in the twentieth century as psychoanalysis and existentialism and in the radical views of the anti-psychiatry movement led by Szasz and Laing, who saw mental illness as a social construct (Kingma, 2013, pp. 365–366). Humanism facilitated patient participation in decision-making. The pressure of folk formulation had facilitated the survival of patient involvement when humanism was marginalized in the eighteenth century (Porter, 1997, p. 286). This foreshadowed the contemporary emphasis on involving the patient in creating working hypotheses on which their individualized treatment will be designed (Tinetti et al., 2012). This requires that the tacit *nous* of patients and carers be brought to consciousness and its development facilitated, in the same way that Engel argued was necessary for physicians.

Uptake of these various models broadened the scope of data collection in psychiatry. The reductionist models of behaviourism and cognitivism narrowed it again, as did the strengthening prioritization of biologism, in the second half of the twentieth century. The emergence of systems theory as espoused in medicine by Engel, and now of complexity theory, has revived the place of holism in the model of illness, requiring multiple vantage points and therefore broadening the scope of data collection by those favouring a patient-centred formulation. Rethinking biopsychosocial psychiatry needs understanding of the history of how one selects data in seeking an understanding of a patient's presentation.

The history of clinical reasoning

Formulation is a central component of clinical reasoning, the term now used to embrace all aspects of making sense of data in medicine (Loughlin et al., 2012). Such reasoning was addressed formally by Galen, the second century CE Roman doctor/philosopher, who boldly applied to the empirical art of medicine the methodical principles of logic developed by classical Greek philosophers for the physical sciences (Barnes, 1991, p. 66). This aspect of Hippocratic/Galenic medicine has persisted ever since. Barnes (1991, p. 102) describes it as glorified common sense organized and regimented; the commonly used expression 'clear thinking' captures it well. One method, that of taking observations as axiomatic or given, 'dividing' them into syndromes, labelling them as diagnoses, and classifying them into systems, had been in use since ancient Mesopotamian times (Scurlock and Andersen, 2005, p. 549). Psychiatry's adoption of that method is strongly contested by those who argue that an operationalized diagnosis is an insufficient proxy for formulating presentations of mental illness (Poland and Von Eckardt, 2013; Boyle and Johnstone, 2014). The *Diagnostic and Statistical Manual of Mental Disorders* psychiatric classification tried to address this by being multiaxial, and has now added dimensional ratings (American Psychiatric Association, 2013). However, this falls short of producing a holistic and humanist formulation, that is, an inference that does not involve deduction from the statistical abstraction of diagnosis.

Nous as the highest form of reason

Aristotle, in the third century BCE, argued that human experience is rich and powerful enough to enable it to be used productively to reach conclusions by simple analogy, even in medicine (Frede, 1996a, p. 160). However, to achieve true knowledge, he argued, to grasp the essence of how a thing comes to be the way that it is, of why something is the case and not just that it is the case, requires something that he regarded as the highest form of reason, *nous* (Frede, 1996b, p. 162). Frede argues that most of our scientific explanations do not achieve this level. Holistic, humanist formulation and practice requires this ability.

The concept of *nous* is difficult to put into words. Nowadays, it is often equated with the term 'intuition', but even that does not convey completely its meaning. It is reflected better in common language terms such as 'grasp', 'gut feeling', 'feeling in one's bones', and '*savoir-faire*'. A formulation that captures such essence has been described as 'making a bull's-eye hit'. Socrates' conceptualization of reason in this sense was that of a function of the soul or mind that has its own needs and desires (Frede, 1996b, pp. 5–6). It determines the course of action we take, indeed the course of our life, by making us do what it wants us to do (Frede, 1996b, pp. 12–13). The concept thus adumbrates the dynamic unconscious proposed by Freud and Jasper's concept of grasping the meaning of the patient's experience (Schwartz and Wiggins, 1986). Polanyi (1966, pp. 55–56) used a similar concept, that of 'tacit knowledge', to describe the process whereby comprehension of knowledge in general and of another human being in particular is achieved by indwelling.[10] Aristotle argued that humans were born with the innate capacity of the soul to perform such a mental action, but that it required 'thinking about thinking' in order for this capacity to be developed. It could not be acquired by learning, but rather by opening oneself to experience (Frede, 1996a, p. 171).

There is abundant evidence that a major stream of practitioners of Hippocratic medicine engaged in such processes. Development of the capacity for *nous* took place in open dialogue among all disciplines in the development of theories and practices, using the new arts of rhetoric and proof (Porter, 1997, pp. 56–57). This is a clue to what might be useful in teaching the art of formulation. Galen also considered the features of the ideal doctor to be those of intuition and judgement (Nutton, 2013, p. 251–252). He made the important point that physicians who developed such capacity could use it without being aware of what they were doing (Nutton, 2013, p. 228). Engel agreed with him, but argued that contemporary physicians did not use this tacit knowledge well enough; use of his biopsychosocial model was meant to facilitate this (Engel, 1977a). Subsequent studies on clinical reasoning have confirmed that intuitive or non-analytic reasoning, including pattern recognition, is part of the repertoire in use in medicine, especially by psychiatrists (Bhugra et al., 2011; Holmes et al., 2011). The extensive literature on procedural unconscious knowledge confirms its distinct qualities, which include holism and robustness (Augusto, 2010).

---

[10] See Thornton (2013) for a critical analysis of Polanyi's argument and a review of the contemporary debate about skilled recognitional clinical judgement as a form of tacit knowledge.

Holism

Holism was defined earlier in this chapter as a model in which properties of individual elements are taken to be determined by relations they bear to other elements (Heil, 2005). Aristotle's dictum that 'the totality is not, as it were, a mere heap, but the whole is something besides the parts' (Cohen, 2012) pithily conveys the essence of holism, and shows how old the concept is. Hippocratic/Galenic medicine was holistic (Nutton, 2013, pp. 56–57), and Western medicine remained so until the seventeenth century when reductionism characterized by dualism became its dominant model, and what was known later as logical positivism its methodology (Porter, 1997, pp. 245-254).

Reductionism

Ontological reductionism holds that one kind of entity is no more than a structure of other kinds of entity (Bennett and Hacker, 2003, p. 355) and that organisms are no more (nor less) than complex functioning machines (Ruse, 2005).

Dualism

Humanism's subjectivity was relegated to a realm outside medicine when the Hippocratic/Galenic model of illness, and thus of formulation, was revised drastically by the 'new philosophy' of the late seventeenth century that made latent dualism overt. Descartes played a pivotal role in this movement. He regarded the body as a machine; 'Madness, he taught, could not lie in the immortal soul or mind but had to be in the body' (Porter, 1997, p. 142). Dualism has dominated reasoning in medicine ever since, resulting in an abstracted, reductionist view of mental illness which privileges the biological.

Reasoning in psychiatry in the nineteenth century

When psychiatry emerged as a discipline within medicine in the nineteenth century, it attempted to use the prevailing model of hypothesis testing based on an increasingly broad range of experimentally derived theories of physical aetiology of physical conditions (Porter, 1997, pp. 320–448). Lacking such theories for mental symptoms, psychiatrists speculated, notably with the functionalist theories, the most pertinent of which is 'associationism' (Berrios, 2014). Associationism addressed the nature and sources of ideas and the relation among sensations and ideas in the mind, and although speculative, it stimulated experimental psychology (Gustafson, 2005). The dualist concept of psychogenesis, of ideas interacting to produce mental symptoms, is the basis of contemporary cognitive behavioural therapy.

Unlike medicine in general, psychiatry was slow to incorporate the holistic concept of Claude Bernard. His physiological investigations on the interaction of bodily systems led him to propose that higher organisms are able to create their own sustaining internal environment (*milieu intérieur*) and thereby achieve a degree of autonomy (Porter, 1997, p. 338–341). It was not until the 1930s, when this concept was elaborated into that of homeostasis by Walter Cannon and extrapolated by him and others to social systems, that psychiatry embraced systems theories, as will be discussed later in this chapter (Cannon, 1939; Gregory, 2004). Psychiatry as a discipline privileged the model epitomized by the German psychiatrist, Griesinger's aphorism that 'mental illnesses are brain diseases' (Porter, 1997, pp. 508–509). Nevertheless, it seems that *nous* may have predominated in practice: 'Most doctors swore by the tacit knowledge at their fingers' ends, and in their heads, which they acquired in going about the quotidien business of attending the sick' (Porter, 1997, p. 525). Engel noted that they still did so in the mid-twentieth century when he proposed his model that he hoped would formalize this.

Modernism and psychoanalysis

Towards the end of the nineteenth century some in medicine were posing the questions that Engel later addressed. They raised issues of the underlying philosophy of medical practice; of how subjectivity was becoming formalized, of whether medicine should be reductionist and 'hence blind to the power of organization and the spark of life' (Porter, 1997, p. 527), of how specialization in medicine was eroding the capacity of a single physician to comprehend a patient completely, of how medicine should be integrated with other bodies of knowledge, and of the inadequacy of the clinicopathological model (Porter, 1997, pp. 525–527). This was an example of modernist thinking that was having a profound effect on reasoning in Western culture generally. Modernism challenged assumptions and sought new models; 'Modernists ... shared two defining attributes ... First, the lure of heresy ... and, second, a commitment to a principled self-scrutiny' (Gay, 2007, pp. 3–4).[11] Modernism was a reaction to what was seen as the Enlightenment's descent into sterility, characterized in medicine's prioritization of logical positivism and the decline of humanism (Zaretsky, 2004; Gay, 2007).

The new theories and models that emerged in the psychosocial field included the humanist psychoanalytic and existentialist ones, the holistic Gestaltism and systems theories, and the reactionary, reductionist behaviourism. Crises in the epidemiology of mental disorder were used to explore the role of social factors in symptom formation, for example, shell shock in the First World War. These developments permitted psychiatry to address seriously what now is known as formulation, and to do so in a humanist and holistic way. They eased the pressure on psychiatry to conform to the medical model which prioritized biology. Psychoanalysis took a lead in this by introducing the concept of formulation as being the answer to the question of how a person comes to be presenting in this way at this time. However, psychoanalysts were aiming at an understanding only of the patient's mental processes—what they called the dynamic unconscious—rather than creating a logical basis for treatment. The psychoanalytic model acknowledged that 'non-dynamic' factors, including physical and social ones, were in play in their patients but it did not incorporate other pertinent models. They had no need to develop multiple hypotheses and hence no need to consider integration.

---

[11] There are many different definitions of modernism, but Gay's one is pertinent to the topic of formulation.

General system theory

It seems extraordinary that the ancient concept of holism came to be ignored in nineteenth-century science. The concept of vitalism, which postulated some vital force of organization, a ghost in the machine, was not sufficiently formulated for it to be regarded as holistic (Porter, 1997, pp. 217–218). However, the various systems[12] theories developed in the early twentieth century addressed the issue of holism formally. They were revolutionary, as were the findings in physics that inspired them. GST[13] emerged as the most comprehensive of these theories, greatly appealing to those in the mental health and social disciplines dissatisfied with the ability of a reductionist approach to address problems of behaviour and organization. The principles of GST are described in von Bertalanffy's summaries of his publications from 1928 to 1971 (von Bertalanffy, 1969, 1975). Reviewing the principles as they relate to formulation will help understand its appeal to Engel, and help prepare for the discussion of complexity theory.

GST was based on the new perspective philosophy that rejected logical positivism and acknowledged the concept of relativity developed in physics; it implied that we cannot grasp the ultimate (von Bertalanffy, 1975, pp. 29–30). That 'new philosophy' drew on the work of Schelling and other philosophers in Germany in the late eighteenth and early nineteenth centuries who had challenged Kant's defence of Newtonian mechanics (Gare, 2000; 2013). Those who developed systems theories realized that the findings of physics applied to biological and cultural systems as well, albeit with different explanatory principles because of their organic and social nature (Cannon, 1939; von Bertalanffy, 1960/1975, pp. 40–41). Von Bertalanffy's answer to those who claimed that this was a metaphorical extrapolation[14] was that the test of a model is not a theoretical one but rather the pragmatic one of whether it is useful: 'whether it leads to explanation of facts, the synthesis of otherwise unconnected data, and to verifiable predictions' (von Bertalanffy, 1975/1975, pp. 76–77). GST was to be a transdisciplinary model that embraced all components of the classical hierarchy of systems, and thus offered both a humanist and holistic concept of man: 'How could one reduce human culture, science, art, ethics, and religion to ... biological factors?' (von Bertalanffy, 1960/1975, pp. 48–49).

Von Bertalanffy acknowledged the legitimacy of using classical science on closed systems where only two to three variables were examined. He did not exclude the possibility that one day logical-positivist methods may converge with those of systems theories. However, he regarded reductionists' attempts to date to accommodate the new philosophy as being inadequate. Therefore a new model was necessary, based on understanding of organisms as organized things; he designated it 'organismic' (von Bertalanffy, 1960/1975, p. 41). A fundamental concept is that living organisms are open systems characterized by continuous import and export of substance; inanimate

---

[12] A system is defined as a set of elements standing in inter-relation among themselves and with the environment (von Bertalanffy 1972/1975, p. 159).

[13] General system theory is von Bertalanffy's preferred term (von Bertalanffy 1969, p. xix).

[14] See Sharpe (2005) and Doll and Trueit (2010) for discussion of this.

objects are closed systems governed by different laws (von Bertalanffy, 1960/1975, pp. 43–46). Open systems restrain interactions in a way that facilitates both their independence and survival. The mechanisms available can include the 'suprabiolgical' (non-biological) ideas that constitute meaning structures, as proposed by Jaspers (Schwartz and Wiggins, 1986). Von Bertalanffy's aim was to establish general principles for organismic systems, irrespective of their physical, biological, or sociological nature:

> The properties and modes of action of higher levels are not explicable by the summation of the properties and modes of action of their components taken in isolation. If, however, we know the ensemble of the components and the relations existing between them, then the higher levels are derivable from the components. (von Bertalanffy, 1972, p. 411)

This implies acceptance of the ancient concept of hierarchy of levels, one which has almost the status of an Aristotelian 'first principle', so difficult is it to deduce. Von Bertalanffy used the concept, but called for better understanding of it, citing for example the promising work of Koestler.

Von Bertalanffy's approach to integration was that of finding isomorphies (similarities in form or structure) in organized entities, and deriving general laws and principles for them in mathematical terms (von Bertalanffy, 1972). Each discipline was to work out additional particular principles using appropriate models. The prediction that the principles of a system could be described in mathematical terms was qualified and guarded. He accepted that narrative description was also valid and appropriate in some cases.

Pertinent to the argument that a formulation requires multiple hypotheses is the general principle of equifinality established by GST:

> It is characteristic of organic processes that the same goal may be achieved from different starting points and in different ways … It is characterized by the fact that the system reaches its final state by means of processes which may vary according to the initial conditions … The mechanistic view that the organism is passively determined and can only react to external influences had to be replaced by a viewpoint which admits the primacy of action over reaction. (von Bertalanffy, 1937/1975, p. 100)

Von Bertalanffy revived the valuing of our immediate, lived experience; 'the only reality known to us directly' (von Bertalanffy, 1928/1975, pp. 70–71). He used the concept of symbolization to generalize findings in physics to all systems, and to underpin his project of describing their common principles and laws in mathematical form. He argued that symbolic activity gave humans their specificity, and he argued for inclusion of psychiatry and psychology in GST (von Bertalanffy, 1965/1975, pp. 111–113). He saw the pertinence of his organismic theory, as he called it, to the relations between body and mind, on the basis that the concept of matter in the old sense disappeared in the new philosophy (von Bertalanffy, 1928/1975, p. 72). He saw the need for the spirited expressions of mythical feeling, metaphors and allegories of the ineffable to complement scientific knowledge to prevent civilization becoming meaningless;

> The great world-poems ... are not statements of rational relations that can be examined and verified by experiment and theory, but projections of one's self into reality by way of empathic experience ... It is true that ... science must eliminate emotional values and mythical thought. If, however, this attitude is taken to be the only valid one then our unilaterally intellectual and technological civilization becomes meaningless. (von Bertalanffy, 1928/1975, p. 73)

Such noble statements help to account for Engel's embracing of his theory. GST is both holistic and humanist; it supports both the person- and process-based forms of formulation.

Complexity theory and formulation

The subsequent emergence and development of complexity theory[15] illuminates and offers help in meeting the challenge of formulation. It provides a theoretical basis for embracing rather than factoring out the uncertainty that characterizes complex presentations.

Complexity theory evolved in a way that addresses the criticism that despite its apparent openness, GST's assertion that higher levels are derivable from the components, and that the principles of such laws are describable in mathematical form, perpetuated the mechanistic view. It dealt with the complicated rather than the complex, risking perpetuation of the notion of 'the mind as machine' (M'Pherson, 1974/2003, pp. 120, 128). Complexity theory gives new meaning to the concept of humanism by establishing it as a particular example of the general principle of self-organization and adaptation.

Complexity theory seeks to understand the laws and mechanisms of complex adaptive systems, ones that are dynamic[16] and capable of undergoing self-organization to become more ordered (Gare, 2000). It postulates the existence of a regime, a condition, within those systems in which such adaptation can take place. It calls this the 'edge of chaos' (Gare, 2000; Doll and Trueit, 2010). Given that such systems are postulated to operate in individuals and their cultural relationships (Gare, 2000; Kurtz and Snowden, 2003), complexity theory is arguably able to be applied clinically, to individuals and systems, especially in the field of integrated care (Plsek and Greenhalgh, 2001; Smith, 2009; Paley, 2010; Doll and Trueit, 2010; Jayasinghe, 2012).

---

[15] The specific sense in which the term complexity is used within these theories is captured by the following quotation: 'When things become complex, the patterns can be perceived but not predicted, because the number of agents and the number of relationships defy categorisation or statistical analytic techniques. Other laws appear to be operating, though they are indiscernible' (Kurtz and Snowden, 2003). Importantly, this differs from the common usage in clinical and other domains when indicating that things are more complicated than usual, are 'in the too-hard basket'.

[16] The concept of dynamic systems has been used in formulation in psychiatry throughout the twentieth century, for example, in Freud's concept of the mind as a dynamic system, sustained in the term 'dynamic psychotherapy'.

Emergent behaviour

Highly pertinent to the concept of formulation is that of unpredictable, emergent behaviour resulting from self-organization. This is a concept that deserves a fuller explication than is possible here. However, most pertinently it proposes a break in the nexus of cause and effect. It is 'the idea that there are properties at a certain level of organization which cannot be predicted from the properties found at lower levels' (Emmeche et al., 1997/2003, p. 141). It thus challenges von Bertalanffy's proposal discussed earlier that higher levels are derivable from the components:

> Complex systems are examples of a kind of order which is not the result of plans, intentions, goals or values. This is what 'self-organisation' ... means ... Complex systems mimic design, they are not instances of it. (Paley, 2010, p. 60)

This is pertinent to the concept that a formulation is the basis of a management plan and to the implication of predictability that this involves. This will be discussed further later.

Implications for formulation

In the practise of medicine in general, one can often get away with abstracted, partial formulations represented by the process-based definition of formulation, and even with diagnoses alone, in seeking a logical basis for interventions. But in psychiatry, where no diagnosis is based on proven aetiology, where factors from across the spectrum determine the pattern of presentation, its timing, and often the selection of the clinician, such abstracted thinking is insufficient. The patient-centred question, 'Why does this person present with these problems at this time?' must be addressed. Complexity theory can be validly applied to this because the objects of attention in psychiatry, mental symptoms, have characteristics that permit them to be regarded as the products of adaptive, self-organizing behaviour occurring in a dynamic system, producing unpredictable, emergent behaviour (Marková and Berrios, 2009, 2012). Cramer and colleagues (2010) give the example of the set of depression symptoms, 'connected through a dense set of strong causal relations', a network the understanding of which will require resource to dynamical complexity theory. Mental symptoms, in this theory, are the product of a complex adaptive system. This can be said without privileging any biological, psychological, or social mechanism. However, complexity theory argues for description rather than causal explanation. It leaves the answer to the question open; it argues for recognition of the fact that any attempt at an answer must be an incomplete one.

It has been observed that the clinician employing Engel's hypothesis-driven interview technique begins the process of formulating—of developing, prioritizing, integrating, and testing multiple hypotheses—at the moment of first encounter with the patient (Holmes et al., 2011). This is supported by complexity theory's principle of equifinality, which advocates the use of multiple vantage points in seeking to describe the behaviour of complex adaptive systems. The presentation under consideration may have been reached by many different pathways, some of which may represent the unpredictable emergent behaviour of a dynamic complex adaptive system. This makes prediction difficult also. The following comment embraces these issues:

> Understanding this space requires us to gain multiple perspectives on the nature of the system. This is the time to 'stand still' (but pay attention) and gain new perspective on the situation rather than 'run for your life,' relying on the entrained patterns of past experience to determine our response ... Narrative techniques are particularly powerful in this space ... You need a different type of ability, one that is uncannily mysterious, sometimes even to its owner. (Kurtz and Snowden, 2003, p. 469)

This 'uncanny ability' is Aristotle's non-abstracted *nous*. Engel recognized the importance of it, but was not able to argue for it sufficiently well to enable his biopsychosocial model to survive the challenge of the evidence-based medicine movement and the new wave of biologism. Arguing for the importance of *nous* is as difficult as conveying a sense of what it is by defining it.

Development of the capacity for *nous* requires creation of situations in which thinking about thinking occurs. In the mental health disciplines, there is plenty of opportunity for this. Psychiatry's emphasis on the importance of supervision and peer review sets an example. Medicine provides it to a much more limited extent in reflective processes such as those of the Balint group (Balint, 1963/2000). Facilitation is required rather than didactic teaching for it seems that, as Aristotle said of metaphor, the use of *nous* cannot be learned from anyone else. What sort of mental structure is required in order to exercise its use? Perhaps it is the same as that which permits 'psychological mindedness', a construct that includes the concepts of self-consciousness, insight, empathy, and emotional intelligence, many of which are culture bound (Kirmayer, 2007; Nyklicek and Denollet, 2009; Bhugra et al., 2011; Smith, 2014b).

In practice, use of the process-based type of formulation in which the question is broken down into domains is common, particularly when students are learning to formulate. Grids are often used as a way of organizing the data and beginning the process of considering interactions and development of multiple hypotheses. However, even when an abduction to the most plausible and useful hypotheses is performed, it may leave out ones based on dimensions not included in the grid. Furthermore, this 'spirit of abstraction' can militate against integration. Using the term 'totality' rather than 'biopsychosocial' for the model would help ensure that as many domains as seems pertinent to the case are included in the grid. Achieving full integration may not be possible given our present state of knowledge. However, it must be kept in mind as a goal.

Conclusion

The practise of psychiatry and of medicine in general faces challenges that require rethinking of the clinical reasoning required by the biopsychosocial model. The first is epidemiological. A growing number of people presenting to healthcare professionals have multiple illnesses and problems and are on multiple prescribed and other medications (Smith, 2009; Doessing and Burau, 2015). Evidence-based guidelines based on studies of patients without multimorbidity have unproven validity for many such presentations (Lugtenberg et al., 2011). This is particularly so in psychiatry, given the added problems presented by the nature of its target symptoms and the absence of biological markers. These issues are of growing concern to healthcare funders and administrators, and also to consumers. Systems and complexity theories offer a way of understanding the reasons for unpredictability of outcome in complex systems and accepting the challenge involved. They provide justification for clinicians and patient/consumers seeking better outcomes to formulate in a holistic and humanist paradigm, in order to produce multiple justifiable hypotheses as a basis for prioritized, integrated interventions.

This is pertinent to the second challenge, that of increased patient participation. Encouraged by entrepreneurs of the business model of value-based choice, the citizens' revolution forecast by healthcare theorists such as Muir Gray (2008) is upon us. Patient/consumers and their carers are already accessing and sharing knowledge electronically in a way that has challenged doctors' traditional authoritarian practice. These citizens are formulating without knowing it. Engel made the same observation about doctors; they were using their everyday experience and tacit knowledge without reflecting on that and without adequate training in its use. As the so-called disruptive electronic knowledge practice develops and becomes formalized, patient/consumers and their carers will need to be helped to formulate rather than abstractly diagnose, particularly about mental health problems. This would complement the thrust of the proposed revolution in the paradigm for the production of evidence-based guidelines (Boyd and Kent, 2014). However, formulation makes heavy epistemological demands. Healthcare professionals will need to have a sound understanding of the issues of formulation discussed in this chapter as a basis for development of the capacity to help patient/consumers and carers with their newly specialized role.

Integrated care poses a third challenge. It will become obvious to patient/consumers and their carers that evaluating the efficacy and effectiveness of integrated care using the logical-positivist paradigm has produced inconclusive results (Smith, 2009; Nolte and Pitchforth, 2014). Only gradually is the field beginning to draw on complexity theory and the broader bodies of knowledge integration that can help direct its studies more pertinently. These include knowledge integration, wisdom theory, integrative thinking, adult knowledge and clinical reasoning (Kallio, 2011). The methods available include qualitative research; it is more capable of addressing the patient-focused question of why a person presents in a particular way at a particular time. Its acceptance as being able to contribute to the evidence base is epitomized by the formation of the Cochrane Collaboration Qualitative Methodology Group.[17]

Rethinking biopsychosocial psychiatry and medicine with this focus on formulation would advance Engel's unfinished project. Formulation demands dialectical resolution of competing paradigms; it may help if the term 'biopsychosocial' was replaced by one derived from complexity theory such as 'totality'. There will need to be more emphasis on how to foster the capacity for *nous* and judgement by creating professional spaces in which thinking about thinking is facilitated. Psychiatrists and psychologists will start from a more advanced position in addressing these challenges than that of medical colleagues for whom diagnosis has been sufficient in the past, and who have not had the same opportunities in supervision to think about thinking. Provided that

---

[17] See Gupta (2011) for a review of revisions in the evidence-based movement model.

psychiatry continues to value highly formulation in its broadest sense, it can set an example to other disciplines of how to reason well.

Acknowledgements

The generous contribution of Dr Jocelyn Dunphy-Blomfield over many years to the development and expression of these ideas is gratefully acknowledged, as is that of Dr Traill Dowie.

References

Augusto, L.M. (2010). Unconscious knowledge; a survey. *Advances in Cognitive Psychology*, **6**, 116–141.

American Psychiatric Association (2013). *Diagnostic and Statistical Manual of Mental Disorders* (5th ed.). Washington, DC: American Psychiatric Association.

Balint, M. (1963/2000). *The Doctor, His Patient and the Illness* (2nd ed.). London: Churchill Livingstone.

Barnes, J. (1991). Galen on logic and therapy. In: F. Kudlien and R.J. Durling (Eds.), *Galen's Method of Healing: Proceedings of the 1982 Galen Symposium*, pp. 50–102. New York: EJ Brill.

Beitman, B.D., Goldfried, M.R., and **Norcross, J.C.** (1989). The movement toward integrating the psychotherapies: an overview. *American Journal of Psychiatry*, **146**(2), 138–147.

Bennett, M.R. and **Hacker, P.M.S.** (2003). *Philosophical Foundations of Neuroscience*. Oxford: Blackwell Publishing.

Berrios, G.E. (2014). Defining and classifying mental illness. In: S. Bloch, S.A. Green, and J. Holmes (Eds.), *Psychiatry: Past, Present, and Prospect* (pp. 180–195). Oxford: Oxford University Press.

Bhugra, D., Easter, A., Mallaris, Y. and **Gupta, S.** (2011). Clinical decision making in psychiatry by psychiatrists. *Acta Psychiatrica Scandinavica*, **124**(5), 403–411.

Boyd, C. and **Kent, D.** (2014). Evidence-based medicine and the hard problem of multimorbidity. *Journal of General Internal Medicine*, **29**(4), 552–553.

Boyle, M. and **Johnstone, L.** (2014). Alternatives to psychiatric diagnosis. *Lancet Psychiatry*, **1**(6), 409–411.

Cannon, W.B. (1939). *The Wisdom of the Body*. New York: Norton & Company.

Cohen, S.M. (2012). Aristotle's metaphysics (1045a8–10). In: E.N. Zalta (Ed.), *The Stanford Encyclopedia of Philosophy*, Summer 2012 ed. http://plato.stanford.edu/archives/sum2012/entries/aristotle-metaphysics/

Cramer, A.O.J., Waldorp, L.J., Van Der Maas, H.L.J. and **Borsboom, D.** (2010). Comorbidity: a network perspective. *Behavioral and Brain Sciences*, **33**(2–3). 137–150.

Doessing, A. and **Burau, V.** (2015). Care coordination of multimorbidity: a scoping study. *Journal of Comorbidity*, **5**, 15–28.

Doll, W.E. and **Trueit, D.** (2010). Complexity and the health care professions. *Journal of Evaluation in Clinical Practice*, **16**(4), 841–848.

Eells, T.D. (1997). History and current status of psychotherapy case formulation. In: T.D. Eells (Ed.), *Handbook of Psychotherapy Case Formulation* (pp. 1–32). New York: Guildford Press.

Emmeche, C., Koppe, S. and Stjernfelt, F. (1997/2003). Explaining emergence: towards an ontology of levels. In: G. Midgley (Ed.), *Systems Thinking. Volume 1 General Systems Theory, Cybernetics and Complexity* (pp. 141–170). London: Sage publications,

Engel, G.L. (1954a). Studies of ulcerative colitis. I. Clinical data bearing on the nature of the somatic process. *Psychosomatic Medicine*, **16**(6), 496–501.

Engel, G.L. (1954b). Studies of ulcerative colitis. II. The nature of the somatic processes and the adequacy of psychosomatic hypotheses. *American Journal of Medicine*, **16**(3), 416–433.

Engel, G.L. (1955). Studies of ulcerative colitis. III. The nature of the psychologic processes. *American Journal of Medicine*, **19**(2), 231–256.

Engel, G.L. (1958). Studies of ulcerative colitis. V. Psychological aspects and their implications for treatment. *American Journal of Digestive Disorders*, **3**(4), 315–337.

Engel, G.L. (1960). A unified concept of health and disease. *Perspectives in Biology and Medicine*, **3**, 459–485.

Engel, G.L. (1965). Clinical observation. *JAMA*, **192**, 157–160.

Engel, G.L. (1971). The deficiencies of the case presentation as a method of clinical teaching. Another approach. *New England Journal of Medicine*, **284**(1), 20–24.

Engel, G.L. (1973). Enduring attributes of medicine relevant for the education of the physician. *Annals of Internal Medicine*, **78**(4), 587–593.

Engel, G.L. (1977a). The need for a new medical model: a challenge for biomedicine. *Science*, **196**(4286), 129–136.

Engel, G.L. (1977b). The care of the patient: art or science? *The Johns Hopkins Medical Journal*, **140**(5), 222–232.

Engel, G.L. (1978). The biopsychosocial model and the education of health professionals. *Annals of the New York Academy of Sciences*, **310**, 169–187.

Engel, G.L. (1980). The clinical application of the biopsychosocial model. *American Journal of Psychiatry*, **137**(5), 535–544.

Engel, G.L. (1986). Foreword. In: J.O. Beahrs, *Limits of Scientific Psychiatry–the Role of Uncertainty in Mental Health* (p. xviii). New York, NY: Brunner–Mazel.

Engel, G.L. (1987). Physician-scientists and scientific physicians. Resolving the humanism-science dichotomy. *The American Journal of Medicine*, **82**(1), 107–111.

Engel, G.L. (1992). How much longer must medicine's science be bound by a 17th century world view? *Psychotherapy and Psychosomatics*, **57**(1–2), 3–16.

Engel, G.L. (1997). From biomedical to biopsychosocial. 1. Being scientific in the human domain. *Psychotherapy and Psychosomatics*, **66**(2), 57–62.

Faulkner, L.R., Kinzie, J.D., Angell, R., U'Ren, R.C., and Shore, J.H. (1985). A comprehensive psychiatric formulation model. *The Journal of Psychiatric Education*, **9**, 189–203.

Frede, M. (1996a). Aristotle's rationalism. In: M. Frede and G. Striker (Eds.), *Rationality in Greek Thought* (pp. 157–174). Oxford: Clarendon Press.

Frede, M. (1996b). Introduction. In: M. Frede and G. Striker (Eds.), *Rationality in Greek Thought* (pp. 1–28). Oxford: Clarendon Press.

Gare, A. (2000). Systems theory and complexity: introduction. *Democracy & Nature*, **6**(3), 327–339.

Gare, A. (2013). Overcoming the Newtonian paradigm: the unfinished project of theoretical biology from a Shellingian perspective. *Progress in Biophysics and Molecular Biology*, **113**(1), 5–24.

Gay, P. (2007). *Modernism: The Lure of Heresy: From Baudelaire to Beckett and Beyond.* London: William Heinemann.

Ghaemi, S.N. (2011). The biopsychosocial model in psychiatry: a critique. *Existenz*, **6**(1). http://www.bu.edu/paidea/existenz/volumes/Vol.6-1Ghaemi.html

Greenberg, M., Szmukler, G. and Tantam, D. (1981). Guidelines on formulation. *Bulletin of the Royal College of Psychiatrists*, **5**, 160–162.

Gregory, R.L. (2004). Homeostasis. In: R. L. Gregory (Ed.), *The Oxford Companion to the Mind* (2nd ed., p. 401). Oxford: Oxford University Press.

Grinker, R.R. (1964). Psychiatry rides madly in all directions. *Archives of General Psychiatry*, **10**, 228–237.

Gupta, M. (2003). A critical appraisal of evidence-based medicine: some ethical considerations. *Journal of Evaluation in Clinical Practice*, **9**(2), 111–121.

Gupta, M. (2011). Improved health or improved decision making? The ethical goals of EBM. *Journal of Evaluation in Clinical Practice*, **17**(5), 957–963.

Gustafson, D. (2005). Associationism. In: T. Honderich (Ed.), *The Oxford Companion to Philosophy* (2nd ed., pp. 63–64). Oxford: Oxford University Press.

Haig, B.D. (2005). An abductive theory of scientific method. *Psychological Methods*, **10**(4), 371–378.

Heil, J. (2005). Holism. In: T. Honderich (Ed.), *The Oxford Companion to Philosophy* (2nd ed., pp. 397–398). Oxford: Oxford University Press.

Haslam, N. (2013). Reliability, validity, and the mixed blessings of operationalism. In: K.W.M. Fulford, M. Davies, R.G.T. Gipps, G. Graham, J.Z. Sadler, G. Stranghellini and T. Thornton (Eds.), *The Oxford Handbook of Philosophy and Psychiatry* (pp. 987–1002). Oxford: Oxford University Press.

Holmes, A., Singh, B. and McColl, G. (2011). Revisiting the hypothesis-driven interview in a contemporary context. *Australasian Psychiatry*, **19**(6), 484–488.

Hookway, C.J. (2005). Abduction. In: T. Honderich (Ed.), *The Oxford Companion to Philosophy* (2nd ed., p. 1). Oxford: Oxford University Press.

Jayasinghe, S. (2012). Complexity science to conceptualize health and disease: is it relevant to clinical medicine? *Mayo Clinic Proceedings*, **87**(4), 314–319.

Johnstone, L. and Dallos, R. (Eds.) (2013). *Formulation in Psychology and Psychotherapy: Making Sense of People's Problems* (2nd ed.). New York: Routledge.

Kallio, E. (2011). Integrative thinking is the key: an evaluation of current research into the development of adult thinking. *Theory & Psychology*, **21**(6), 785–801.

Kingma, E. (2013). Naturalist accounts of mental disorder. In: K.W.M. Fulford, M. Davies, R.G.T. Gipps, G. Graham, J.Z. Sadler, G. Stranghellini and T. Thornton (Eds.), *The Oxford Handbook of Philosophy and Psychiatry*, pp. 365–366. Oxford: Oxford University Press.

Kirmayer, L.J. (2007). Psychotherapy and the cultural concept of the person. *Transcultural Psychiatry*, **44**(2), 232–257.

Kurtz, F. and Snowden, D.J. (2003). The new dynamics of strategy: sense-making in a complex and complicated world. *IBM Systems Journal*, **42**(3), 462–483.

Lacey, A. (2005). Humanism. In: T. Honderich (Ed.), *The Oxford Companion to Philosophy* (2nd ed., pp. 481–482). Oxford: Oxford University Press.

Loughlin, M., Bluhm, R., Buetow, S., Upshur, R.E.G., Goldenberg, M.J., Borgerson, K., Entwisle, V. and Kingma, E. (2012). Reason and value: making reasoning fit for practice. *Journal of Evaluation in Medical Practice*, **18**(5), 929–937.

Lugtenberg, M., Burgers, J.S., Clancy, C., Westert, G.P. and Schneider, E.C. (2011). Current guidelines have limited applicability to patients with comorbid conditions: a systematic analysis of evidence-based guidelines. *PLoS One*, **6**(10). E25987.

M'Pherson, P.K. (1974/2003). A perspective on systems science and systems philosophy. In: G. Midgley (Ed.), *Systems Thinking. Volume 1 General Systems Theory, Cybernetics and Complexity* (pp. 119–140). London: Sage Publications.

Marková, I.S. and Berrios, G.E. (2009). Epistemology of mental symptoms. *Psychopathology*, **42**(6), 343–349.

Marková, I.S. and Berrios, G.E. (2012). Epistemology of psychiatry. *Psychopathology*, **45**(4), 220–227.

Muir Gray, J.A. (2008). Viva the revolution. *Health Information and Libraries Journal*, **25** (Suppl. 1), 96–98.

Nolte, E. and Pitchforth, E. (2014). *What is the Evidence on the Economic Impacts of Integrated Care?* Copenhagen: World Health Organization. http://www.euro.who.int/__data/assets/pdf_file/0019/251434/What-is-the-evidence-on-the-economic-impacts-of-integrated-care.pdf

Nutton, V. (2013). *Ancient Medicine* (2nd ed.). Abingdon: Routledge.

Nyklicek, I. and Denollet, J. (2009). Development and evaluation of the Balanced Index of Psychological Mindedness (BIPM). *Psychological Assessment*, **21**(1), 32–44.

Paley, J. (2010). The appropriation of complexity theory in health care. *Journal of Health Services Research & Policy*, **15**(1), 59–61.

Parsons, T. (1977a). On building social system theory: a personal history. In: *Social Systems and the Evolution of Action Theory* (pp. 22–76). New York: The Free Press.

Parsons, T. (1977b). Some problems of general theory in sociology. In: *Social Systems and the Evolution of Action Theory* (pp. 229–269). New York: The Free Press.

Perry, S., Cooper, A.M. and Michels, R. (1987). The psychodynamic formulation: its purpose, structure, and clinical application. *American Journal of Psychiatry*, **144**(5), 543–550.

Plsek, P.E. and Greenhalgh, T. (2001). The challenge of complexity in health care. *BMJ*, **323**(7313), 625–628.

Poland, J. and Von Eckardt, B. (2013). Mapping the domain of mental illness. In: K.W.M. Fulford, M. Davies, R.G.T. Gipps, G. Graham, J.Z. Sadler, G. Stranghellini and T. Thornton (Eds.), *The Oxford Handbook of Philosophy and Psychiatry* (pp. 735–752). Oxford: Oxford University Press.

Polanyi, M. (1966). *The Tacit Dimension*. London: Routledge & Kegan Paul.

Porter, R. (1997). *The Greatest Benefit to Mankind: A Medical History of Humanity from Antiquity to the Present*. London: HarperCollins.

Ruse, R. (2005). Reductionism. In: T. Honderich (Ed.), *The Oxford Companion to Philosophy* (2nd ed., pp. 793–794). Oxford: Oxford University Press.

Sanford, D.H. (2005). Inference to the best explanation. In: T. Honderich (Ed.), *The Oxford Companion to Philosophy* (2nd ed., p. 434). Oxford: Oxford University Press.

Sharpe, R. (2005). Metaphor. In: T. Honderich (Ed.), *The Oxford Companion to Philosophy* (2nd ed., p. 589). Oxford: Oxford University Press.

Schwartz, M.A. and Wiggins, O. (1985). Science, humanism, and the nature of medical practice: a phenomenological view. *Perspectives in Biology and Medicine*, **28**(3), 231–261.

Schwartz, M.A. and Wiggins, O.P. (1986). Systems and structuring of meaning: contributions to biopsychosocial medicine. *American Journal of Psychiatry*, **143**(10), 1213–1221.

Scurlock, J.A. and **Andersen, B.R.** (2005). *Diagnoses in Assyrian and Babylonian Medicine: Ancient Sources, Translations, and Modern Medical Analyses.* Urbana, IL: The University of Illinois Press.

Smith, G.C. (2009). From consultation-liaison psychiatry to integrated care for multiple and complex needs. *Australian and New Zealand Journal of Psychiatry*, **43**(1), 1–12.

Smith, G.C. (2014a). Revisiting formulation Part 1. The tasks of formulation: their rationale and philosophic basis. *Australasian Psychiatry*, **22**(1), 23–27.

Smith, G.C. (2014b). Revisiting formulation. Part 2. The task of addressing the concept of the unique individual. Remediating problems with formulation. *Australasian Psychiatry*, **22**(1), 28–31.

Smith, G.C. and **Strain, J.J.** (2002). George Engel's contribution to clinical psychiatry. *Australian and New Zealand Journal of Psychiatry*, **36**(4), 458–466.

Sperry, L., **Gudeman, J.E.**, **Blackwell., B.** and **Faulkner, L.R.** (1992). *Psychiatric Case Formulations.* Washington, DC: American Psychiatric Press.

The British Psychological Society Division of Clinical Psychology (2011). Good practice guidelines on the use of psychological formulation. https://www.canterbury.ac.uk/social-and-applied-sciences/salomons-centre-for-applied-psychology/docs/resources/DCP-Guidelines-for-Formulation.pdf

Thornton, T. (2013). Clinical judgement, tacit knowledge, and recognition in psychiatric diagnosis. In: K.W.M. Fulford, M. Davies, R.G.T. Gipps, G. Graham, J.Z. Sadler, G. Stranghellini and T. Thornton (Eds.), *The Oxford Handbook of Philosophy and Psychiatry* (pp. 1047–1062). Oxford: Oxford University Press.

Tinetti, M.E., **Fried, T.R.** and **Boyd, C.M.** (2012). Designing health care for the most common chronic condition—multimorbidity. *JAMA*, **307**(23), 2493–2494.

von Bertalanffy, L. (1928/1975). The heritage of Cusamus. In: L. von Bertalanffy (edited by E. Taschdjian), *Perspectives on General System Theory: Scientific-Philosophical Studies* (pp. 53–66). New York: George Braziller.

von Bertalanffy, L. (1937/1975). The organismic conception. In L. von Bertalanffy (edited by E. Taschdjian), *Perspectives on General System Theory: Scientific-Philosophical Studies* (pp. 97–102). New York: George Braziller.

von Bertalanffy, L. (1960/1975). New patterns in biological and medical thought. In L. von Bertalanffy (edited by E. Taschdjian), *Perspectives on General System Theory: Scientific-Philosophical Studies* (pp. 40–53). New York: George Braziller.

von Bertalanffy, L. (1965/1975). Theoretical models in biology. In L. von Bertalanffy (edited by E. Taschdjian), *Perspectives on General System Theory: Scientific-Philosophical Studies* (pp. 103–114). New York: George Braziller.

von Bertalanffy, L. (1969). *General System Theory: Foundations, Development, Applications*, revised edn. New York: George Braziller.

von Bertalanffy, L. (1972). The history and status of general systems theory. *Academy of Management Journal*, **December**, 407–426.

von Bertalanffy, L. (1972/1975). The history and development of General System Theory. In: L. von Bertalanffy (edited by E. Taschdjian), *Perspectives on General System Theory: Scientific-Philosophical Studies* (pp. 149–169). New York: George Braziller.

von Bertalanffy, L. (edited by E. Taschdjian) (1975). *Perspectives on General System Theory: Scientific-philosophical Studies.* New York: George Braziller.

von Bertalanffy, L. (1975/1975). Cultures as systems. In L. von Bertalanffy (edited by E. Taschdjian), *Perspectives on General System Theory. Scientific-Philosophical Studies* (pp. 74–84). New York: George Braziller.

Walsh, B.W. and Peterson, L.E (1985). Philosophical foundations of psychological theories: the issue of synthesis. *Psychotherapy*, **22**(2), 145–153.

Zaretsky, E. (2004). *Secrets of the Soul: A Social and Cultural History of Psychoanalysis.* New York: Alfred A. Knopf.

Part 3

Risk and Resilience

Chapter 10

Developmental risk and resilience: The challenge of translating multilevel data to concrete interventions

Essi Viding

Introduction

Poor mental health is one of the leading causes of the overall disease burden in the world and touches all of us, either directly or through the experiences of our friends and family. It has been estimated that 25% of the adults in the UK suffer from a diagnosable mental health problem at any one time (McManus et al., 2009). The majority of mental illnesses have their roots in childhood, with 50% of lifetime cases of diagnosable mental illness beginning by 14 years of age and 75% before the age of 18 (Kim-Cohen et al., 2003; Kessler et al., 2007). The most recent national surveys of child and adolescent mental health, in 1999 and 2004, found that 10% of children and young people (aged 5–16 years)—three in every average classroom—had a clinically diagnosable mental health problem (Green at al., 2005). Childhood mental health problems can adversely affect emotional and social development, educational achievement, physical health, and later chances of employment (Odgers et al., 2007; MQ: Transforming Mental Health, 2016).

We are still a long way from effectively treating mental health problems in childhood or adulthood. Even the best treatments are relatively limited (helping at most 50% of the sufferers) and a significant proportion of individuals who suffer from mental health problems either do not improve or relapse following treatment (e.g. Thase et al., 2009). There is a clear need for a better evidence base on the causal risk factors that precipitate the development of mental ill health, as well as interventions that work to prevent and treat mental illness in children and young people. We need to delineate how causal mechanisms at different levels of analyses unfold across development and we need to understand the role of different environmental ecologies in canalizing particular vulnerabilities to disordered outcomes. Why has this task been so complicated and why has the progress been so slow to date?

Equifinality and multifinality

We measure mental health outcomes by charting behavioural symptom criteria. Yet, it is no surprise to mental health practitioners that two individuals qualifying for the same diagnosis can present with remarkably different histories or core difficulties, even if they share certain aspects of their presentation. The term 'equifinality' refers to the notion that a particular outcome/end state (e.g. diagnosis) can be reached by many potential means. In other words, just because two individuals qualify for the same behaviourally defined diagnosis, we cannot assume that the aetiology of their presentation is identical. They may present with comparable behaviours for different underlying reasons. If these individuals are treated with a single intervention, possibly targeting the underlying causal factors important for person A, it is by no means inevitable that person B will be helped. The recognition of the problems of relying on behavioural diagnoses has led to initiatives such as the US National Institute of Mental Health's Research Domain Criteria (RDoC), which encourages researchers to focus on basic dimensions of functioning (e.g. threat reactivity variously specified) rather than diagnostic criteria. The aim of such initiatives is to elucidate how individual differences in a particular domain/construct, such as negative valence representation probed by paradigms targeting the functioning of threat circuitry, may increase the risk of developing psychiatric disorder.

The research focus advocated by the RDoC initiative is important, but has its own set of challenges. Most practitioners recognize that particular shared traits or difficulties can characterize two individuals who in fact qualify for different diagnoses or may even be present in some individuals who appear largely free from mental health problems. In their seminal article on equifinality and multifinality in developmental psychopathology, Cicchetti and Rogosch (1996, pp. 597–598) wrote: 'The principle of multifinality (Wilden, 1980) suggests that any one component may function differently depending on the organization of the system in which it operates.' Individuals who share particular characteristics, for example the degree to which their amygdala originally responds to threat, can differ in their genetic and environmental endowments. This in turn may spell individual differences in the ability to regulate the amygdala response and in the range of likely choices and behaviours available to that particular person. In other words, developmental outcomes for people with similar amygdala responsivity in childhood may vary considerably, a phenomenon known as 'multifinality'.

Both equi- and multifinality pose substantial challenges to our attempts to understand dynamic development of risk and resilience across the lifespan. Cicchetti and Rogosch wrote the following over 20 years ago:

> This attention to diversity in origins, processes, and outcomes in understanding developmental pathways does not suggest that prediction is futile as a result of the many potential individual patterns of adaptation (Sroufe, 1989). There are constraints on how much diversity is possible, and not all outcomes are equally likely (Cicchetti & Tucker, 1994a; Sroufe et al., 1990). Nonetheless, the appreciation of equifinality and multifinality in development encourages theorists and researchers to entertain more complex and varied approaches to how they conceptualize and investigate development and psychopathology. (Cicchetti and Rogosch, 1996, p. 599)

Although progress has been made, it has been slow. In part this may be because not everyone in the field has heeded Cicchetti and Rogosch's counsel and in part because developmental psychopathology is only now starting to get the attention that it deserves. In the following section of this chapter, I will use my own area of research, the development of antisocial behaviour (conduct problems) in children and youth, to illustrate how we can use multiple levels of analyses to study heterogeneity within a diagnostic category. I will also use this area of research to illustrate the challenges of integrating multilevel data to understand the development of psychopathology.

Conduct problems as an 'illustration'

Diagnosis of conduct disorder

Conduct problems refer to antisocial behaviour in children and in young people, behaviours that constitute violations of age-appropriate societal norms and rights of other people. In order to be diagnosed with conduct disorder, a child/young person has to present with at least three conduct problem behaviours during a sustained (12-month) period of time to the level that causes clinically significant impairment in social, educational, or occupational functioning (American Psychiatric Association, 2013). Symptoms of conduct disorder include bullying and threatening other people, violence, cruelty to people or animals, physical fights, robbery, coercion, running away, destruction of property, and truanting (American Psychiatric Association, 2013).

Heterogeneity

Unsurprisingly, children who present with conduct problems form a heterogeneous population. They do not all have an identical presentation or identical risk factors for their conduct problems and as such, this population illustrates the inherent challenge of uncovering underlying mechanisms for a disorder identified with behavioural symptom criteria. How should we go about our research efforts in a sensible way?

Typically, when we try to study mechanisms that are related to disordered outcome, we select individuals based on their behavioural symptoms and try to find an underlying cause. There is a clear circularity of argument here. We already know that children and young people who qualify for a conduct disorder diagnosis are unlikely to all present within this diagnostic category for the same underlying reason. Yet we use behaviourally defined diagnostic criteria to select individuals to take part in our research, then try and look for mechanisms. If we accept that in all likelihood there are conduct disorders, rather than a conduct disorder, then such an approach is not likely to take us very far.

One way to potentially get around this problem is to use subtle differences in behaviour to provide clues for subsequent systematic investigation at different levels of analyses. This approach is clearly not ideal as we are still starting with behaviour and we cannot assume that the behavioural indicators we have chosen, or our ability to observe them, are always entirely accurate. But it is perhaps the best we have as a starting point and once the data accumulate, they will indicate to us how reasonable this starting point has been. We can assess whether the behavioural indicators that we have used provide meaningful differentiation at multiple levels of analyses.

Callous-unemotional traits as a subtyping indicator for children with conduct problems

One of the ways in which we can differentiate the children who present with conduct problems is by charting so-called callous–unemotional (CU) traits in these children. After 20 years of research using multiple methodologies, these traits have now been included as the 'limited prosocial emotions' specifier to the *Diagnostic and Statistical Manual of Mental Disorders*, fifth edition, conduct disorder diagnosis (American Psychiatric Association, 2013). Behaviourally, children with conduct problems and high levels of CU traits (henceforth CP/HCU) show a marked lack of empathy or guilt (Frick et al., 2014; Viding and McCrory, 2015). They are capable of engaging in proactive, instrumentally aggressive acts to get what they want, seem impervious to sanctions, and do not appear to exhibit the affiliative needs and goals that characterize typical children (Frick et al., 2014; Viding and McCrory, 2015). In contrast, children who have conduct problems and low levels of CU traits (henceforth CP/LCU) often aggress when they feel under threat or are frustrated, are capable of feeling guilt and empathy, and form strong affiliative bonds with other people (Frick and Viding, 2009).

Behavioural experimental data on CU subtyping indicator

Many of the experimental studies on children with CP/HCU have focused on how they process emotions, whether they empathize with others, how they attend to caregivers, and whether they change their behaviour following punishment (e.g. see Kimonis et al., 2008; Marsh and Blair, 2008; Jones et al., 2010; Dadds et al., 2011, 2012; Sylvers et al., 2011; Schwenck et al., 2012; de Wied et al., 2012; Blair et al., 2014; Hodsoll et al., 2014; Bedford et al., 2015; White et al., 2016; Martin-Key et al., 2017). The majority of these studies have documented that, compared with typically developing children, those with CP/HCU are less likely to attend to, react to, and recognize affective stimuli, including distress cues such as fearful and sad expressions of other people; are more likely to show blunted empathy towards others; are less likely to direct attention to the eyes of attachment figures; have difficulty learning from punishment; and adapt less well to changes in reward–punishment contingencies. I and others (see e.g. Blair, 2017) think that this presentation explains why children with CP/HCU are so difficult to socialize and explains their reduced threshold in engaging in instrumental aggression. When we socialize young children, we deploy empathy induction. We ask the children to imagine how someone else is feeling, particularly if the child has done something hurtful to the other person. We also give sanctions when a child behaves in a way we do not approve of. If someone's distress does not impact a child and if sanctions do not matter, two powerful and typical tools of socialization are no longer effective.

We have less experimental data specifically pertaining to CP/LCU children. Like children with CP/HCU, they have difficulties in adapting to changes in reward–punishment contingencies, which may explain frustration-based aggression in this group (Blair et al., 2018). Children with CP/LCU also appear typical on many measures of empathy (e.g. Jones et al., 2010) and can show heightened (rather than reduced) responsivity to emotional stimuli (e.g. Penton-Voak et al., 2013).

Neural correlates on CP/HCU and CP/LCU

Several functional magnetic resonance imaging (fMRI) studies have indicated a neural activity profile consistent with low emotional responsiveness to others' distress/pain and poor ability to learn from reinforcement information in children with CP/HCU (Blair et al., 2014; Viding and McCrory, 2015).[1] For example, reduced amygdala activity to fearful faces CP/HCU children—relative to CP/LCU children, typically developing children, or children with attentional difficulties—has been reported in a number of studies using both incidental affective processing and attention to emotion paradigms (e.g. see Marsh et al., 2008; Jones et al., 2009; Viding et al., 2012; White et al., 2012; Blair et al., 2014). One study found that the association between CU traits and proactive aggression is partially mediated by low amygdala reactivity to fearful faces (Lozier et al., 2014). Reduced amygdala and insula activity in the CP/HCU group is also seen when these children engage in more complex forms of social judgement regarding other people's distress, such as categorization of legal and illegal behaviours in moral judgement tasks (Marsh et al., 2011), making decisions about appropriate responses to the distress of others (Sebastian et al., 2012), or making decisions about whether to benefit self by harming others (Sakai et al., 2017). Finally, five recent studies of children exhibiting conduct problems and varying levels of CU traits (four involving fMRI, and the other brain event-related potential measurement) have reported atypical neural reactivity to other people's pain (Cheng et al., 2012; Lockwood et al., 2013; Marsh et al., 2013; Michalska et al., 2015; Yoder et al., 2016). Collectively, these studies implicate reduced activity and altered connectivity in children with CP/HCU, in a network of brain areas known to be associated with empathy for other people's pain in healthy individuals. This network encompasses a number of brain regions including the anterior insula, posterior insula, anterior cingulate cortex, and the amygdala. Importantly, this profile of reduced neural activity to expressions of pain is not coupled with difficulty in understanding intentionality on the part of others (Cheng et al., 2012).

Interestingly, children with CP/LCU appear to either show exaggerated, rather than reduced, amygdala activity to emotional stimuli (Viding et al., 2012; Sebastian et al., 2013) or do not appear different from typically developing children (Hwang et al., 2016). All children with conduct problems appear to show compromised sensitivity to early reinforcement information in the ventromedial prefrontal cortex/orbitofrontal cortex and caudate, and compromised sensitivity to reward outcome information in the ventromedial prefrontal cortex/orbitofrontal cortex (e.g. White et al.,

---

[1] A number of other neuroimaging methodologies (both structural and functional) have been used to interrogate the neural correlates of conduct problems. I focus on fMRI studies here for illustrative purposes, because they represent the most common functional neuroimaging studies of conduct problems and report data that are most readily comparable with behavioural experimental findings.

2013, 2014)—with the degree of dysfunction tracking the levels of conduct disorder symptoms (White et al., 2016). If, as is the case for individuals with CP/HCU, you do not automatically orient to and resonate with other people's distress, it will be easier (less distressing) to commit aggression against other people. If, furthermore, you are not able to optimally compute the potential consequences of your own behaviour, you make poor choices—even if you end up worse off because of them. If, as is the case for individuals with CP/LCU, you sometimes find neutral or potentially threatening stimuli particularly salient, you are more likely to prime a defensive 'fight' response and engage in reactive aggression. If you are also poor at computing reward–punishment contingencies, your ability to plan ahead is compromised and you are more likely to experience frustration. Interestingly, the pattern of neural activity we have observed for the CP/LCU children is very similar to what our group has also reported in studies of children who have experienced family violence and childhood maltreatment (e.g. McCrory et al., 2011, 2013). It may be that the pattern of emotional responsiveness (behavioural and neural) seen in CP/LCU children represents adaptation to stimuli that signal the potential for physical or emotional abuse. In other words, some individuals sadly grow up in environments where it pays to be hypervigilant to potential threat.

Collectively, these functional neuroimaging findings are largely in line with findings from studies of psychopathic and antisocial adults (e.g. Kiehl et al., 2001; Birbaumer et al., 2005; for a comprehensive review, see Seara-Cardoso and Viding, 2014) and suggest functional neural bases for (1) why children with CP/HCU appear relatively unaffected by other people's distress, readily aggress against others to fulfil their own needs, and often make and repeat disadvantageous decisions; and (2) why children with CP/LCU may present with frustration-based aggression or reactive aggression and behave impulsively.

Genetic and environmental risk

Studies by our group suggest that CP/HCU and CP/LCU differ aetiologically (Viding et al., 2005, 2008). Conduct problems in the presence of HCU are strongly heritable (81% of group difference in conduct problems between CP/HCU and typically developing children is due to genetic influences), whereas environmental factors more readily explain the group difference in conduct problems between CP/LCU and typically developing children (for these children only about one-third of the group difference in conduct problems is due to genetic factors). Our findings do not mean that children with CP/HCU are genetically destined to become antisocial. In interpreting findings from genetically informative studies, it is of critical importance to keep in mind that *there are no genes that directly give rise to CU traits or conduct problems*. Genes code for proteins that influence characteristics such as neurocognitive vulnerabilities that may in turn increase *risk for* developing CU traits or conduct problems. We know that the neurocognitive vulnerabilities associated with CP/HCU and CP/LCU are at least partially distinct, with the former group displaying reduced and the latter heightened neural activity to affective stimuli (as mentioned previously). This suggests that the risk alleles for CP/HCU may not always be the same as risk alleles for CP/LCU.

At the current time, the evidence base does not enable us to reliably identify specific genetic risk factors for CP/HCU and CP/LCU. This is in part because most studies to date have focused on undifferentiated antisocial behaviour phenotypes. A handful of candidate gene-association studies to date have focused on CU traits in children or adolescents, and these studies have tentatively implicated variants of genes related to the serotonin and oxytocin systems (e.g. Fowler et al., 2009; Beichtman et al., 2012; Malik et al., 2012; Dadds et al., 2013; Moul et al., 2013). These associations need to be investigated in larger samples to evaluate whether they reflect true replicable findings. Increasingly, researchers in psychiatric genetics are focusing on genome-wide association (GWA), rather than candidate gene studies. The GWA studies systematically scan the genome with hundreds of thousands of DNA markers, made possible by DNA arrays. GWA studies focusing specifically on CU traits suggest that much larger samples will be needed to detect novel associations with common single nucleotide polymorphisms that account for far less than 1% of the variance (Viding et al., 2010, 2013). Furthermore, one genome-wide complex trait analysis study suggests that most of the genetic variance that is important for explaining genetically driven individual differences in CU traits (or conduct problems for that matter) is not due to the additive effects of common genetic variants (Trzaskowski et al., 2013). This means that the search for genetic influences on CP/HCU and CP/LCU is likely to be complicated by the presence of gene–gene interactions and rare variants, as well as gene–environment interplay.

Although an individual's genome likely limits a 'range for phenotypic expression', it does not pre-specify how an individual will turn out. The specific developmental trajectory of any individual is determined by a complex interplay between genetic propensities and other factors that constrain how those genetic propensities are expressed at several different levels of analyses, across development. Genetic variants that are implicated as risk genes for conduct problems and/or CU traits may include several genes that confer advantages, as well as disadvantages, depending on the environmental context. It is also of critical importance to remember that an individual's genetic predisposition influences the types of environments the individual will encounter, a phenomenon known as gene–environment correlation (rGE). For example, an individual's genetic predisposition may influence behaviours that will in turn evoke different reactions in others. In order to understand how environmental risk operates in relation to the development of CP/HCU and CP/LCU it is thus important to conduct research into environmental risk within genetically informative study designs.

Studies into the development of conduct problems, including those executed within genetically informative designs, identify maltreatment, harsh discipline, and negative parental affect as environmental risk factors for conduct problems (e.g. Moffitt, 2005). Research also indicates that while conduct problems of CP/LCU show a dose–response association with harsh/negative parenting, conduct problems of CP/HCU children do not show this dose–response association (Frick and Viding, 2009). To date, only three genetically informative longitudinal studies have investigated parenting and development of CU traits (Viding et al., 2009; Hyde et al., 2016; Waller et al., 2016). Results from the first of these studies, capitalizing on a monozygotic-twin differences design, suggest that the association between harsh and negative parenting and higher levels of

CU traits in children may, at least in part, reflect genetic vulnerability within families (Viding et al., 2009). This could either reflect a shared genetic vulnerability for poor parenting and CU temperament, or an effect of CU temperament in evoking negative/harsh parenting. Does this mean that we should feel pessimistic about intervention prospects for CP/HCU children? Recent findings from an adoption cohort suggest otherwise (Hyde et al., 2016; Waller et al., 2016). Two studies based on this cohort showed that levels of antisocial behaviour and fearlessness in the *biological mother* predicted early CU behaviours in toddlers who had been adopted—in line with our twin study findings of genetic risk for CU traits and CP/HCU. However, high levels of *adoptive mother* positive reinforcement were able to buffer the effects of heritable risk for CU behaviours (Hyde et al., 2016; Waller et al., 2016). These findings are extremely encouraging, although it is important to bear in mind that parents in adoptive families are typically very motivated to undertake the challenges of parenting and are also often relatively well resourced. By contrast, in biological families, parents of children with CU traits are more likely to have a host of genetic and contextual risk factors (including socioeconomic disadvantage), which can make it more difficult to deliver interventions that seek to increase positive reinforcement behaviours by parents towards a behaviourally challenging child.

Clinical implications

We now have an emerging evidence base regarding the different aetiology and presentation of children with CP/HCU and CP/LCU. We can demonstrate differentiation between these groups at multiple levels of analyses. This offers an example of how particular differences in behavioural presentation can be used to motivate systematic investigation of different pathways to a disordered outcome. The challenge over the next decade will be to more comprehensively delineate what precisely works for CP/HCU and CP/LCU children and how current intervention and prevention programmes can be optimized in ways that improve engagement as well as clinical outcomes. To optimize existing interventions (as well as engagement), we may need a better understanding of rGE processes. Such research has the potential to inform clinical approaches that promote warm and consistent parenting. For example, a child with CU traits is more likely to evoke negative parenting responses (as well as a sense of parental inadequacy) and will furnish more infrequent occasions for parental praise or reward. This in turn increases the likelihood that the pattern of parent–child interaction becomes largely negative in tone. Furthermore, the biological parents of such a child may themselves share some of the same vulnerabilities that characterize their child and may find it harder to implement many aspects of typical parenting intervention programmes. Biological families of children with CU traits may need additional (or different forms of) clinical support in order to facilitate a shift towards more positive patterns of parent–child interaction. These could include intensive and supported reward token-economy adjuncts and extensive support in increasing warm parent–child interactions (see Armstrong and Kimonis, 2013 for a promising case study).

In addition, it will be important to examine the degree to which the neurocognitive biases associated with CP/HCU and CP/LCU are malleable as this will help inform the development of adjuncts to existing parenting or family focused clinical interventions. If it transpires (for example) that a given bias is not malleable, it may be more fruitful to focus on the development of compensatory processes that can have the effect of normalizing behaviour. Relatedly, we also need to investigate whether there are particularly sensitive developmental periods during which the neurocognitive functioning may be most responsive to intervention. Given that the child's processing of the world around them is likely to impact their social interactions, development of treatment adjuncts can also be seen as providing extra scaffolding for a positive parent–child (or child–peer) relationship and attenuating rGE processes that might otherwise unfold over development.

Conduct problems as a 'case study': summary

I have used the study of children with conduct problems as an illustration of how we can use data from multiple levels of analyses to investigate heterogeneity within a diagnostic criterion. Despite all the exciting data that have accumulated in the past 20 years alone, a number of challenges remain. These are not challenges that are unique to the study of conduct problems, but apply to other developmental psychopathology phenotypes as well.

1. *How should we best define our phenotypes?* To date, we have mainly worked backwards from behaviour. We need more work with putative risk mechanisms as a starting point, but we need to be mindful of multifinality and devise incisive ways of meaningfully studying that phenomenon.

2. *How can we find genes associated with disorder risk or resilience?* These are likely to at least partly differ for subtypes of any given disorder (e.g. CP/HCU vs CP/LCU) and the quest will be further complicated by genes of small effect size, rare variants, gene–environment interactions, gene–gene interactions, and developmentally specific genetic effects.

3. *How can we better understand environmental contributions to maladaptive or resilient outcomes?* Again, environmental factors influencing an outcome may not be equal for all individuals who get the same diagnosis (e.g. CP/HCU vs CP/LCU) and are likely to include a variety of pre- and postnatal factors. For most mental health conditions, environmental risk factors come in multiples. This means that the impact of a single risk factor may be difficult to isolate and is likely vary depending on the presence versus absence of other risk factors. There also needs to be more work directed at understanding protective factors, both those that occur naturally and those that can be delivered via interventions designed to promote resilience. Interventions afford a degree of experimental control that is not possible to achieve when quantifying naturally occurring risk and resilience factors and provide means to quantify possible sensitive windows for environmental impact.

4. *How does brain development unfold for individuals who develop a disorder, for individuals who are resilient, or for individuals whose symptoms remit?* Relatively small cross-sectional studies are the mainstay of current developmental psychopathology neuroimaging studies. We need more longitudinal studies. Currently, we do not have a precise idea how malleable neural development is on different domains, how

that may differ according to a specific subtype of a disorder, or to what degree malleability might depend on a particular developmental window.

5. *To what degree may environmental risk and protective factors reflect family-wide or individual genetic endowment?* Many of the parenting, family peer variables that are associated with disordered outcomes (e.g. conduct disorder) have a genetic component. They can reflect genetic vulnerability or protective factors within families, such as the reactions that an individual's genetically influenced temperament evoke in those around them. We desperately need more genetically informative research that helps us elucidate how environmental risk operates.

6. *To what degree is an individual's developmental trajectory a reasonable adaptation to their environmental circumstances?* What may appear disordered could in fact be an accommodation to a particular social ecology. A child growing up in a home environment characterized by domestic violence may be hypervigilant to potential threat and may aggress more readily than their peers. Their behaviour can appear maladaptive, but may have in fact kept them safer in the home environment they grew up in.

7. *How reasonable are translational recommendations based on individual differences or group differences data when treating a single individual?* I am yet to meet a developmental psychopathology researcher who does not sincerely hope that their findings will have tangible benefits for vulnerable children, but we need better mechanisms for translation and systematic development of evidence-based interventions.

In the remaining sections of this chapter I will elaborate on the challenges highlighted here and briefly outline some practical and ethical issues that need to be actively considered by the field.

Longitudinal multilevel research: we need it, why is there so little of it?

Any individual developmental trajectory is an emergent product of the interplay between various different levels of analyses: genetic, neural, cognitive, behavioural, and environmental (Figure 10.1). We have only a limited understanding pertaining to each level of analysis. The sheer scale of what we do not yet know becomes particularly clear when we try to think about the different levels of analyses interacting with and influencing each other (including via reverse causation), across development. However, exciting new data are constantly emerging that provide some pieces to the vast mental health developmental puzzle and also help focus the 'search space' for future studies.

To progress our understanding of how psychopathology develops, we need to combine different analytical approaches and measurement at different levels of analyses, within a longitudinal, developmental framework.

For example, twin study designs have been used to examine why disordered behaviour initially emerges, why it is maintained, and whether the aetiological influences for the initial risk versus developmental course overlap. Pingault and colleagues (2015) studied these questions in relation to attention deficit hyperactivity disorder

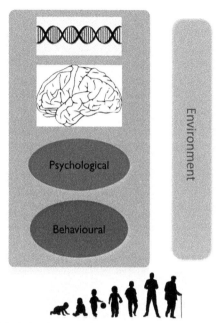

Figure 10.1 An individual developmental trajectory is an emergent product of the interplay between various different levels of analyses: genetic, neural, cognitive, behavioural, and environmental.

(ADHD) symptomatology from early childhood to adolescence. They found that genetic influences on the emergence of ADHD symptoms and those which contributed to symptom maintenance (or change) were largely independent. In other words, new genetic influences came into play in early adolescence and made an important contribution to shaping the developmental course of ADHD symptomatology. The same study also demonstrated that environmental influences on ADHD symptomatology were mostly specific to a particular time point under study. These data suggest that future molecular genetic investigations of ADHD might not expect identical genetic risk factors to be implicated at different points in development. The findings also suggest that protective environmental influences (e.g. the type of treatment or treatment adjuncts) may need not only to be repeated, but may need to vary across the development in order to have a sustained impact on behaviour.

We can supplement genetically informative analyses by looking at longitudinal neuroimaging data. Such studies can provide additional pieces to the puzzle of what drives initial disorder risk and what explains differences in the course of symptom development. Philip Shaw and colleagues (2006) have done some very elegant work on longitudinal structural brain development in both typical and disordered populations. For example, they found that compared with typically developing children, children with ADHD show relative cortical thinning in prefrontal regions that are important for attentional control. They also found that the children who had the worst clinical outcomes had 'fixed' thinning of the left medial prefrontal cortex, which Shaw and colleagues proposed accounted for a failure to develop age-appropriate attentional control and explained resistance to clinical improvement. Their study also showed that for the children whose ADHD symptoms reduced over time, there was normalization of parietal cortical thickness measures, with these children looking increasingly like their typically developing peers on these measures as time went on. Shaw and colleagues interpreted this finding as potentially indicating maturation of components of the attentional network through adolescence for children with ADHD who had better outcomes. The outstanding question that we have is, of course, to what extent this sort of cortical 'normalization' reflects the impact of developmental genetic or environmental inputs and what those inputs are. We can extrapolate from the findings of Pingault and colleagues (2015) and speculate that neurodevelopmental genetic effects that account for individual differences in the maturation of parietal cortex in part explain individual differences in the developmental course of ADHD symptomatology. This hypothesis awaits testing and before it is possible to do so, it is necessary to find a reliable set of genetic variants associated with initial symptomatology and another set associated with developmental course of ADHD.

A further challenge that faces us when we attempt to combine multiple levels of analyses is incorporating measurement of different environmental contexts over the course of development. Pioneering work by Andersen and colleagues (2008) has shown that the effect of childhood sexual abuse on regional brain development varies as a function of the point of development during which the abuse occurred. If the abuse occurred very early on, the brain region that was maximally impacted was the hippocampus. If the abuse occurred later on in life, it was more likely to impact the development of frontal cortex. These findings are consistent with the view that different brain regions have their own unique sensitive periods, or windows of vulnerability, with regard to the effects of environmental risk factors and we need substantially more data regarding these sensitive periods as we try to understand the emergence of mental ill health and resilience. Interventions delivered at different developmental periods can also further our understanding of the sensitive periods in brain development.

Particular environmental risk factors are also likely to be more or less important at different stages in development. For infants and toddlers, parents provide the critical environmental context in which the child either thrives or fails to reach their potential (McCrory et al., 2017). For adolescents, peers are increasingly important and are thought to provide a very important context for the 'social brain' development (Kilford et al., 2016). We know that adolescents are easily worried about what other people think about them, whether they are 'cool' or whether someone is laughing at them. Obviously infants do not worry about such things. Conversely, adolescents are less dependent on their parents for meeting their basic needs.

There is clear interest and drive to bring together multiple levels of analyses to study the development of mental ill health and resilience, but the progress has been relatively slow to date. There are very few longitudinal cohort studies (which are representative of both genetic and environmental risk burden of a population) that have a rich set of longitudinal biomarker (e.g. neuroimaging) data. We are also far from identifying reliable combinations of genetic and environmental risk factors and how they specifically influence neural development and particular outcomes. The task is further complicated by the fact that many of the environmental risk (and protective) variables we study, in part reflect genetic confounding (Jaffee and Price, 2012).

Gene–environment correlation

As already alluded in earlier sections of this chapter, risk factors that are commonly thought to be 'environmental', may in part reflect genetic endowment. Children, as well as the adults who interact with them, have substantial, in part heritable, individual differences in their social information-processing capacities and behaviour. This clearly impacts how the children behave and what they best respond to, as well as how the adults behave and how they respond to the child or meet his/her needs. In typical biological families, the parents and children share genetic endowments and information processing styles. This is likely to constrain the range of 'inputs' and learning outcomes that are probable for a particular child and may explain why behaviours canalize in certain ways in particular family ecologies. For example, an individual's genetic predisposition may influence behaviours, which will in turn evoke different reactions in others or lead to that individual making specific choices that limit their range of experiences. We can imagine an adolescent prone to depression finding it harder to retain friends (who find it a 'downer' to be around him/her) or choosing to stay at home when others go out, thus missing out on positive interactions. That adolescent would score low on measures of social support, but without a genetically informative study design, it would not be possible to disentangle to what extent a lack of social support has led to depression compared to the possibility that it has been the depression that has led to lack of social support. Similarly, without genetically informative longitudinal studies it is not possible to tell to what extent an association between harsh parenting and antisocial behaviour in the offspring reflect passive rGE (the same genes that predispose to harsh parenting also predispose to antisocial behaviour) or evocative rGE (children who are genetically vulnerable to oppositional and aggressive behaviour are more likely to evoke harsh parenting).

Environment is not just something that 'happens to us'. Individuals create, select, and modify their own environment. This has implications for understanding development of mental ill health and resilience, as well as for designing interventions. Without accounting for rGE, we cannot be sure as to how 'environmental risk' operates or the degree to which such risk factors reflect genetic confounding. Given that children often reside among biological relatives who can share some of the same vulnerabilities that affect the child, we may need to consider modified delivery models that take into account some of the challenges that are inherent in those family ecologies (e.g. how much and what kind of support a parent may need to be able to regulate their emotions while dealing with a very difficult child).

Adaptation

When we try to understand the emergence of mental ill health, it is also important to consider the degree to which some of the information-processing biases that we may see in individuals who are vulnerable to (or have) certain disorders, may represent reasonable adaptations to particular environmental contexts, but which do not serve the individual well in a different (more normative) environmental context, predisposing him/her to mental ill health. This point can be illustrated by an elegant experimental demonstration. Inability to wait when faced with a desirable treat (typically marshmallows) has been attributed to poor self-control and those young children who are unable to delay gratification have been shown to be less successful in later life (e.g. Shoda et al., 1990). It is difficult to argue that the ability to delay gratification does not serve you well. However, it would be wrong to assume that an inability to wait is always an inherently maladaptive strategy. In this 'marshmallow test', the child is typically told that they can either eat the marshmallows placed in front of them immediately, or they can wait for a certain time and get more marshmallows. However, when researchers manipulate how reliable the adult giving the marshmallows is (by having the adult deliver on their promise of rewards in a pre-experiment task or not) this will modulate the child's behaviour on the marshmallow task (Kidd et al., 2012). In other words, the performance on this task may not only reflect differences in the children's self-control abilities, but also differences in their beliefs about the stability of the world. In an environment where resources are scarce and unpredictable, it pays off to eat the marshmallows (or grab any other goodies) straight away. Such behaviour may not serve an individual well in the wider world, but it may represent a useful adaptation in an environment where he/she grows up.

We have recently proposed the theory of 'latent vulnerability' to examine such potential adaptations (McCrory and Viding, 2015; McCrory et al., 2017). We have suggested that these adaptations constitute latent vulnerabilities that may increase risk for mental ill health in at least two ways. First, there may be direct effects on immediate processing of the internal and external world. For example, increased allocation of attention to threat cues, which we have demonstrated to occur in individuals with maltreatment experiences (McCrory et al., 2011) may reduce the attentional capacity available to be invested in more normative aspects of social and cognitive development, reducing the degree to which an individual is able to process other potentially helpful cues in their environment. Second, there may be indirect effects that serve— over time—to compromise the development of the social support network around the child or adolescent and increase the likelihood of experiencing stressor events. For example, altered patterns of threat vigilance may increase the risk of conflictual social interactions making it more difficult for the child to build stable friendships that can help buffer the impact of future stressors (McCrory et al., 2017) or lead to breakdown of relationships or school exclusion. Such latent vulnerability effects (adaptations) will over time reduce the degree of resilience shown by an individual in the face of a future stressor, thereby increasing the probability of poor mental health outcomes.

An emerging body of work indicates that altered neurocognitive functioning following maltreatment (which we think of as an adaptation to particular circumstances) can be observed even in the absence of overt psychopathology, looks similar to the perturbations seen in individuals presenting with psychiatric disorder, and can predict future psychiatric symptomatology (McCrory et al., 2017). Currently most of our intervention resources are focused on treating manifest clinical disorders. But the theory of latent vulnerability proposes that we should think about a shift towards a preventative psychiatry model, which is in line with many of the campaigns for physical health and well-being. In order to deliver such interventions appropriately, we need to develop tools to accurately index latent vulnerability so that we can identify those children who are not yet overtly symptomatic but who are at most risk of future psychiatric disorder. We also need to work together with ethicists to ensure that any preventative interventions are implemented in such a way that they do not label or stigmatize children who have already had extremely adverse early experiences.

Translating findings from basic science to the clinic

Can individual differences and group-level basic science data inform the treatment of a single individual? It is very unlikely that we can map the precise developmental trajectory across multiple levels of analyses for a single individual. We are unlikely to have the data available to do so and there will more than likely to be stochastic factors that make it complicated to fully understand how any single individual has arrived at a particular outcome. However, as we improve our understanding of different pathways to mental ill health at the population level, we reduce the problem space in a way that can improve clinical formulation and clinical hypothesis testing in relation to individual clients.

Well formulated treatment studies can also be used to inform basic science and subsequent translation to new treatments. Are there certain developmental periods during which certain information processing capacities are particularly malleable? Treatment settings enable control over (protective) environmental factors in a way that is not possible to achieve in naturalistic settings. It is possible to systematically deliver an input and see if the impact of that input varies at different time periods or in different social contexts. This can inform our understanding of neural and cognitive development, as well as optimal delivery windows or settings for particular interventions.

Conclusion

It will be challenging, but not impossible, to combine multiple levels of analyses to improve our understanding of developmental risk and resilience. Some of this research can only be accomplished when new methodological advances are achieved or discoveries in one field (e.g. genetic findings that enable the generation of polygenic risk scores) make it more feasible to bring together different approaches (e.g. genetics and developmental neuroimaging). We need to be mindful of equi- and multifinality as we conduct this work and we should expect that for every discovery that advances our knowledge base, there will probably be a few blind alleys that seemed like a good idea at the time, but end up leading us down a cul-de-sac. This is inevitable as our understanding of mechanisms of mental ill health is still relatively rudimentary and our starting point is often imprecise (behavioural presentation). However, the field of developmental psychopathology has seen some exciting advances in the past 10 years and I am confident that this trend will continue.

References

Andersen, S.L., Tomada, A., Vincow, E.S., Valente, E., Polcari, A., and Teicher, M.H. (2008). Preliminary evidence for sensitive periods in the effect of childhood sexual abuse on regional brain development. *The Journal of Neuropsychiatry and Clinical Neurosciences*, **20**(3), 292–301.

Armstrong, K. and Kimonis, E.R. (2013). Parent-child interaction therapy for the treatment of Asperger's disorder in early childhood: a case study. *Clinical Case Studies*, **12**(1), 60–72.

American Psychiatric Association (2013). *Diagnostic and Statistical Manual of Mental Disorders* (5th ed.). Washington, DC: American Psychiatric Association.

Bedford, R., Pickles, A., Sharp, H., Wright, N., and Hill, J. (2015). Reduced face preference in infancy: a developmental precursor to callous-unemotional traits? *Biological Psychiatry*, **78**(2), 144–150.

Beitchman, J.H., Zai, C.C., Muir, K., Berall, L., Nowrouzi, B., Choi, E., and Kennedy, J.L. (2012). Childhood aggression, callous-unemotional traits and oxytocin genes. *European Child & Adolescent Psychiatry*, **21**(3), 125–132.

Birbaumer, N., Veit, R., Lotze, M., Erb, M., Hermann, C., Grodd, W., and Flor, H. (2005). Deficient fear conditioning in psychopathy: a functional magnetic resonance imaging study. *Archives of General Psychiatry*, **62**(7), 799–805.

Blair, R.J.R. (2017). Emotion-based learning systems and the development of morality. *Cognition*, **167**, 38–45.

Blair, R.J.R., Leibenluft, E., and Pine, D.S. (2014). Conduct disorder and callous–unemotional traits in youth. *New England Journal of Medicine*, **371**(23), 2207–2216.

Blair, R.J.R., Veroude, K., and Buitelaar, J.K. (2018). Neuro-cognitive system dysfunction and symptom sets: a review of fMRI studies in youth with conduct problems. *Neuroscience & Biobehavioral Reviews*, **91**, 69–90.

Cheng, Y., Hung, A.Y., and Decety, J. (2012). Dissociation between affective sharing and emotion understanding in juvenile psychopaths. *Development and Psychopathology*, **24**(2), 623–636.

Cicchetti, D. and Rogosch, F.A. (1996). Equifinality and multifinality in developmental psychopathology. *Development and Psychopathology*, **8**(3), 597–600.

Dadds, M.R., Allen, J.L., Oliver, B.R., Faulkner, N., Legge, K., Moul, C., Woolgar, M., and Scott, S. (2012). Love, eye contact and the developmental origins of empathy v. psychopathy. *The British Journal of Psychiatry*, **200**(3), 191–196.

Dadds, M.R., Jambrak, J., Pasalich, D., Hawes, D.J., and Brennan, J. (2011). Impaired attention to the eyes of attachment figures and the developmental origins of psychopathy. *Journal of Child Psychology and Psychiatry*, **52**(3), 238–245.

Dadds, M.R., Moul, C., Cauchi, A., Hawes, D.J., and Brennan, J. (2013). Replication of a ROBO2 polymorphism associated with conduct problems but not psychopathic tendencies in children. *Psychiatric Genetics*, **23**(6), 251–254.

de Wied, M., van Boxtel, A., Matthys, W., and Meeus, W. (2012). Verbal, facial and autonomic responses to empathy-eliciting film clips by disruptive male adolescents with high versus low callous-unemotional traits. *Journal of Abnormal Child Psychology*, **40**(2), 211–223.

Fowler, T., Langley, K., Rice, F., van den Bree, M.B., Ross, K., Wilkinson, L.S., Owen, M.J., O'Donovan, M.C., and Thapar, A. (2009). Psychopathy trait scores in adolescents with childhood ADHD: the contribution of genotypes affecting MAOA, 5HTT and COMT activity. *Psychiatric Genetics*, **19**, 312–319.

Frick, P.J., Ray, J.V., Thornton, L.C., and Kahn, R.E. (2014). Can callous-unemotional traits enhance the understanding, diagnosis, and treatment of serious conduct problems in children and adolescents? A comprehensive review. *Psychological Bulletin*, **140**(1), 1–57.

Frick, P.J. and **Viding, E.** (2009). Antisocial behavior from a developmental psychopathology perspective. *Development and Psychopathology*, **21**(4), 1111–1131.

Green, H., McGinnity, A., Meltzer, H., Ford, T., and **Goodman, R.** (2005). *Mental Health of Children and Young People in Great Britain, 2004*. New York: Palgrave Macmillan.

Hodsoll, S., Lavie, N., and **Viding, E.** (2014). Emotional attentional capture in children with conduct problems: the role of callous-unemotional traits. *Frontiers in Human Neuroscience*, **8**, 570.

Hwang, S., Nolan, Z.T., White, S.F., Williams, W.C., Sinclair, S., and **Blair, R.J.R.** (2016). Dual neurocircuitry dysfunctions in disruptive behavior disorders: emotional responding and response inhibition. *Psychological Medicine*, **46**(7), 1485–1496.

Hyde, L.W., Waller, R., Trentacosta, C.J., Shaw, D.S., Neiderhiser, J.M., Ganiban, J.M., Reiss, D., and **Leve, L.D.** (2016). Heritable and nonheritable pathways to early callous-unemotional behaviors. *American Journal of Psychiatry*, **173**(9), 903–910.

Jaffee, S.R. and **Price, T.S.** (2012). The implications of genotype–environment correlation for establishing causal processes in psychopathology. *Development and Psychopathology*, **24**(04), 1253–1264.

Jones, A.P., Happé, F.G., Gilbert, F., Burnett, S., and **Viding, E.** (2010). Feeling, caring, knowing: different types of empathy deficit in boys with psychopathic tendencies and autism spectrum disorder. *Journal of Child Psychology and Psychiatry*, **51**(11), 1188–1197.

Jones, A.P., Riley, R.D., Williamson, P.R., and **Whitehead, A.** (2009). Meta-analysis of individual patient data versus aggregate data from longitudinal clinical trials. *Clinical Trials*, **6**, 16–27.

Kessler, R.C., Amminger, G.P., Aguilar-Gaxiola, S., Alonso, J., Lee, S., and **Ustun, T.B.** (2007). Age of onset of mental disorders: a review of recent literature. *Current Opinion in Psychiatry*, **20**(4), 359–364.

Kidd, C., Palmeri, H., and **Aslin, R.N.** (2013). Rational snacking: young children's decision-making on the marshmallow task is moderated by beliefs about environmental reliability. *Cognition*, **126**(1), 109–114.

Kiehl, K.A., Smith, A.M., Hare, R.D., Mendrek, A., Forster, B.B., Brink, J., and **Liddle, P.F.** (2001). Limbic abnormalities in affective processing by criminal psychopaths as revealed by functional magnetic resonance imaging. *Biological Psychiatry*, **50**(9), 677–684.

Kilford, E.J., Garrett, E., and **Blakemore, S.J.** (2016). The development of social cognition in adolescence: an integrated perspective. *Neuroscience & Biobehavioral Reviews*, **70**, 106–120.

Kimonis, E.R., Frick, P.J., Munoz, L.C., and **Aucoin, K.J.** (2008). Callous-unemotional traits and the emotional processing of distress cues in detained boys: testing the moderating role of aggression, exposure to community violence, and histories of abuse. *Development and Psychopathology*, **20**(2), 569–589.

Kim-Cohen, J., Caspi, A., Moffitt, T.E., Harrington, H., Milne, B.J., and **Poulton, R.** (2003). Prior juvenile diagnoses in adults with mental disorder: developmental follow-back of a prospective-longitudinal cohort. *Archives of General Psychiatry*, **60**(7), 709–717.

Lockwood, P.L., Sebastian, C.L., McCrory, E.J., Hyde, Z.H., Gu, X., De Brito, S.A., and **Viding, E.** (2013). Association of callous traits with reduced neural response to others' pain in children with conduct problems. *Current Biology*, **23**(10), 901–905.

Lozier, L.M., Cardinale, E.M., VanMeter, J.W., and **Marsh, A.A.** (2014). Mediation of the relationship between callous-unemotional traits and proactive aggression by amygdala response to fear among children with conduct problems. *JAMA Psychiatry*, **71**(6), 627–636.

Malik, A.I., Zai, C.C., Abu, Z., Nowrouzi, B., and Beitchman, J.H. (2012). The role of oxytocin and oxytocin receptor gene variants in childhood-onset aggression. *Genes, Brain and Behavior*, **11**(5), 545–551.

Marsh, A.A. and Blair, R.J.R. (2008). Deficits in facial affect recognition among antisocial populations: a meta-analysis. *Neuroscience & Biobehavioral Reviews*, **32**(3), 454–465.

Marsh, A.A., Finger, E.C., Fowler, K.A., Adalio, C.J., Jurkowitz, I.T., Schechter, J.C., Pine, D.S., Decety, J., and Blair, R.J.R. (2013). Empathic responsiveness in amygdala and anterior cingulate cortex in youths with psychopathic traits. *Journal of Child Psychology and Psychiatry*, **54**(8), 900–910.

Marsh, A.A., Finger, E., Mitchell, D.G.V., Reid, M.E., Sims, C., Kosson, D.S., Towbin, K.E., Leibenluft, E., Pine, D.S., and Blair, R.J. (2008). Reduced amygdala response to fearful expressions in children and adolescents with callous-unemotional traits and disruptive behavior disorders. *American Journal of Psychiatry*, **165**(6), 712–720.

Marsh, A.A., Finger, E.C., Schechter, J.C., Jurkowitz, I.T., Reid, M.E., and Blair, R.J.R. (2011). Adolescents with psychopathic traits report reductions in physiological responses to fear. *Journal of Child Psychology and Psychiatry*, **52**(8), 834–841.

Martin-Key, N., Brown, T., and Fairchild, G. (2017). Empathic accuracy in male adolescents with conduct disorder and higher versus lower levels of callous-unemotional traits. *Journal of Abnormal Child Psychology*, **45**(7), 1385–1397.

McCrory, E.J., De Brito, S.A., Kelly, P.A., Bird, G., Sebastian, C.L., Mechelli, A., Samuel, S., and Viding, E. (2013). Amygdala activation in maltreated children during pre-attentive emotional processing. *British Journal of Psychiatry*, **202**(4), 269–276.

McCrory, E.J., De Brito, S.A., Sebastian, C.L., Mechelli, A., Bird, G., Kelly, P.A., and Viding, E. (2011). Heightened neural reactivity to threat in child victims of family violence. *Current Biology*, **21**(23), 947–948.

McCrory, E.J., Gerin, M.I., and Viding, E. (2017). Childhood maltreatment, latent vulnerability and the shift to preventative psychiatry–the contribution of functional brain imaging. *Journal of Child Psychology and Psychiatry*, **58**(4), 338–357.

McCrory, E.J. and Viding, E. (2015). The theory of latent vulnerability: Reconceptualizing the link between childhood maltreatment and psychiatric disorder. *Development and Psychopathology*, **27**(2), 493–505.

McManus, S., Meltzer, H., Brugha, T.S., Bebbington, P.E., and Jenkins, R. (2009). *Adult Psychiatric Morbidity in England, 2007: Results of a Household Survey*. Leeds: The NHS Information Centre for Health and Social Care.

Michalska, K.J., Zeffiro, T.A., and Decety, J. (2015). Brain response to viewing others being harmed in children with conduct disorder symptoms. *Journal of Child Psychology and Psychiatry*, **57**(4), 510–519.

Moffitt, T.E. (2005). The new look of behavioral genetics in developmental psychopathology: gene-environment interplay in antisocial behaviors. *Psychological Bulletin*, **131**(4), 533–554.

Moul, C., Dobson-Stone, C., Brennan, J., Hawes, D., and Dadds, M. (2013). An exploration of the serotonin system in antisocial boys with high levels of callous-unemotional traits. *PloS One*, **8**(2), e56619.

MQ: Transforming Mental Health (2016). MQ manifesto for young people's mental health. https://www.mqmentalhealth.org/articles/mq-manifesto-for-young-peoples-mental-health

Odgers, C.L., Caspi, A., Broadbent, J.M., Dickson, N., Hancox, R.J., Harrington, H., Poulton, R., Sears, M.R., Thomson, W.M., and Moffitt, T.E. (2007). Prediction of differential adult health burden by conduct problem subtypes in males. *Archives of General Psychiatry*, **64**(4), 476–484.

Penton-Voak, I.S., Thomas, J., Gage, S.H., McMurran, M., McDonald, S., and Munafò, M.R. (2013). Increasing recognition of happiness in ambiguous facial expressions reduces anger and aggressive behavior. *Psychological Science*, **24**(5), 688–697.

Pingault, J.B., Viding, E., Galéra, C., Greven, C.U., Zheng, Y., Plomin, R., and Rijsdijk, F. (2015). Genetic and environmental influences on the developmental course of attention-deficit/hyperactivity disorder symptoms from childhood to adolescence. *JAMA Psychiatry*, **72**(7), 651–658.

Sakai, J.T., Dalwani, M.S., Mikulich-Gilbertson, S.K., Raymond, K., McWilliams, S., Tanabe, J., Rojas, D., Regner, M., Banich, M.T., and Crowley, T.J. (2017). Imaging decision about whether to, or not to, benefit self by harming others: adolescents with conduct and substance problems, with or without callous-unemotionality, or developing typically. *Psychiatry Research: Neuroimaging*, **263**, 103–112.

Schwenck, C., Mergenthaler, J., Keller, K., Zech, J., Salehi, S., Taurines, R., Romanos, M., Schecklmann, M., Schneider, W., Warnke, A., and Freitag, C.M. (2012). Empathy in children with autism and conduct disorder: Group-specific profiles and developmental aspects. *Journal of Child Psychology and Psychiatry*, **53**(6), 651–659.

Seara-Cardoso, A. and Viding, E. (2014). Functional neuroscience of psychopathic personality in adults. *Journal of Personality*, **83**(6), 723–737.

Sebastian, C.L., McCrory, E.J., Cecil, C.A., Lockwood, P.L., De Brito, S.A., Fontaine, N.M., and Viding., E. (2012). Neural responses to affective and cognitive theory of mind in children with conduct problems and varying levels of callous-unemotional traits. *Archives of General Psychiatry*, **69**(8), 814–822.

Sebastian, C.L., McCrory, E.J., Dadds, M.R., Cecil, C.A., Lockwood, P.L., Hyde, Z.H., De Brito, S.A., and Viding, E. (2014). Neural responses to fearful eyes in children with conduct problems and varying levels of callous-unemotional traits. *Psychological Medicine*, **44**(1), 99–109.

Shaw, P., Lerch, J., Greenstein, D., Sharp, W., Clasen, L., Evans, A., Giedd, J., Castellanos, F.X., and Rapoport, J. (2006). Longitudinal mapping of cortical thickness and clinical outcome in children and adolescents with attention-deficit/hyperactivity disorder. *Archives of General Psychiatry*, **63**(5), 540–549.

Shoda, Y., Mischel, W., and Peake, P.K. (1990). Predicting adolescent cognitive and self-regulatory competencies from preschool delay of gratification: identifying diagnostic conditions. *Developmental Psychology*, **26**(6), 978–986.

Sylvers, P.D., Brennan, P.A., and Lilienfeld, S.O. (2011). Psychopathic traits and preattentive threat processing in children: a novel test of the fearlessness hypothesis. *Psychological Science*, **22**(10), 1280–1287.

Thase, M.E., Gaynes, B., Papakostas, G.I., Shelton, R.C., and Trivedi, M.H. (2009). Tackling partial response to depression treatment. *Primary Care Companion to The Journal of Clinical Psychiatry*, **11**(4), 155–162.

Trzaskowski, M., Dale, P.S., and Plomin, R. (2013). No genetic influence for childhood behavior problems from DNA analysis. *Journal of American Academy of Child and Adolescent Psychiatry*, **52**, 1048–1056.

Viding, E., Blair, R.J.R., Moffitt, T.E., and Plomin, R. (2005). Evidence for substantial genetic risk for psychopathy in 7-year-olds. *Journal of Child Psychology and Psychiatry*, **46**(6), 592–597.

Viding, E., Hanscombe, K.B., Curtis, C.J., Davis, O.S., Meaburn, E.L., and Plomin, R. (2010). In search of genes associated with risk for psychopathic tendencies in children: a two-stage genome-wide association study of pooled DNA. *Journal of Child Psychology and Psychiatry*, **51**(7), 780–788.

Viding, E., Jones, A.P., Paul, J.F., Moffitt, T.E., and Plomin, R. (2008). Heritability of antisocial behaviour at 9: do callous-unemotional traits matter? *Developmental Science*, **11**(1), 17–22.

Viding, E., Price, T.S., Jaffee, S.R., Trzaskowski, M., Davis, O.S., Meaburn, E.L., Haworth, C.M., and Plomin, R. (2013). Genetics of callous-unemotional behavior in children. *PLoS One*, **8**(7), e65789.

Viding, E., Sebastian, C.L., Dadds, M.R., Lockwood, P.L., Cecil, C.A., De Brito, S.A., and McCrory, E.J. (2012). Amygdala response to preattentive masked fear in children with conduct problems: the role of callous-unemotional traits. *American Journal of Psychiatry*, **169**(10), 1109–1116.

Viding, E., Simmonds, E., Petrides, K.V., and Frederickson, N. (2009). The contribution of callous-unemotional traits and conduct problems to bullying in early adolescence. *Journal of Child Psychology and Psychiatry*, **50**(4), 471–481.

Waller, R., Dishion, T.J., Shaw, D.S., Gardner, F., Wilson, M.N., and Hyde, L.W. (2016). Does early childhood callous-unemotional behavior uniquely predict behavior problems or callous-unemotional behavior in late childhood? *Developmental Psychology*, **52**(11), 1805–1819.

White, S.F., Brislin, S., Sinclair, S., Fowler, K.A., Pope, K., and Blair, R.J.R. (2013). The relationship between large cavum septum pellucidum and antisocial behavior, callous-unemotional traits and psychopathy in adolescents. *Journal of Child Psychology and Psychiatry*, **54**(5), 575–581.

White, S.F., Fowler, K.A., Sinclair, S., Schechter, J.C., Majestic, C.M., Pine, D.S., and Blair, R.J. (2014). Disrupted expected value signaling in youth with disruptive behavior disorders to environmental reinforcers. *Journal of American Academy of Child and Adolescent Psychiatry*, **53**(5), 579–588.

White, S.F., Williams, W.C., Brislin, S.J., Sinclair, S., Blair, K.S., Fowler, K.A., Pine, D.S., Pope, K., and Blair, J.R. (2012). Reduced activity within the dorsal endogenous orienting of attention network to fearful expressions in youth with disruptive behavior disorders and psychopathic traits. *Development and Psychopathology*, **24**(3), 1105–1116.

White, S.F., Tyler, P.M., Erway, A.K., Botkin, M.L., Kolli, V., Meffert, H., Pope, K., and Blair, J.R. (2016). Dysfunctional representation of expected value is associated with reinforcement-based decision-making deficits in adolescents with conduct problems. *Journal of Child Psychology and Psychiatry*, **57**(8), 938–946.

Yoder, K.J., Lahey, B.B., and Decety, J. (2016). Callous traits in children with and without conduct problems predict reduced connectivity when viewing harm to others. *Scientific Reports*, **6**, 20216.

Chapter 11

The case for a preventative approach to mental health: Childhood maltreatment, neuroimaging, and the theory of latent vulnerability

Eamon J. McCrory

The link between maltreatment and psychiatric risk

There is now an overwhelming body of evidence that childhood maltreatment significantly increases the risk of psychiatric disorder in adolescence and throughout adulthood (Gilbert et al., 2009). It is important to note that such an association is probabilistic: maltreatment experience serves to significantly increase the likelihood of poor outcome (e.g. Widom et al., 2007; Koenen and Widom, 2009). This impact on psychological health is one of a broader set of maladaptive outcomes that have been associated with maltreatment in longitudinal prospective studies, including poorer physical health (Widom et al., 2012), economic productivity (Currie and Widom, 2010), educational attainment, and social functioning (Nikulina et al., 2011).

Despite the well-established association between childhood maltreatment and increased risk for psychopathology (Gilbert et al., 2009; Vachon et al., 2015), there is a surprising lack of precision in our understanding of the neurocognitive mechanisms through which increased psychiatric vulnerability becomes instantiated. In other words, how do experiences of early adversity alter psychological and neurobiological functioning in ways that increase risk of mental health problems? This gap in our understanding leaves clinicians and professionals without the necessary resources and knowledge that would allow them to identify and provide support for those individuals most likely to develop mental health difficulties in the future (McCrory et al., 2017). The dominant focus on service provision organized around a medical diagnostic model has arguably impeded progress. Mental health research has largely tended to privilege the study of manifest disorders with much less attention given to understanding the mechanisms associated with the *emergence* of disorders during childhood. In other words, although we know a lot about the risk factors associated with mental health problems, we still have a relatively poor understanding of the *mechanisms* that shape how psychiatric disorders develop.

I believe that this current approach is failing many children. Despite the fact that we know maltreatment is associated with a significantly elevated risk of psychiatric disorder, the received wisdom is to wait until full-blown disorders emerge before treatment is offered. Such an approach is increasingly at odds with a recent shift towards pre-emptive psychiatry (e.g. Insel, 2009; McGorry, 2013). The challenge is to find ways of identifying those individuals who are most vulnerable to later poor outcome, and to offset their risk trajectory by developing a form of preventative intervention that can reduce the likelihood of a mental illness in the future.

The theory of latent vulnerability

In an effort to shift the focus on prevention and the developmental mechanisms associated with the emergence of mental health problems following childhood maltreatment, McCrory and Viding have proposed the theory of latent vulnerability (McCrory and Viding, 2015; McCrory et al., 2017). This theory offers a system-level approach that places emphasis on the neurocognitive mechanisms that link childhood maltreatment to subsequent mental health problems (see Figure 11.1 for a graphical illustration of the latent vulnerability model). According to this account, childhood maltreatment leads to measurable alterations that can be characterized at neurobiological and cognitive levels. These changes can be understood as developmental recalibrations to negative early experiences. Rather than conferring brain 'damage', such changes may be adaptive within the context of maltreatment and confer short-term functional advantages, such as faster detection of threat or reduced expectation of reward. However, such alterations are also thought to incur long-term costs (e.g. increased risk of psychological problems or re-victimization) as an individual may not be optimized to cope with the demands of more normative environments, such as the school setting or a stable foster placement. Importantly, maltreatment-related patterns of adaptation are understood to be 'latent' as they may appear *before* the emergence of mental health problems and are not necessarily manifest symptoms or precursors of any future condition.

The theory of latent vulnerability focuses on maltreatment-related neurocognitive processes that increase, non-deterministically, the risk of future difficulties. In doing so, it complements a wider research literature demonstrating that a variety of maltreatment-related emotional states (such as shame), self and other representations (such as abuse-related self-blame), and psychological states (such as dissociation) also confer risk for future difficulties (e.g. Feiring and Taska, 2005; Feiring and Cleland, 2007; Yates et al., 2008; Hanson, 2016). By focusing attention on the maltreatment-related processes and alterations that precede the emergence of more overt difficulties, this framework has the potential to increase the application of research to practice. First, a systematic investigation of the neurocognitive processes associated with increased vulnerability may help inform the development of a screening tool that could be used by frontline practitioners to identify those individuals at most risk of developing later mental health problems. Second, understanding the processes that instantiate increased vulnerability may inform the development of interventions that

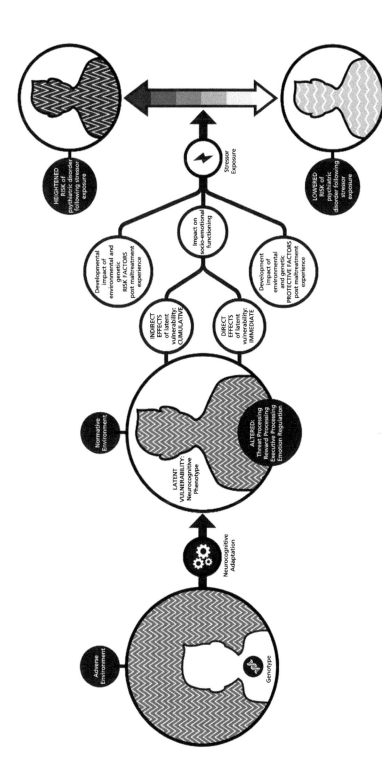

Figure 11.1 A schematic displaying the embedding of latent vulnerability at the neurocognitive level and differential outcome in relation to psychiatric risk depending on protective factors, stressor exposure, and genotypes.

Reproduced from McCrory, E.J., Gerin, M.I., and Viding, E. (2017). Annual research review: childhood maltreatment, latent vulnerability and the shift to preventative psychiatry—the contribution of functional brain imaging. *Journal of Child Psychology and Psychiatry*, 58(4), 338–357. doi: 10.1111/jcpp.12713.

most effectively help to prevent maltreated children developing subsequent mental health difficulties. Third, this understanding provides a clear rationale for rethinking service design and delivery, with a much greater focus on the prevention of mental health problems.

Three key features characterize the construct of latent vulnerability:

◆ Indicators of latent vulnerability are not necessarily *symptoms* of any future disorder. Rather, they refer to cognitive processes or representations and associated patterns of neural activation that are implicated in the pathogenesis of a disorder. For example, as discussed later in greater length, an altered response to reward cues at the neurocognitive level may increase vulnerability to depression (e.g. Hanson et al., 2015; Dennison et al., 2016), but this pattern of altered reward processing does not in itself constitute a symptom of depression.

◆ Latent vulnerability is best understood at a *systems level*. In other words, it likely reflects a complex phenotype that can be thought of as a 'maladaptive calibration' in higher-order systems important for socioemotional and cognitive functioning, such as an increase in threat vigilance that may be adaptive in a violent family home but poorly optimized for functioning within a school setting. Given the heterogeneity of poor (and resilient) outcomes associated with maltreatment across psychiatric disorders (Gilbert et al., 2009), it would be reasonable to hypothesize that a limited but varied set of candidate neurocognitive systems are altered in a way that increases or reduces psychiatric vulnerability following maltreatment exposure.

◆ Any indicators of latent vulnerability should be present *prior* to the onset of a psychiatric disorder and help predict the level of future risk. That latent vulnerability is present does not necessarily inform us of the timing of disease onset; such vulnerability could theoretically be present for months or years, but clinical symptoms may only manifest under certain conditions characterized by stress or developmental challenge, or indeed may never manifest given adequate intrinsic and extrinsic protective factors (e.g. resilient genotypes, social support; see Figure 11.1), and the absence of future stressors, despite the enduring presence of latent vulnerability. In other words, the emergence of a psychiatric disorder can be understood as the interaction between latent vulnerability and stressor exposure.

Functional magnetic resonance imaging studies of childhood maltreatment

Latent vulnerability can be characterized across multiple levels. I believe that investigation at the neurocognitive level is likely to offer the most promise in relation to real-world application with regard to policy and practice. For this reason, this review will focus on the functional neuroimaging literature, as this method has greater potential to refine our understanding of how neurocognitive processes may be altered following childhood abuse and neglect. In brief, the studies discussed here support the notion that individuals with histories of childhood maltreatment, even in the absence of manifest clinical symptoms, present with changes in brain function across several cognitive, social, and emotional domains. Remarkably, these changes are often consistent with neural signatures observed in individuals with psychiatric disorders commonly associated with maltreatment. I will review the child studies relating to threat and reward processing; however, other domains of functioning (including emotional regulation, executive processing, and memory) are all likely to be relevant (see McCrory et al., 2017). To help put these findings into context, I first provide a brief description of each system and then summarize how each has been implicated in common mental health disorders associated with maltreatment experience.

Threat processing

What is threat processing?

Survival is dependent on the ability to detect and respond to dangerous and aversive stimuli in the environment. For this reason, it is not surprising that both animal and human studies have revealed that a large amount of cognitive resources and neurobiological systems are dedicated to threat detection (Ledoux, 2000; Öhman, 2009). Within the central nervous system, the amygdala is one of the core structures dedicated to the processing of danger and to the detection of salient information more broadly (Ledoux, 2000; Phelps and LeDoux, 2005). Crucially, the amygdala is part of an integrated network comprising several cortical and subcortical brain regions involved in fear conditioning, stress responses, and salience detection, such as the hippocampus, the striatum, the anterior insula, and the dorsal anterior cingulate cortex (Shin and Liberzon, 2010).

How is altered threat processing implicated in mental health disorders?

In recent years, neuroimaging findings have shown that alterations in amygdala and anterior insula activation are implicated in several disorders, including post-traumatic stress disorder (PTSD), mood and anxiety disorders (Etkin and Wager, 2007; Patel et al., 2012; Kerestes et al., 2014), drug addiction (Sripada et al., 2011), and conduct problems (Viding et al., 2012). Crucially, recent longitudinal studies of healthy individuals exposed to various environmental stressors have shown that baseline hyper-responsiveness to a threat in the brain is associated not just with current, but also with future symptoms (Admon et al., 2009, 2013; Swartz et al., 2015).

What have we learnt from functional neuroimaging studies of threat processing in children and adolescents exposed to maltreatment?

Animal studies have established a strong link between early adverse experiences (such as early separation from a caregiver, social isolation, or reduced maternal care and sensitivity) and long-lasting alterations in the central and peripheral nervous system involved in threat processing and stress responses (Rosenblum et al., 1994; Caldji et al., 1998; Meaney, 2001; Caldji et al., 2003). Behavioural and electrophysiological studies with humans also suggest that abuse and neglect are associated with long-lasting alterations in threat processing that can be detected even during infancy. These changes include heighted electrophysiological responses to negative stimuli, as well as preferential attention and enhanced perceptual ability for cues associated with threat, such as angry or fearful faces (Pollak and Sinha, 2002; Pollak and Tolley-Schell, 2003; Pollak et al., 2005; Curtis and Cicchetti, 2013).

These behavioural and neurophysiological findings have been extended by a series of functional magnetic resonance imaging studies with children and adolescents that have shown a pattern of increased neural response during the processing of threat cues (e.g. angry faces), in both the amygdala and other subcortical neighbouring regions, such as the anterior insula and hippocampus (Maheu et al., 2010; McCrory et al., 2011, 2013; Tottenham et al., 2011). Such neural alterations seem to be shared across individuals with different experiences of early adversity, ranging from severe institutional neglect (Maheu et al., 2010; Tottenham et al., 2011), to substantiated maltreatment in community settings (McCrory et al., 2011, 2013), to more normative experiences of neglect (White et al., 2012). Importantly, by using well-matched control groups, these studies suggest that increased threat-related neural responses among maltreated children and adolescents are independent of potentially confounding factors, such as IQ, socioeconomic status, pubertal status, and concurrent psychopathology (e.g. Maheu et al., 2010; McCrory et al., 2013). Moreover, by showing that both amygdala and insula hyperactivity have a dose-dependent relation with the severity and duration of maltreatment (Maheu et al., 2010; McCrory et al., 2011, 2013), these findings suggest a pattern of neural calibration in line with the degree of exposure to early adversity. Finally, it is worth noting that a similar pattern of findings comes from studies with adults with a history of maltreatment, suggesting that abuse and neglect can have a long-lasting impact on the threat-processing system (e.g. Dannlowski et al., 2012).

Summary

It has been shown that different forms of early adversity alter the neural reactivity of the threat system, especially amygdala activation, even in children and adolescents who are not presenting with overt psychiatric symptomatology. Crucially, this association seems to be directly related to the degree of severity of the maltreatment experience (Maheu et al., 2010; McCrory et al., 2011; White et al., 2012). Interestingly, similar findings have been reported in adults who experienced maltreatment during childhood (see Hein and Monk, 2016), suggesting that such alterations are long lasting. It should be noted, however, that a number of studies have also reported *reduced* amygdala reactivity to threat cues in maltreated children, which may reflect an avoidant response that can arise in some contexts (see McCrory et al., 2017 for a discussion of this issue). Given that increased and decreased reactivity of the amygdala and anterior insula have been associated with several psychiatric conditions, including depression, anxiety, and PTSD, it is possible that altered threat processing may represent an index of latent vulnerability to future mental health problems. However, longitudinal studies are required to test this hypothesis.

Reward processing

What is reward processing?

Learning what stimuli and actions are associated with attaining rewarding objects, experiences, or events is essential to motivate and guide goal-directed behaviour and adaptive decision-making. The main network underpinning the processing of reward is the mesocorticolimbic dopaminergic neural pathway. This includes brainstem regions, such as the ventral tegmental area, which project to basal ganglia nuclei, especially the striatum, and terminate in prefrontal regions, including the orbitofrontal cortex (Valentin and O'Doherty, 2009; O'Doherty, 2011; Clithero and Rangel, 2013; Tanaka et al., 2016).

How is altered reward processing implicated in mental health disorders?

Neural alterations in the reward system have been associated with suboptimal decision-making and maladaptive outcomes, including the emergence and maintenance of anxiety, mood, conduct, and substance abuse disorders (Eshel and Roiser, 2010; Hartley and Phelps, 2012; White et al., 2013; Zhang et al., 2013; Balodis and Potenza, 2015; Stringaris et al., 2015). For example, neuroimaging findings show a consistent pattern of reduced activation in the striatum during reward processing among depressed individuals (Pizzagalli et al., 2009; Forbes and Dahl, 2012; Ubl et al., 2015). Interestingly, this predicts not only current but also future clinical status and symptoms level (Bress et al., 2012; Morgan et al., 2013; Olino et al., 2014; Telzer et al., 2014), even in previously 'healthy' individuals (Stringaris et al., 2015). Model-based neuroimaging studies seem to suggest that this pattern of blunted neural activation may be associated with difficulties in performing the necessary computations underlying outcome representation/reward anticipation and prediction-error signalling (i.e. the ability to detect the difference between the expected outcome and the reward actually received). In the context of mood disorders, this might entail reduced sensitivity to rewards and limited motivational response (i.e. anhedonia) (Gotlib et al., 2010; Stringaris et al., 2015; Ubl et al., 2015); in the context of conduct disorder, this may suggest difficulties in integrating and updating reward (and punishment) information (White et al., 2013, 2016).

What have we learnt from functional neuroimaging studies of reward processing in children and adolescents exposed to maltreatment?

Researchers have been motivated to investigate reward processing in individuals who have experienced maltreatment for two reasons. First, the clinical literature previously described suggests that altered reward processing may be associated not just with current mental health symptoms, but may play a role in the risk of developing a disorder. Second, we know that the familial environment experienced by maltreated children is often characterized by erratic and infrequent availability of rewards. To date, most neuroimaging studies of maltreatment have found reduced activation during reward processing, especially in the striatum and the orbitofrontal cortex (McCrory et al., 2017). This pattern of findings has been shown in both individuals who have experienced extreme forms of institutional deprivation (Mehta et al., 2010; Goff et al., 2013) and individuals who have experienced maltreatment in community settings—especially neglect (Hanson et al., 2015; Gerin et al., 2017). Dennison and colleagues did not show this effect but nevertheless found that a higher neural response to reward was linked to better future mental health outcomes, suggesting that increased activation in the striatum may represent a marker of resilience to psychopathology (Dennison et al., 2016). Therefore, the pattern of lower neural response in individuals who experienced early adversity may reflect neural calibration to reduced opportunities for reward-based contingency learning. Such alterations may represent adaptive regulatory mechanisms that reduce disappointment in the context of inconsistent and insensitive parenting (McCrory et al., 2017). However, these neurocognitive alterations may also hamper functioning in more normative situations. For example, they may hinder exploratory behaviour of novel environments, thus decreasing opportunities for learning and for motivating the search of alternative sources of reward outside the (maladaptive) home environment.

Summary

Overall, these findings suggest that maltreatment—especially neglect and institutional deprivation—is associated with blunted neural response to reward cues in the orbitostriatal network. This neural profile, which may be shaped by familial environments characterized by erratic and infrequent availability of rewards, is also known to be associated with common mental health problems, particularly depression and conduct disorder. Therefore, alterations in reward processing may represent a potential neurocognitive mechanism through which the experience of maltreatment leads to increased psychiatric vulnerability. Some preliminary longitudinal evidence suggests that higher levels of neural response in this network may be a potential marker of *resilience* to future psychopathology.

Clinical implications

The functional neuroimaging literature suggests that the experience of abuse and neglect can influence the development of specific aspects of cognitive and affective functioning, which may increase vulnerability to future mental health problems. From a clinical perspective, three aspects of the findings reviewed merit particular attention. First, maltreatment-related changes resemble the neurocognitive profile associated with increased risk and maintenance of mental health disorders commonly associated with maltreatment, such as anxiety and depression. Second, these alterations are already present before a *manifest* clinical disorder emerges. As such, they can be considered markers of latent vulnerability to psychiatric disorder since they have prognostic value, but do not reflect overt symptomatology. Third, despite the link with mental health problems, these neurocognitive changes should not be automatically interpreted as a sign of 'damage'. Rather, in line with the theory of latent vulnerability, they may in many instances be understood as the outcome of a complex set of adaptive processes, which may confer short-term advantages for the child in the context of abusive and neglectful environments (McCrory and Viding, 2015; McCrory et al., 2017). However, they may equally incur long-term costs as such adaptations may be poorly optimized for more normative environments.

We have suggested that these neurocognitive changes can confer latent vulnerability either directly or indirectly (McCrory et al., 2017) (Figure 11.1). *Direct effects* can be understood as the way in which maltreatment-related neurocognitive changes alter how an individual perceives, processes, and responds to the social world around them. For example, altered emotional regulation may have a direct effect on psychological functioning, increasing the degree to which new stressors or indeed everyday challenges burden and tax an individual (Tottenham and Gabard-Durnam, 2017); this can be understood as an increase in 'stress susceptibility'. Equally, neurocognitive changes may alter how an individual influences their own social experience. Direct effects here capture how an individual may act in ways that precipitate the likelihood of stressor events occurring; this can be considered a form of 'stress generation'. By contrast, *indirect effects* refer to how maltreatment-related neurocognitive changes influence how an individual cumulatively shapes their own social ecology over time. Childhood maltreatment history is associated with an increased likelihood of reduced social support in adulthood, even decades after abuse is experienced (Sperry and Widom, 2013). This can be conceptualized as a process of 'social thinning'. Over time, reduced social support will make individuals more vulnerable to stressors when they occur. For example, alterations of the threat system may compromise the child's ability to develop positive peer friendships and social support networks that can help buffer their experiences of future stressors. For instance, heightened threat reactivity may lead to more conflictual interactions as the child may misinterpret neutral cues, and over-respond to negative cues. It is not difficult to imagine how this pattern of interaction could, over time, affect their ability to cultivate social support networks and positive peer friendships.

Currently, interventions mainly occur at two stages. Once the maltreatment has been substantiated, professionals seek to ensure safety and the stability of the child's placement. Then, if an individual meets clinical criteria for a mental health problem, referral is made to mental health services. Arguably, the evidence reviewed here is providing the motivation and the rationale to pursue a 'third' stage of preventative care where help is offered to those individuals that are at most risk of a *future* mental health disorder. It seems important to explore whether it is possible, in real-world settings, to index those neurocognitive systems that show alterations following maltreatment. Ideally, such a tool would identify those individuals with the highest levels of latent vulnerability (i.e. those at most risk of future mental health problems following maltreatment).

We now know that treatments as usual (Nanni et al., 2011) and general parental caring (Rothman and Silverman, 2007) may not be enough to ameliorate symptoms and prevent re-victimization among individuals who suffered early abuse and neglect. If we are able to accurately delineate which neurocognitive systems are altered following maltreatment experiences, an important next question is to understand the factors that can promote malleability in these systems in order to inform the development of an effective model of preventative intervention (McCrory et al., 2017). What might such a preventative model look like? While systematic research is needed, our preliminary view is that any preventative approach will include a focus on promoting more effective social functioning, stabilizing and enhancing the social network around the child. This social network is likely to be the most effective buffer to protect the child from future stressors.

What factors might be implicated in promoting malleability and change in the functioning of the neurocognitive systems associated with latent vulnerability? One framework that takes a developmental perspective focuses on the child's relationship with a sensitive and warm caregiver, who understands the child to be an intentional agent capable of representing their mental states. Such caring and sensitive parenting promotes the development of *epistemic trust*, the ability to use others (e.g. a parent, a friend) to acquire new knowledge about the internal and external world. However, in the case of maltreatment, caregivers often show an absence of mentalizing, parental affective reactions may be erratic, and behavioural responses may not be contingent with environmental events or the behaviour of others. In such situations, the development of epistemic trust is jeopardized as the child mistrusts the information conveyed by caregivers. This can limit the ability to learn from the world more broadly and especially from interpersonal relationships (even when others can be trusted). Therefore, promoting the development of healthy and supportive relationships may be a necessary condition for any future change to occur. If the channels through which new knowledge can be acquired are closed (i.e. if epistemic trust is broken), then we would speculate that system-level neurocognitive alterations that follow the experience of early adversity are less likely to recalibrate to more benign social environments. Thus, as a starting point towards the development of preventative psychiatric interventions for maltreated individuals, it may be useful to draw from evidence-based interpersonally focused therapies (Toth et al., 2013). However, the potential role of epistemic trust remains a hypothesis. Systematic research is still required to formally test any model of preventative intervention and to identify factors important in promoting malleability of those neurocognitive changes implicated in latent vulnerability.

Conclusion

Recent functional magnetic resonance imaging research has demonstrated that childhood maltreatment is associated with altered functioning in a range of neurocognitive systems, including threat and reward processing. Such changes are observable even in the absence of psychiatric disorder and in some cases, predict future symptomatology. According to the theory of latent vulnerability they are thought, in part, to reflect adaptations to early adverse environments. The evidence from clinical studies suggests that these changes are strikingly consistent with those observed in individuals presenting with psychiatric disorder, suggesting such neurocognitive 'adaptations' embed latent vulnerability to future psychiatric disorder. This growing body of work is establishing a compelling case to develop a more precise, mechanistic understanding of the pathogenesis of psychiatric disorder following maltreatment, and the need to invigorate efforts to build a preventative clinical approach. Although this chapter has focused on threat and reward processing, other domains have also been implicated including autobiographical memory functioning and emotion regulation (Gerin et al., 2017). In the longer term, it is hoped that delineating the range of neurocognitive systems implicated in latent vulnerability will inform the development of a screening tool to identify those most at risk, and provide clues as to the kinds of preventative approaches that could effectively promote resilience. The success of this endeavour will in part depend on our ability to specify how alterations in neurocognitive systems impact social functioning in ways that increase vulnerability, including in relation to stress susceptibility, but also in how such alterations can contribute to stress generation and social thinning across the lifespan.

Acknowledgements

This work was supported by an Economic and Social Research Council grant (ES/K005723/1). Many of the ideas expressed in this chapter have been shaped by the work within the Developmental Risk and Resilience Unit at University College London. I am especially grateful to Essi Viding for her important contribution to the ideas presented here and to Mattia Gerin for his helpful input to earlier versions of this chapter. Thanks also to Vivien Vuong for bibliographic assistance and careful proof reading of the manuscript.

References

Admon, R., Lubin, G., Stern, O., Rosenberg, K., Sela, L., Ben-Ami, H., and Hendler, T. (2009). Human vulnerability to stress depends on amygdala's predisposition and hippocampal plasticity. *Proceedings of the National Academy of Sciences of the United States of America*, *106*(33), 14120–14125.

Admon, R., Milad, M.R., and Hendler, T. (2013). A causal model of post-traumatic stress disorder: disentangling predisposed from acquired neural abnormalities. *Trends in Cognitive Sciences*, **17**(7), 337–347.

Balodis, I.M. and Potenza, M.N. (2015). Anticipatory reward processing in addicted populations: a focus on the monetary incentive delay task. *Biological Psychiatry*, **77**(5), 434–444.

Bress, J.N., Smith, E., Foti, D., Klein, D.N., and Hajcak, G. (2012). Neural response to reward and depressive symptoms in late childhood to early adolescence. *Biological Psychology*, **89**(1), 156–162.

Caldji, C., Diorio, J., and Meaney, M.J. (2003). Variations in maternal care alter GABA(A) receptor subunit expression in brain regions associated with fear. *Neuropsychopharmacology*, **28**(11), 1950–1959.

Caldji, C., Tannenbaum, B., Sharma, S., Francis, D., Plotsky, P.M., and Meaney, M.J. (1998). Maternal care during infancy regulates the development of neural systems mediating the expression of fearfulness in the rat. *Proceedings of the National Academy of Sciences*, **95**(9), 5335–5340.

Clithero, J.A. and Rangel, A. (2013). Informatic parcellation of the network involved in the computation of subjective value. *Social Cognitive and Affective Neuroscience*, **9**(9), 1289–1302.

Currie, J. and Widom, C.S. (2010). Long-term consequences of child abuse and neglect on adult economic well-being. *Child Maltreatment*, **15**(2), 111–120.

Curtis, W.J. and Cicchetti, D. (2013). Affective facial expression processing in 15-month-old infants who have experienced maltreatment: an event-related potential study. *Child Maltreatment*, **18**(3), 140–154.

Dannlowski, U., Stuhrmann, A., Beutelmann, V., Zwanzger, P., Lenzen, T., Grotegerd, D., Domschke, K., Hohoff, C., Ohrmann, P., Bauer, J., Lindner, C., Postert, C., Konrad,

C., **Arolt, V., Heindel, W., Suslow, T.,** and **Kugel, H.** (2012). Limbic scars: long-term consequences of childhood maltreatment revealed by functional and structural magnetic resonance imaging. *Biological Psychiatry*, **71**(4), 286–293.

Dennison, M.J., Sheridan, M.A., Busso, D.S., Jenness, J.L., Peverill, M., Rosen, M.L., and **McLaughlin, K.A.** (2016). Neurobehavioral markers of resilience to depression amongst adolescents exposed to child abuse. *Journal of Abnormal Psychology*, **125**(8), 1201–1212.

Eshel, N. and **Roiser, J.P.** (2010). Reward and punishment processing in depression. *Biological Psychiatry*, **68**(2), 118–124.

Etkin, A. and **Wager, T.D.** (2007). Functional neuroimaging of anxiety: a meta-analysis of emotional processing in PTSD, social anxiety disorder, and specific phobia. *American Journal of Psychiatry*, **164**(10), 1476–1488.

Feiring, C. and **Cleland, C.** (2007). Childhood sexual abuse and abuse-specific attributions of blame over 6 years following discovery. *Child Abuse & Neglect*, **31**(11–12), 1169–1186.

Feiring, C. and **Taska, L.S.** (2005). The persistence of shame following sexual abuse: a longitudinal look at risk and recovery. *Child Maltreatment*, **10**(4), 337–349.

Forbes, E.E. and **Dahl, R.E.** (2012). Altered reward function in adolescent depression: what, when and how? *Journal of Child Psychology and Psychiatry*, **53**(1), 3–15.

Gerin, M.I., Puetz, V., Blair, J., White, S., Sethi, A., Hoffmann, F., Palmer, A., Viding, E., and **McCrory, E.** (2017). A neurocomputational investigation of reinforcement-based decision making as a candidate latent vulnerability mechanism in maltreated children. *Development and Psychopathology*, **29**(5), 1689–1705.

Gilbert, R., Widom, C.S., Browne, K., Fergusson, D., Webb, E., and **Janson, S.** (2009). Burden and consequences of child maltreatment in high-income countries. *The Lancet*, **373**(9657), 68–81.

Goff, B., Gee, D.G., Telzer, E.H., Humphreys, K.L., Gabard-Durnam, L., Flannery, J., and **Tottenham, N.** (2013). Reduced nucleus accumbens reactivity and adolescent depression following early-life stress. *Neuroscience*, **249**, 129–138.

Gotlib, I.H., Hamilton, J.P., Cooney, R.E., Singh, M.K., Henry, M.L., and **Joormann, J.** (2010). Neural processing of reward and loss in girls at risk for major depression. *Archives of General Psychiatry*, **67**(4), 380–387.

Hanson, E. (2016). Understanding and preventing re-victimisation. In: L. Smith (Ed.), *Clinical Practice at the Edge of Care* (pp. 197–227). Cham: Palgrave Macmillan.

Hanson, J.L., Hariri, A.R., and **Williamson, D.E.** (2015). Blunted ventral striatum development in adolescence reflects emotional neglect and predicts depressive symptoms. *Biological Psychiatry*, **78**(9), 598–605.

Hartley, C.A. and **Phelps, E.A.** (2012). Anxiety and decision-making. *Biological Psychiatry*, **72**(2), 113–118.

Hein, T.C. and **Monk, C.S.** (2016). Neural response to threat in children, adolescents, and adults after child maltreatment—a quantitative meta-analysis. *Journal of Child Psychology and Psychiatry*, **58**(3), 222–230.

Insel, T.R. (2009). Translating scientific opportunity into public health impact: a strategic plan for research on mental illness. *Archives of General Psychiatry*, **66**, 128–133.

Kerestes, R., Davey, C.G., Stephanou, K., Whittle, S., and **Harrison, B.J.** (2014). Functional brain imaging studies of youth depression: a systematic review. *NeuroImage: Clinical*, **4**, 209–231.

Koenen, K.C. and **Widom, C.S.** (2009). A prospective study of sex differences in the lifetime risk of post-traumatic stress disorder among abused and neglected children grown up. *Journal of Traumatic Stress*, **22**(6), 566–574.

Ledoux, J.E. (2000). Emotion circuits in the brain. *Annual Review of Neuroscience*, **23**, 155–184.

Maheu, F.S., Dozier, M., Guyer, A.E., Mandell, D., Peloso, E., Poeth, K., Jenness, J., Lau, J.Y.F., Ackerman, J.P., Pine, D.S., and Ernst, M. (2010). A preliminary study of medial temporal lobe function in youths with a history of caregiver deprivation and emotional neglect. *Cognitive, Affective & Behavioral Neuroscience*, **10**(1), 34–49.

McCrory, E.J., De Brito, S.A., Kelly, P.A., Bird, G., Sebastian, C.L., Mechelli, A., Samuel, S., and Viding, E. (2013). Amygdala activation in maltreated children during pre-attentive emotional processing. *British Journal of Psychiatry*, **202**(4), 269–276.

McCrory, E.J., De Brito, S.A., Sebastian, C.L., Mechelli, A., Bird, G., Kelly, P.A., and Viding, E. (2011). Heightened neural reactivity to threat in child victims of family violence. *Current Biology*, **21**(23), 947–948.

McCrory, E.J., Gerin, M.I., and Viding, E. (2017). Childhood maltreatment, latent vulnerability and the shift to preventative psychiatry—the contribution of functional brain imaging. *Journal of Child Psychology and Psychiatry*, **58**(4), 338–357.

McCrory, E.J. and Viding, E. (2015). The theory of latent vulnerability: reconceptualizing the link between childhood maltreatment and psychiatric disorder. *Development and Psychopathology*, **27**(2), 493–505.

McGorry, P. (2013). Prevention, innovation and implementation science in mental health: the next wave of reform. *British Journal of Psychiatry Supplement*, **202**, S3–S4.

Meaney, M.J. (2001). Maternal care, gene expression, and the transmission of individual differences in stress reactivity across generations. *Annual Review of Neuroscience*, **24**, 1161–1192.

Mehta, M.A., Gore-Langton, E., Golembo, N., Colvert, E., Williams, S.C.R., and Sonuga-Barke, E. (2010). Hyporesponsive reward anticipation in the basal ganglia following severe institutional deprivation early in life. *Journal of Cognitive Neuroscience*, **22**(10), 2316–2325.

Morgan, J.K., Olino, T.M., McMakin, D.L., Ryan, N.D., and Forbes, E.E. (2013). Neural response to reward as a predictor of increases in depressive symptoms in adolescence. *Neurobiology of Disease*, **52**, 66–74.

Nanni, V., Uher, R., and Danese, A. (2011). Childhood maltreatment predicts unfavorable course of illness and treatment outcome in depression: a meta-analysis. *American Journal of Psychiatry*, **169**(2), 141–151.

Nikulina, V., Widom, C.S., and Czaja, S.J. (2011). The role of childhood neglect, and childhood poverty in predicting mental health, academic achievement and crime in adulthood. *American Journal of Community Psychology*, **48**(3–4), 309–321.

O'Doherty, J.P. (2011). Contributions of the ventromedial prefrontal cortex to goal-directed action selection. *Annals of the New York Academy of Sciences*, **1239**(1), 118–129.

Öhman, A. (2009). Of snakes and faces: an evolutionary perspective on the psychology of fear. *Scandinavian Journal of Psychology*, **50**(6), 543–552.

Olino, T.M., McMakin, D.L., Morgan, J.K., Silk, J.S., Birmaher, B., Axelson, D.A., Williamson, D.E., Dahl, R.E., Ryan, N.D., and Forbes, E.E. (2014). Reduced reward anticipation in youth at high-risk for unipolar depression: a preliminary study. *Developmental Cognitive Neuroscience*, **8**, 55–64.

Patel, R., Spreng, R.N., Shin, L.M., and Girard, T.A. (2012). Neurocircuitry models of posttraumatic stress disorder and beyond: a meta-analysis of functional neuroimaging studies. *Neuroscience and Biobehavioral Reviews*, **36**(9), 2130–2142.

Phelps, E.A. and LeDoux, J.E. (2005). Contributions of the amygdala to emotion processing: from animal models to human behavior. *Neuron*, **48**(2), 175–187.

Pizzagalli, D.A., Holmes, A.J., Dillon, D.G., Goetz, E.L., Birk, J.L., Bogdan, R., Dougherty, D.D., Iosifescu, D.V, Rauch, S.L., and Fava, M. (2009). Reduced caudate and nucleus accumbens response to rewards in unmedicated individuals with major depressive disorder. *American Journal of Psychiatry*, **166**(6), 702–710.

Pollak, S.D. and Sinha, P. (2002). Effects of early experience on children's recognition of facial displays of emotion. *Developmental Psychology*, **38**(5), 784–791.

Pollak, S.D. and Tolley-Schell, S.A. (2003). Selective attention to facial emotion in physically abused children. *Journal of Abnormal Psychology*, **112**(3), 323–338.

Pollak, S.D., Vardi, S., Putzer Bechner, A.M., and Curtin, J.J. (2005). Physically abused children's regulation of attention in response to hostility. *Child Development*, **76**(5), 968–977.

Rosenblum, L.A., Coplan, J.D., Friedman, S., Bassoff, T., Gorman, J.M., and Andrews, M.W. (1994). Adverse early experiences affect noradrenergic and serotonergic functioning in adult primates. *Biological Psychiatry*, **35**(4), 221–227.

Rothman, E. and Silverman, J. (2007). The effect of a college sexual assault prevention program on first-year students' victimization rates. *Journal of American College Health*, **55**(5), 283–290.

Shin, L.M. and Liberzon, I. (2010). The neurocircuitry of fear, stress, and anxiety disorders. *Neuropsychopharmacology*, **35**(1), 169–191.

Sperry, D.M. and Widom, C.S. (2013). Child abuse and neglect, social support, and psychopathology in adulthood: a prospective investigation. *Child Abuse & Neglect*, **37**(6), 415–425.

Sripada, C.S., Angstadt, M., McNamara, P., King, A.C., and Phan, K.L. (2011). Effects of alcohol on brain responses to social signals of threat in humans. *Neuroimage*, **55**(1), 371–380.

Stringaris, A., Vidal-Ribas Belil, P., Artiges, E., Lemaitre, H., Gollier-Briant, F., Wolke, S., Vulser, H., Miranda, R., Penttilä, J., Struve, M., Fadai, T., Kappel, V., Grimmer, Y., Goodman, R., Poustka, L., Conrod, P., Cattrell, A., Banaschewski, T., Bokde, A.L.W., Bromberg, U., Büchel, C., Flor, H., Frouin, V., Gallinat, J., Garavan, H., Gowland, P., Heinz, A., Ittermann, B., Nees, F., Papadopoulos, D., Paus, T., Smolka, M.N., Walter, H., Whelan, R., Martinot, J.L., Schumann, G., and Paillère-Martinot, M.L. (2015). The brain's response to reward anticipation and depression in adolescence: dimensionality, specificity, and longitudinal predictions in a community-based sample. *American Journal of Psychiatry*, **172**(12), 1215–1223.

Swartz, J.R., Knodt, A.R., Radtke, S.R., and Hariri, A.R. (2015). A neural biomarker of psychological vulnerability to future life stress. *Neuron*, **85**(3), 505–511.

Tanaka, S.C., Doya, K., Okada, G., Ueda, K., Okamoto, Y., and Yamawaki, S. (2016). Prediction of immediate and future rewards differentially recruits cortico-basal ganglia loops. In: S. Ikeda, H.K. Kato, F. Ohtake, and Y. Tsutsui (Eds.), *Behavioral Economics of Preferences, Choices, and Happiness* (pp. 593–616). Japan: Springer.

Telzer, E.H., Fuligni, A.J., Lieberman, M.D., and Galvan, A. (2014). Neural sensitivity to eudaimonic and hedonic rewards differentially predict adolescent depressive symptoms over time. *Proceedings of the National Academy of Sciences*, **111**(18), 6600–6605.

Toth, S.L., Gravener-Davis, J.A., Guild, D.J., and Cicchetti, D. (2013). Relational interventions for child maltreatment: past, present, and future perspectives. *Developmental Psychopathology*, **25**(402), 1601–1617.

Tottenham, N. and Gabard-Durnam, L.J. (2017). The developing amygdala: a student of the world and a teacher of the cortex. *Current Opinion in Psychology*, **17**, 55–60.

Tottenham, N., Hare, T.A., Millner, A., Gilhooly, T., Zevin, J.D., and Casey, B.J. (2011). Elevated amygdala response to faces following early deprivation. *Developmental Science*, **14**(2), 190–204.

Ubl, B., Kuehner, C., Kirsch, P., Ruttorf, M., Diener, C., and Flor, H. (2015). Altered neural reward and loss processing and prediction error signalling in depression. *Social Cognitive and Affective Neuroscience*, **10**(8), 1102–1112.

Vachon, D.D., Krueger, R.F., Rogosch, F.A., and Cicchetti, D. (2015). Assessment of the harmful psychiatric and behavioral effects of different forms of child maltreatment. *JAMA Psychiatry*, **72**(11), 1135–1142.

Valentin, V.V. and O'Doherty, J.P. (2009). Overlapping prediction errors in dorsal striatum during instrumental learning with juice and money reward in the human brain. *Journal of Neurophysiology*, **102**(6), 3384–3391.

Viding, E., Sebastian, C.L., Dadds, M.R., Lockwood, P.L., Cecil, C.A.M., De Brito, S.A., and McCrory, E.J. (2012). Amygdala response to preattentive masked fear in children with conduct problems: the role of callous-unemotional traits. *American Journal of Psychiatry*, **169**(10), 1109–1116.

White, M.G., Bogdan, R., Fisher, P.M., Muñoz, K.E., Williamson, D.E., and Hariri, A.R. (2012). FKBP5 and emotional neglect interact to predict individual differences in amygdala reactivity. *Genes, Brain, and Behavior*, **11**(7), 869–878.

White, S., Pope, K., Sinclair, S., Fowler, K.A., Brislin, S.J., Williams, W.C., Pine, D.S., and Blair, R.J.R. (2013). Disrupted expected value and prediction error signaling in youths with disruptive behavior disorders during a passive avoidance task. *American Journal of Psychiatry*, **170**(3), 315–323.

White, S., Tyler, P., Erway, A.K., Botkin, M.L., Kolli, V., Meffert, H., Pope, K., and Blair, J.R. (2016). Dysfunctional representation of expected value is associated with reinforcement-based decision-making deficits in adolescents with conduct problems. *Journal of Child Psychology and Psychiatry*, **57**(8), 938–946.

Widom, C.S., Czaja, S.J., Bentley, T., and Johnson, M.S. (2012). A prospective investigation of physical health outcomes in abused and neglected children: new findings from a 30-year follow-up. *American Journal of Public Health*, **102**(6), 1135–1144.

Widom, C.S., Dumont, K., and Czaja, S.J. (2007). A prospective investigation of major depressive disorder and comorbidity in abused and neglected children grown up. *Archives of General Psychiatry*, **64**(1), 49–56.

Yates, T.M., Carlson, E.A., and Egeland, B. (2008). A prospective study of child maltreatment and self-injurious behavior in a community sample. *Development and Psychopathology*, **20**(2), 651–671.

Zhang, W.N., Chang, S.H., Guo, L.Y., Zhang, K.L., and Wang, J. (2013). The neural correlates of reward-related processing in major depressive disorder: a meta-analysis of functional magnetic resonance imaging studies. *Journal of Affective Disorders*, **151**(2), 531–539.

Chapter 12

Biopsychosocial pathways to mental health and disease across the lifespan: The emerging role of epigenetics

Charlotte A.M. Cecil

Introduction

The biopsychosocial (BPS) model was first proposed by Engel (1980) in an effort to bridge the rift between biomedical and psychosocial perspectives on disease, and counteract the mind–body dualism prevailing in medicine and psychiatry at the time. Over the past three decades, major advances in biological psychiatry, neuroscience, epidemiology, and developmental psychopathology—among others—have contributed to a more complete and layered understanding of mental health and disease, supporting the idea of mental illness as a complex and multi-determined construct. Indeed, growing collaboration between disciplines has begun to break down the silos of knowledge traditionally confined to purely biological versus psychosocial views, paving the way for a more holistic, dimensional, and multilevel approach to psychiatry. Despite this progress, interdisciplinary BPS work remains the exception rather than the rule in psychiatry. It has been suggested that this may stem in part from a failure of the BPS model to articulate a clear agenda for research and clinical practice, providing few details as to *how* exactly biological, social, and psychological factors jointly influence risk for psychiatric disorders (Davies and Roache, 2017).

In this chapter, I discuss how the rapidly growing field of epigenetics is emerging as a promising unifying framework for the integration of biological and psychosocial research, by shedding new light on BPS pathways to mental health and disease. I first begin the chapter with a brief overview of gene–environment (GE) research, and discuss how the knowledge generated in this area has provided key support for the BPS model, by documenting the importance of *both* biological and psychosocial factors in the development of psychiatric disorders. I then argue that, despite this important contribution, it has been difficult to translate knowledge from GE studies into a fully interdisciplinary psychiatric research programme due to the lack of an empirically testable mechanism explaining how genes and the environment interact. Following this, I introduce epigenetics, and discuss how seminal work in this area is beginning to shed new light into the biology underlying GE interplay on development, health, and disease across the lifespan. Finally, I conclude with a discussion of the implications of epigenetics for BPS psychiatry, as well as outlining current challenges and future directions for the field.

Gene–environment interplay in the aetiology of psychiatric disorders

Support for the BPS model is perhaps best evidenced in the widespread recognition that psychiatric disorders, like most other complex phenotypes (i.e. observable characteristics), result from the interplay of *both* genetic and environmental factors. Data from genetic studies indicate that the heritability of psychiatric disorders is moderate to high (37% for major depression vs 81% in schizophrenia; Sullivan et al., 2012), reflecting the contribution of many genetic variants with small effect, as well as rare variants of large effect (Gratten et al., 2014). At the same time, epidemiological studies have underscored the importance of the social environment, identifying a large number of risk factors for psychiatric disorders, including prenatal stress, parental psychopathology, childhood maltreatment, family conflict, low socioeconomic status, and violence exposure (Schilling et al., 2007). Importantly, studies examining GE interplay have demonstrated that these factors combine in complex ways, jointly influencing trajectories of development, health, and disease across the lifespan (Rutter et al., 2006).

Notably, GE research has taught us three key lessons about the extent to which biological and psychosocial factors co-act. First, it has demonstrated that individuals play an *active* role in shaping and selecting their environment, and that this is partly driven by their own genetic makeup—a phenomenon termed *gene–environment correlation* (rGE; Knafo and Jaffee, 2013). For example, individuals with a genetic vulnerability towards aggression may be more likely to behave antisocially, evoking negative reactions from people around them (i.e. evocative rGE), and actively seeking relationships with other antisocial individuals (i.e. active rGE). This suggests that, rather than being randomly distributed across the population, social exposures may be more likely to occur to certain individuals, partly because of their genetic background. Thus, what can appear to be purely 'psychosocial' risk factors for psychiatric illness may actually contain a 'biological' component.

Second, GE research has shown that genes and the environment not only correlate with one another, but can also interact. In other words, genes can influence how sensitive we are to our environment, and in turn, our environment can influence the degree to which our genes are expressed. In one of the first examples of such *gene–environment interactions* (G×E), Caspi and colleagues (2002) found that, among children with a history of maltreatment, those who carried the 'low-activity' allele of the monoamine oxidase A (*MAOA*) gene—conferring a reduced ability to break down neurotransmitters, such as dopamine and serotonin—showed the most severe levels of antisocial behaviour compared to children who carried the 'high-activity' genotype. Since this early report of G×E, a large body of research has provided empirical support for the idea that an individual's genetic makeup can moderate his or her response to external events, partially explaining why people exposed to the same stressor can react in very different ways (Manuck and McCaffery, 2014). Importantly, the converse has also been shown to be true, in that the environment can constrain or potentiate genetic influences as well. For example, individuals with a genetic vulnerability towards alcoholism will be less likely to develop the disorder within societies that prohibit alcohol use (McCutcheon, 2006).

Third, this research has highlighted the fundamental role of *developmental context* in GE interplay. Half of diagnosable mental health problems start by the age of 14 years (Kessler et al., 2005), and often manifest earlier in childhood as internalizing (e.g. anxiety, depression) and externalizing (e.g. conduct problems, hyperactivity) problems, pointing to an important role of early vulnerabilities. Indeed, genetic influences have been shown to interact with environmental factors as early as in the womb (Gordon et al., 2012), and be dynamic across development, with new genetic influences coming 'online' at different periods, perhaps in response to changing environmental exposures (Lacourse et al., 2014). Similarly, the impact of an environmental exposure can vary greatly depending on its timing. In particular, environmental exposures (both positive and negative) that occur during critical, sensitive windows of biological development—such as the prenatal period, early life, and adolescence—can exert a more profound and lasting impact on individual characteristics, compared to exposures that occur after the affected organs (e.g. brain) have fully matured and are therefore less plastic (Bornstein, 2014). An example of this 'environmental programming' is the observed link between prenatal undernutrition, low birthweight, and lifelong risk of coronary heart disease in the offspring (Godfrey and Barker, 2001). Another well-documented example is the impact of prenatal (but not postnatal) folate deficiency on infant mortality and neural tube defects (Blencowe et al., 2010). In relation to mental health, a growing body of research has begun to delineate the role of pre- and postnatal exposures in shaping neuroendocrine, metabolic, and immune development, with lasting effects on stress reactivity, behaviour, and risk for adult psychiatric disorders (Davis et al., 2011, Sullivan et al., 2014). Together, this evidence suggests that, in concert with genetic factors, environmental experiences during sensitive developmental periods may 'program' calibrated biological responses that, while potentially beneficial in promoting short-term adaptation, may engender latent vulnerability to disease in the long-term (McCrory and Viding, 2015).

Gene–environment interactions: the 'black box' of biology

Largely as a result of the knowledge generated by the GE studies reviewed earlier in this chapter, current scientific opinion holds that 'nature' (i.e. heritable/biological factors) and 'nurture' (i.e. psychosocial factors) are intrinsically interwoven, and that both elements must be taken into account if we are to understand the aetiology of psychiatric disorders. While this represents a considerable step forward in the process of harmonizing biological and psychosocial perspectives on mental illness, as well as providing key support for the BPS model, GE influences continue to be rarely examined together in psychiatric research and practice. For example, although the importance of the environment is often acknowledged within psychiatric genetic studies, data on exposures are not usually examined. Similarly, studies investigating the impact of environmental exposures on psychiatric outcomes tend not to account for genetic influences, despite the knowledge that such outcomes (and the exposures themselves) likely reflect a heritable component. Barriers to GE integration may partly result from the lack of a unifying 'mechanism' in the field capable of explaining *how* genes and environments co-act at a biological level.

Indeed, although GE studies have provided robust evidence for a *statistical* association between genes and the environment—and early molecular studies started identifying environmental triggers for gene expression (e.g. temperature changes, chemical signals) over 50 years ago—the biological mechanisms underlying these associations have remained very much a 'black box'. In other words, how do genes and the environment actually 'communicate' with one another at a biological level? How does the genome 'capture' environmental experiences and propagate their influences? And how can psychosocial experiences become 'biologically embedded', shaping an individual's development, health, and behaviour even long after the exposure itself has ceased? These questions lie at the heart of the BPS model, by probing deep into the mechanisms that enable BPS interactions to occur, with potentially widespread implications for the way we contextualize, assess, and treat psychiatric disorders.

Thanks to recent technological and methodological advances, epigenetic processes that regulate gene expression, such as DNA methylation (DNAm), are rapidly emerging as a potential mechanism of interest. So far, epigenetic processes have been shown to (1) respond to *both* genetic and environmental factors (Feil and Fraga, 2012; Jones et al., 2013); (2) play an essential role in normative development and health across the lifespan (Boland et al., 2014; Jones et al., 2015); and (3) be implicated in the emergence of disease states, including psychiatric and medical disorders (Bergman and Cedar, 2013; Klengel et al., 2014). Consequently, epigenetic processes may begin to explain how G×E operate at a molecular level, shedding new light on the old nature–nurture conundrum, fostering the development of an interdisciplinary research agenda and enabling BPS hypotheses that were previously out of scientific reach to be empirically tested.

Epigenetics: a brief overview

The 'epigenome' refers to a collection of epigenetic processes that regulate *when* and *where* genes are expressed (i.e. switched 'on' or 'off')—primarily via chemical modifications to DNA, histone proteins, and chromatin structure (Jaenisch and Bird, 2003). Whereas the DNA sequence can be thought of as a type of biological 'hardware' that remains mostly unchanged over the lifespan, providing a genetic 'blueprint' for all living things, epigenetic processes can instead be thought of as a type of biological 'software', dictating how this genetic information should be used over time and across tissues. A good example of epigenetic regulation is the process of cellular differentiation: every cell in the human body contains a nearly identical DNA sequence (i.e. the same genetic blueprint), and yet, over 200 different cell types exist. This is possible because epigenetic processes regulate, within each cell, which parts of the DNA sequence (i.e. genes) can be read (i.e. expressed/switched 'on') and which parts must remain silenced (i.e. switched 'off'). As a result of these epigenetic 'instructions', genes that are expressed within a brain cell may differ from genes that are expressed within a liver cell or a muscle cell, enabling these cells to acquire different physical properties and perform specialized functions (Boland et al., 2014). Nowadays, we know that epigenetic modifications are not only fundamental for the establishment and maintenance of cellular identity, but also coordinate a much wider range of biological processes, including genomic imprinting and X chromosome inactivation, as well as processes relevant to psychiatric disorders, such as regulation of stress response, immune function, and neurodevelopment (Suárez-Álvarez et al., 2013; Gapp et al., 2014; Zannas and West, 2014). Although a number of different epigenetic processes exist, this chapter focuses specifically on DNAm, as it is the most extensively studied in the context of mental health. For the interested reader, several high-quality reviews are available covering other epigenetic processes in depth (Peschansky and Wahlestedt, 2014; Non and Thayer, 2015).

DNAm refers to the addition of a methyl group to specific DNA base pairs, primarily in the context of cytosine–guanine (CpG) dinucleotides. The human genome contains in excess of 28 million CpG sites, around 10% of which cluster together to form CpG 'islands', close to gene promoter regions (Eckhardt et al., 2006). These islands are typically unmethylated (i.e. no methyl group attached), enabling transcription factors to bind to the DNA sequence and activate gene expression. In contrast, methylated CpG islands create a 'physical barrier' around the gene, which impedes transcription factors from accessing the DNA sequence, thereby repressing expression. Because of this, higher DNAm of a gene is usually associated with decreased expression of that gene, although exceptions have been noted (Wagner et al., 2014). DNAm patterns can be mitotically passed on during cell division, with around 80% of sites across the genome remaining stable over time, leading to long-term alterations in gene activity (Ziller et al., 2013). However, a sizable minority of DNAm sites can also show a considerable degree of flexibility, enabling cells to respond to changing internal and external inputs (Alabert and Groth, 2012).

In summary, epigenetic processes such as DNAm play a key role in shaping individual characteristics, by regulating how genetic information is used over time and across the different cells in our body. But what factors drive variability in DNAm in the first place? Mounting evidence suggests that, much like the determinants of mental health and disease, DNAm patterns reflect the influence of *both* genetic and environmental factors.

Genetic and environmental influences on DNA methylation

Behavioural genetic studies have reported that identical twin pairs (who share 100% of their DNA) show more similar DNAm patterns compared to non-identical twin pairs (who only share around 50% of their DNA), supporting a role of genetic architecture in DNAm patterns (Kaminsky et al., 2009). Consistent with this, molecular genetic studies have found that a large number of DNAm sites (called 'methylation quantitative trait loci'; mQTLs) are under genetic control—both as a result of common (Gaunt et al., 2016) and rare (Richardson et al., 2016) genetic variants. In particular, genetic influences have been found to be strongest when the variant is in close physical prox-imity to the DNAm site (i.e. located in *cis*), with weaker effects identified instead for distal variants (i.e. located in *trans*; Gibbs et al., 2010). As such, there is convincing evidence from multiple lines of research that DNAm patterns are genetically influ-enced. It is therefore important to keep in mind that observed associations between DNAm and phenotypes of interest, such as psychiatric disorders, may reflect in part underlying, heritable variations in DNA sequence.

It is clear, however, that this is not the only type of influence on DNAm—although the studies mentioned robustly demonstrate that genetic factors are important, they also show that genetic factors do *not entirely* account for variability in DNAm. For example, while it is true that identical twins show more similar DNAm patterns com-pared to non-identical twins, these similarities have been found to decrease with age—a phenomenon termed 'epigenetic drift' (Fraga et al., 2005). It has been sug-gested that—in addition to internal biological inputs and random, stochastic changes in DNAm—this divergence may reflect the influence of non-shared environmental factors (Feil and Fraga, 2012; Teschendorff et al., 2013). In other words, as twins grow older and begin to experience different things (e.g. going to different schools, making different friends, developing different hobbies and habits), the accumulation of these non-shared exposures may contribute not only to differences in twins' physical ap-pearance, individual characteristics, and behaviour, but also in their DNAm patterns.

The idea that *environmental* exposures could potentially influence the activity of genes via epigenetic changes led to a radical re-evaluation of the nature–nurture de-bate. As mentioned previously, environmental effects on gene expression had already been observed many decades earlier. However, the mechanisms underlying these ef-fects were poorly understood. Furthermore, information on gene expression alone could not explain how cells were seemingly able to keep a 'biochemical record' of past environmental exposures, which could alter their long-term function and responsivity to future environmental triggers (Isles, 2015). One of the earliest studies to contribute empirical support for environmental effects on the epigenome was that of Heijmans and colleagues (2008), who examined DNAm in survivors of the Dutch hunger winter, a severe famine at the end of the Second World War. The authors found that, even 60 years after the event had taken place, individuals who had been prenatally exposed to famine showed lower levels of DNAm in the insulin-like growth factor 2 (*IGF2*) gene—a key regulator of fetal development—compared to their unexposed, same-sex sibling. Since then, further evidence has supported a link between early nutri-tional exposures (e.g. undernutrition, maternal obesity) and DNAm changes in the offspring, particularly in genes involved in metabolic, neural and developmental pro-cesses. In turn, these changes in DNAm have been shown to associate with disease-relevant developmental outcomes, such as neonatal birthweight, cholesterol levels, and neurocognitive function (e.g. Peter et al., 2016).

Another environmental exposure that has received extensive scrutiny in relation to DNAm is tobacco smoking. As well as being harmful in adults, tobacco exposure during pregnancy exerts widespread neurotoxic effects on the developing fetus, including restricted blood flow supply to the brain, alterations in neurotransmitter function, and increased risk for psychiatric disorders (Bruin et al., 2010). Epigenetic studies suggest that these effects may be in part mediated by changes in DNAm. In fact, the association between tobacco smoking (whether directly or via prenatal exposure) and DNAm is one of the most replicated in the field of epigenetics, evidencing widespread changes in genes primarily involved in the detoxification of teratogens (see Gao et al. (2015) for a review). While some of these changes have found to be reversible with time, others have been shown to persist into adulthood, indicating that exposure to teratogens early in development can have a lasting impact on epigenetic regulation, with potentially long-term consequences for disease risk (Richmond et al., 2015).

In summary, environmental influences such as dietary and neurotoxic exposures that occur as early as in the womb have been found to associate with changes in DNAm patterns, with implications for long-term health. It is becoming increasingly clear, however, that DNAm may not only respond to such 'direct' or 'physical' exposures, but may also be sensitive to 'social' exposures, including key predictors of psychiatric risk (e.g. childhood maltreatment, trauma). This is of major relevance to the BPS model, as it points to a biological basis for the influence of psychosocial factors on individual development and disease risk.

DNA methylation and the biological embedding of psychosocial experiences: evidence from animal models

The earliest evidence for the impact of psychosocial exposures on the epigenome came from the animal literature. In a series of seminal studies on rodents, Weaver and colleagues (2004, 2005) examined the influence of postnatal maternal care on pups' epigenetic regulation of a specific gene, called the glucocorticoid receptor gene (*GR*, also referred to as *NR3C1*). The selection of this gene was based on extensive work documenting its key role in regulating the hypothalamic–pituitary–adrenal (HPA) axis system, and mediating the effects of stress on neurodevelopmental, metabolic, cardiovascular, and immune function (Nicolaides et al., 2014). Briefly, the *GR* gene codes for glucocorticoid receptors that are located in virtually all cells and that bind to glucocorticoids (e.g. cortisol)—stress hormones centrally involved in neuroendocrine activity (Meaney, 2010). When exposed to stressors, the HPA axis triggers the release of glucocorticoids in the bloodstream, which set in motion a cascade of adaptive physiological responses, including mobilization of glucose reserves for energy, heightened vigilance, and increased heart rate and blood flow to muscles. When glucocorticoid levels become excessively high, they are sensed by these glucocorticoid receptors, which in turn signal the need for reduced secretion of stress hormones—a mechanism called a 'negative feedback loop' that helps to restore homeostasis once the stressor has ceased (Nicolaides et al., 2014). While this system has evolved to cope successfully with short-term/moderate stressors, exposure to periods of prolonged or acute stress (e.g. chronic adversity, childhood maltreatment, trauma) has been found to result in dysregulation of the HPA axis response, leading to long-term physiological alterations, neuronal death, and changes in a number of stress-sensitive brain areas (e.g. hippocampus, amygdala, prefrontal cortex), with downstream consequences for mood, behaviour, and psychiatric risk (e.g. depression, post-traumatic stress disorder (PTSD)).

Based on this evidence, Weaver and colleagues set out to investigate the specific biological pathways through which early psychosocial exposures influence HPA axis function and stress response, using an animal model. The authors capitalized on the fact that, much like humans, female rats show naturally occurring variations in the quality of caregiving towards their pups, measured as levels of *licking and grooming* (LG). As such, the authors examined whether early differences in the social environment—specifically indexed by levels of maternal LG—caused alterations to the pup's stress response via epigenetic changes to the *GR* gene. The authors found that, compared to pups who received *high* levels of LG (i.e. nurturing care), those exposed to *low* levels of LG (i.e. poor/neglectful care) showed higher methylation of the *GR* gene, which in turn resulted in decreased expression of this gene, leading to a lower density of glucocorticoid receptors in the hippocampus. When exposed to future stressors, these pups had a harder time 'bouncing back' compared to pups who had been exposed to high levels of LG, showing slower physiological recovery, higher circulating stress hormones, and greater defensive responses, such as anxious and aggressive behaviour. Remarkably, these biological changes, which could be traced to differences in maternal care *within the first week of life*, were found to be stable over time, influencing stress response and behaviour across the lifespan. When these rats had pups of their own, they were also found to be more likely to engage in low LG behaviour themselves, suggesting an intergenerational transmission of caregiving behaviour (Champagne, 2010).

These studies were groundbreaking for three reasons. First, they were the first to show that *psychosocial* experiences, such as maternal care, could exert a measurable, observable effect on gene expression via changes in epigenetic regulation—thereby delineating a physical basis for GE interplay. Second, these studies showed that epigenetic regulation could, in turn, exert a measurable, observable effect on stress response and behaviour, which persisted long after the initial stressor had taken place—pointing to a mechanism for the biological embedding of psychosocial experiences. At a broader level, this evidence suggested that what may often be considered as a disordered outcome (e.g. anxiety, aggression) could instead be better understood as a calibrated *adaptation* to early environmental conditions, mediated by epigenetic changes. Indeed, for a pup raised in a low-care environment, characteristics such as heightened threat vigilance and enhanced defensive responses may be necessary for maximizing chances of survival, compared to a pup who has been raised in a nurturing environment. Third, these studies showed that the effects of maternal care on DNAm could be *reversed*, either by using a chemical treatment (i.e. methionine infusion; Weaver et al., 2005) or a 'social' intervention (i.e. cross-fostering; Weaver et al., 2004), which in turn led to the normalization of physiological and behavioural function (i.e. low LG pups no longer distinguishable from high LG pups). Together, this evidence not only provided robust evidence for causality between the environment (exposure), DNAm (mediator), and behaviour (outcome), but also suggested that the implementation of social (as well as chemical) intervention strategies may be effective in reversing stress-related epigenetic patterns.

Human studies on early adversity and DNA methylation

Animal studies such as those reviewed in the previous section have a number of important strengths, including the ability to manipulate the type, timing, and severity of environmental exposures, trace the effects of these exposures on DNAm, and measure the downstream consequences of DNAm changes on gene expression and behaviour. Despite these strengths, however, an important question that usually emerges from animal studies is the extent to which findings generalize to humans. Addressing this question is challenging, as experimental manipulation and access to relevant tissues in humans is usually not possible. Postmortem studies represent one important tool for testing the translational potential of animal findings. For example, Weaver and colleagues' *GR* findings were successfully replicated in humans, based on hippocampal tissue from suicide completers. Specifically, the authors found that, among adults who had committed suicide, those retrospectively identified as having experienced maltreatment during childhood showed higher levels of *GR* methylation in the hippocampus—consistent with the findings from low LG pups (McGowan et al., 2009). Importantly, subsequent studies in living individuals, which must rely on peripheral tissues (e.g. saliva, blood, and placenta) as opposed to brain tissue, have also reported increased *GR* methylation in relation to early adversity—not only postnatal, but prenatal as well (e.g. maternal depression during pregnancy; see Turecki and Meaney (2016) for a review). This is particularly promising given that DNAm patterns can differ widely across tissues and cell types, so that the relevance of peripheral epigenetic patterns to the brain is often unclear. Also of interest are recent studies showing that *GR* methylation levels associate with stress-relevant outcomes, including markers of HPA axis function (e.g. cortisol reactivity; van der Knaap et al., 2015) as well as psychiatric outcomes (e.g. borderline personality disorder, PTSD; Dammann et al., 2011; Yehuda et al., 2015)—although null results have also been reported (Turecki and Meaney, 2016).

Together, these studies support animal findings in showing that (1) early psychosocial adversity can influence epigenetic regulation of the *GR* gene; and that (2) changes in *GR* methylation can, in turn, influence physiological and psychiatric outcomes. As a result, *GR* methylation is currently identified as a promising biomarker for stress exposure, stress response, and psychiatric risk. However, as the field moves forward, there is an increasing appreciation that, if we are to gain a more complete picture of how environmental exposures influence epigenetic regulation, we must look beyond the *GR* gene and examine wider changes in DNAm *across the genome*. This is supported by evidence showing that DNAm levels across genes are not independent but interrelated, forming larger co-methylation networks (Spiers et al., 2015). Indeed, emerging epigenome-wide studies have shown that exposure to early adversity (e.g. prenatal maternal stress, poverty, institutionalization, childhood maltreatment) associates with DNAm patterns across a much wider range of genes, involved in numerous processes in addition to stress response, such as neurodevelopment and immune function (Naumova et al., 2012; Lutz and Turecki, 2016). For example, in a recent study, we sought to characterize the epigenome-wide 'signatures' of childhood abuse and neglect, based on a sample of high-risk youth (Cecil et al., 2016b). We found that physical forms of maltreatment associated with widespread changes in DNAm, implicating multiple genes previously associated with psychiatric and neurodevelopmental disorders (e.g. *GABBR1*, *GRIN2D*, *CACNA2D4*, *PSEN2*). We also found that, although maltreatment types showed unique methylation patterns linked to specific biological processes (e.g. physical abuse and cardiovascular function vs physical neglect and nutrient metabolism), they also shared a 'common' epigenetic signature related to neural and developmental processes.

In summary, growing evidence suggests that, in addition to being under genetic control, epigenetic patterns are also sensitive to environmental influences, including psychosocial exposures. It is important to note here that, because epigenetic regulation is developmentally dynamic, the *timing* of an exposure may moderate its effects on DNAm and downstream outcomes, depending on the degree of maturation/plasticity of the affected biological systems. For example, a stressor that occurs prenatally (i.e. a period of major neurodevelopmental growth) may affect DNAm differently than the same stressor occurring during childhood (i.e. when certain brain regions are more mature than others) or in adulthood (i.e. when there is still a degree of plasticity, but neural systems have fully matured). This may help to explain the multifinality of stress exposure—that is, why the same type of stressor can lead to a multitude of different outcomes (Cicchetti and Rogosch, 1996).

The role of DNA methylation in the development of psychiatric disorders

So far, DNAm has been discussed as a potential mechanism for GE interplay, and as a process through which exposures can become biologically embedded. But what bearing does this have for our understanding of psychiatric disorders? Epigenetic regulation is known to be an *essential* part of healthy development and function. As mentioned earlier, DNAm plays a key role in a wide range of processes, including cellular differentiation, genomic imprinting, and X-chromosome inactivation, as well as coordinating hormonal, metabolic, immune, and neural changes across the lifespan. Indeed, if we think once again of DNAm as a mechanism through which the body can 'read' and make use of its genetic blueprint, it is unsurprising that *disruptions* in DNAm patterns would be linked to negative outcomes, both in terms of physical and mental health. This is supported, for example, by strong evidence of genome-wide DNAm alterations in cancer, as well as reported associations with other diseases, including metabolic, cardiovascular, and autoimmune disorders (Bergman and Cedar, 2013).

Although epigenetic research has been slower to permeate the psychiatric literature, recent years have seen an exponential increase in studies in this area. Most of these have been candidate-gene focused, cross-sectional, and based on adult samples, reporting associations between numerous psychiatric disorders (e.g. major depression, suicide risk, PTSD, schizophrenia) and DNAm levels in genes mainly related to stress response (e.g. *GR* and other HPA axis genes) and neurotransmitter function (e.g. dopamine and serotonin pathway genes; Klengel et al., 2014; Nestler et al., 2016). As with the broader field of epigenetics, however, studies are also beginning to move beyond candidate gene analyses, to characterize more systematically epigenome-wide DNAm patterns associated with psychiatric outcomes. This is a promising step forward, given that psychiatric disorders are aetiologically complex and unlikely to result from epigenetic alterations in single genes. However, this research is still in its infancy, so that a consistent picture of *unique* vs *shared* DNAm patterns across psychiatric disorders has yet to emerge.

A related area in which epigenetics is making an increasing contribution is that of developmental psychopathology. Work from our own group, as well as others, has begun to delineate the role of DNAm in the *emergence* of psychiatric symptoms during childhood and adolescence (e.g. externalizing and internalizing difficulties), which in turn are important predictors of mental health across the lifespan (see Barker et al. (2017) for a review). In particular, we have made use of longitudinal data spanning pregnancy to adolescence to test whether epigenome-wide DNAm patterns measured in early life (i.e. *prior* to symptom onset) prospectively associate with psychopathological outcomes later in development. Using this hypothesis-free approach, we have found that, for example, children who follow a high, chronic trajectory of ADHD symptoms show early epigenetic differences in genes involved in fatty acid metabolism and neuron myelination (Walton et al., 2017); that early-onset conduct problems are associated with DNAm of a gene involved in pain perception and endocannabinoid signalling (Cecil et al., 2018); and that adolescent substance use is linked to neonatal DNAm levels across a network of genes implicated in neurodevelopment (Cecil et al., 2016a).

In summary, a growing literature points to a link between alterations in DNAm patterns and the emergence of psychiatric symptoms. However, evidence to date is still preliminary, and more work will be needed to replicate findings and establish whether these links are truly causal. In the following section, I outline some of the key challenges for the field and how these may be addressed, before concluding in the final section with a discussion of the implications of epigenetic research for BPS psychiatry.

Key challenges, recommendations, and future directions

Despite considerable advances over recent years, epigenetic research on psychiatric disorders currently faces a number of challenges that limit the conclusions that can be drawn (see Barker et al. (2017) for a review).

Firstly, our knowledge of DNAm (and other epigenetic processes) is still limited. At present, commonly used technologies only capture a fraction of DNAm in the genome, so that many regions of potential relevance to psychopathology remain largely inaccessible (Non and Thayer, 2015). To complicate matters, DNAm has been shown to vary across multiple factors, including age, sex, tissue, and cell type (Liang and Cookson, 2014), making it difficult to establish what a 'typical' methylation profile looks like, and how far such a profile must deviate in order to contribute to diseased states. Because DNAm can differ across tissues, it has also been unclear to what extent DNAm patterns observed in easily accessible tissues (e.g. saliva, blood) reflect those found in the brain—likely the most relevant (yet most inaccessible) organ for the study of psychiatric disorders. Furthermore, because very few studies have incorporated biological data at multiple levels, it is often unknown whether the identified DNAm patterns significantly affect gene expression levels, and downstream consequences on physiology, neural function, and behaviour. Rapid technological advances, however, are helping to bridge this knowledge gap. For example, the development of novel genome-wide platforms will make it increasingly possible to obtain a more complete picture of DNAm. At the same time, the compilation of reference datasets will be important for providing a normative benchmark against which to compare epigenetic findings (Shakya et al., 2012). In particular, sampling of DNAm across multiple tissues and time points will make it possible to quantify peripheral brain tissue variability and to examine whether longitudinal trajectories of DNAm may be informative in predicting the onset and course of psychiatric disorders. Moreover, strategies for big data integration will help to establish the functional significance of DNAm changes at transcriptomic, neural, and behavioural levels, in order to delineate more clearly the biological pathways through which epigenetic alterations influence psychiatric risk (Gomez-Cabrero et al., 2014).

A second set of challenges relates to research methodology. Existing studies have varied widely in sample characteristics (e.g. age range, clinical vs population based), methodology (e.g. data processing, analysis pipeline, choice of covariates, etc.) and outcomes measured (e.g. type of psychiatric disorder, clinical thresholds used, etc.). Together, these sources of variability have limited comparability across findings, making replication difficult (Barker et al., 2017). Furthermore, because most studies in humans have been cross-sectional, it has not been possible to establish causality—in other words, whether DNAm is indeed a risk factor for, rather than a consequence of, psychiatric disorders. To address these limitations, guidelines for best practice in epigenetic research are continuously being fine-tuned. In particular, the increased availability of standardized procedures and analytic tools will help to maximize convergence across studies (Morris and Beck, 2015), while replication will become increasingly important for identifying robust findings. Studies that examine multiple psychiatric outcomes will also make it possible in future to disentangle DNAm patterns that may be disorder specific versus those that may be shared across multiple psychiatric disorders—potentially shedding light on the biological basis of psychiatric comorbidity. Finally, the use of advanced inference methods (e.g. Mendelian randomization; Relton and Davey Smith, 2012) will make it possible to test causal pathways between GE influences, DNAm, and the emergence of psychiatric disorders.

Implications of epigenetics for biopsychosocial psychiatry

Epigenetic processes are fast emerging as a promising molecular mechanism through which genetic and environmental factors influence development, health, and disease across the lifespan. Yet, as we gain an appreciation of the challenges facing epigenetic research, we must be mindful to manage expectations. Bearing this in mind, the knowledge generated by epigenetic studies may hold important implications for the way that we understand, prevent, and potentially even treat mental disorders. In the first instance, findings may be used to re-evaluate and refine the BPS model, by delineating *how* psychosocial experiences can become biologically embedded, shaping trajectories of psychiatric risk. In other words, epigenetic data may be used as a novel tool for testing hypotheses about the specific pathways through which the 'bio' (e.g. genetic/heritable influences) and the 'social' (e.g. early adversity) combine to influence the 'psycho' (e.g. mood, cognition, behaviour) in the development of psychiatric disorders. With regard to prevention, the use of longitudinal research to investigate the timing of epigenetic effects may identify specific windows of biological vulnerability that could benefit most from preventive action. As the number of replications grow and robust associations are identified, epigenetic variation in specific genes may be employed across clinical and research settings as biomarkers for environmental exposures, psychiatric risk, and response to treatment. This is already the case in oncology, where epigenetic biomarkers within the clinic inform cancer detection, prognosis, and treatment success (Heyn and Esteller, 2012). Furthermore, the comparison of DNAm patterns prior to and post intervention (e.g. environmental enrichment, psychological therapy, medication) may lend insights into the potential reversibility of disorder-related epigenetic patterns and how best to promote resilience. Indeed, tentative evidence that DNAm patterns respond to psychological and pharmaceutical intervention within individuals with psychiatric disorders is already beginning to emerge (Roberts et al., 2014; Ding et al., 2017). Ultimately, establishing causal pathways between environmental risk exposure, epigenetic regulation, and psychiatric disorders could lead to the development of novel strategies for treating mental health problems.

Acknowledgements

The author was supported by the Economic and Social Research Council (grant reference: ES/N001273/1) and by the European Union's Horizon 2020 research and innovation program under the Marie Skłodowska-Curie grant agreement (Grant No. 707404) during the preparation of this manuscript.

References

Alabert, C. and Groth, A. (2012). Chromatin replication and epigenome maintenance. *Nature Reviews; Molecular Cell Biology*, **13**(3), 153–167.

Barker, E.D., Walton, E., and Cecil, C.A.M. (2017). Annual Research Review: DNA methylation as a mediator in the association between risk exposure and child and adolescent psychopathology. *Journal of Child Psychology and Psychiatry*, **59**(4), 303–322.

Bergman, Y. and Cedar, H. (2013). DNA methylation dynamics in health and disease. *Nature Structural & Molecular Biology*, **20**(3), 274–281.

Blencowe, H., Cousens, S., Modell, B., and Lawn, J. (2010). Folic acid to reduce neonatal mortality from neural tube disorders. *International Journal of Epidemiology*, **39**(Suppl.1), i110–i121.

Boland, M.J., Nazor, K.L., and Loring, J.F. (2014). Epigenetic regulation of pluripotency and differentiation. *Circulation Research*, **115**(2), 311–324.

Bornstein, M.H. (2014). *Sensitive Periods in Development: Interdisciplinary Perspectives*. New York: Psychology Press.

Bruin, J.E., Gerstein, H.C., and Holloway, A.C. (2010). Long-term consequences of fetal and neonatal nicotine exposure: a critical review. *Toxicological Sciences*, **116**(2), 364–374.

Caspi, A., McClay, J., Moffitt, T.E., Mill, J., Martin, J., Craig, I.W., Taylor, A., and Poulton, R. (2002). Role of genotype in the cycle of violence in maltreated children. *Science*, **297**(5582), 851–854.

Cecil, C., Walton, E., Smith, R., Viding, E., Mccrory, E., Relton, C., Suderman, M., Pingault, J., McArdle, W., and Gaunt, T. (2016a). DNA methylation and substance-use risk: a prospective, genome-wide study spanning gestation to adolescence. *Translational Psychiatry*, **6**(12), e976.

Cecil, C.A.M., Smith, R.G., Walton, E., Mill, J., Mccrory, E.J., and Viding, E. (2016b). Epigenetic signatures of childhood abuse and neglect: implications for psychiatric vulnerability assessment. *Journal of Psychiatric Research*, **83**, 184–194.

Cecil, C.A.M., Walton, E., Jaffee, S.R., O'Connor, T., Maughan, B., Relton, C.L., Smith, R., McArdle, W., Gaunt, T.R., Ouellet-Morin, I., and Barker, E.D. (2018). Neonatal DNA methylation and early-onset conduct problems: a genome-wide, prospective study. *Development and Psychopathology*, **30**(2), 383–397.

Champagne, F.A. (2010). Epigenetic influence of social experiences across the lifespan. *Development and Psychopathology*, **52**(4), 299–311.

Cicchetti, D. and Rogosch, F.A. (1996). Equifinality and multifinality in developmental psychopathology. *Development and Psychopathology*, **8**(4), 597–600.

Dammann, G., Teschler, S., Haag, T., Altmüller, F., Tuczek, F., and Dammann, R.H. (2011). Increased DNA methylation of neuropsychiatric genes occurs in borderline personality disorder. *Epigenetics*, **6**(12),1454–1462.

Davies, W. and Roache, R. (2017). *Reassessing biopsychosocial psychiatry. The British Journal of Psychiatry*, **210**(1), 3–5.

Davis, E.P., Glynn, L.M., Waffarn, F., and Sandman, C.A. (2011). Prenatal maternal stress programs infant stress regulation. *Journal of Child Psychology and Psychiatry*, **52**(2), 119–129.

Ding, K., Yang, J., Reynolds, G.P., Chen, B., Shao, J., Liu, R., Qian, Q., Liu, H., Yang, R., and Wen, J. (2017). DAT1 methylation is associated with methylphenidate response on oppositional and hyperactive-impulsive symptoms in children and adolescents with ADHD. *The World Journal of Biological Psychiatry*, **18**(4), 291–299.

Eckhardt, F., Lewin, J., Cortese, R., Rakyan, V.K., Attwood, J., Burger, M., Burton, J., Cox, T.V., Davies, R., Down, T.A., Haefliger, C., Horton, R., Howe, K., Jackson, D.K., Kunde, J., Koenig, C., Liddle, J., Niblett, D., Otto, T., Pettett, R., Seemann, S., Thompson, C., West, T., Rogers, J., Olek, A., Berlin, K., and Beck, S. (2006). DNA methylation profiling of human chromosomes 6, 20 and 22. *Nature Genetics*, **38**(12), 1378–1385.

Engel, G.L. (1980). The clinical application of the biopsychosocial model. *American Journal of Psychiatry*, **137**(2), 535–544.

Feil, R. and Fraga, M.F. (2012). Epigenetics and the environment: emerging patterns and implications. *Nature Reviews Genetics*, **13**(2), 97–109.

Fraga, M.F., Ballestar, E., Paz, M.F., Ropero, S., Setien, F., Ballestar, M.L., Heine-Suñer, D., Cigudosa, J.C., Urioste, M., and Benitez, J. (2005). Epigenetic differences arise during the lifetime of monozygotic twins. *Proceedings of the National Academy of Sciences*, **102**(30), 10604–10609.

Gao, X., Jia, M., Zhang, Y., Breitling, L.P., and Brenner, H. (2015). DNA methylation changes of whole blood cells in response to active smoking exposure in adults: a systematic review of DNA methylation studies. *Clinical Epigenetics*, **7**, 113.

Gapp, K., Woldemichael, B., Bohacek, J., and Mansuy, I. (2014). Epigenetic regulation in neurodevelopment and neurodegenerative diseases. *Neuroscience*, **264**, 99–111.

Gaunt, T.R., Shihab, H.A., Hemani, G., Min, J.L., Woodward, G., Lyttleton, O., Zheng, J., Duggirala, A., McArdle, W.L., and Ho, K. (2016). Systematic identification of genetic influences on methylation across the human life course. *Genome Biology*, **17**, 1.

Gibbs, J.R., van der Brug, M.P., Hernandez, D.G., Traynor, B.J., Nalls, M.A., Lai, S.-L., Arepalli, S., Dillman, A., Rafferty, I.P., and Troncoso, J. (2010). Abundant quantitative trait loci exist for DNA methylation and gene expression in human brain. *PLoS Genetics*, **6**(5), e1000952.

Godfrey, K.M. and Barker, D.J. (2001). Fetal programming and adult health. *Public Health Nutrition*, **4**(2B), 611–624.

Gomez-Cabrero, D., Abugessaisa, I., Maier, D., Teschendorff, A., Merkenschlager, M., Gisel, A., Ballestar, E., Bongcam-Rudloff, E., Conesa, A., and Tegnér, J. (2014). Data integration in the era of omics: current and future challenges. *BMC Systems Biology*, **8**(Suppl 2). I1.

Gordon, L., Joo, J.E., Powell, J.E., Ollikainen, M., Novakovic, B., Li, X., Andronikos, R., Cruickshank, M.N., Conneely, K.N., and Smith, A.K. (2012). Neonatal DNA methylation profile in human twins is specified by a complex interplay between intrauterine environmental and genetic factors, subject to tissue-specific influence. *Genome Research*, **22**(8), 1395–1406.

Gratten, J., Wray, N.R., Keller, M.C., and Visscher, P.M. (2014). Large-scale genomics unveils the genetic architecture of psychiatric disorders. *Nature Neuroscience*, **17**(6), 782–790.

Heijmans, B.T., Tobi, E.W., Stein, A.D., Putter, H., Blauw, G.J., Susser, E.S., Slagboom, P.E., and Lumey, L. (2008). Persistent epigenetic differences associated with prenatal exposure to famine in humans. *Proceedings of the National Academy of Sciences*, **105**(44), 17046–17049.

Heyn, H. and Esteller, M. (2012). DNA methylation profiling in the clinic: applications and challenges. *Nature Reviews Genetics*, **13**(10), 679–692.

Isles, A.R. (2015). Neural and behavioral epigenetics; what it is, and what is hype. *Genes, Brain and Behavior*, **14**(1), 64–72.

Jaenisch, R. and Bird, A. (2003). Epigenetic regulation of gene expression: how the genome integrates intrinsic and environmental signals. *Nature Genetics*, **33**(Suppl.), 245–254.

Jones, M.J., Fejes, A.P., and Kobor, M.S. (2013). DNA methylation, genotype and gene expression: who is driving and who is along for the ride? *Genome Biology*, **14**(7), 126.

Jones, M.J., Goodman, S.J., and Kobor, M.S. (2015). DNA methylation and healthy human aging. *Aging Cell*, **14**(6), 924–932.

Kaminsky, Z.A., Tang, T., Wang, S.-C., Ptak, C., Oh, G.H., Wong, A.H., Feldcamp, L.A., Virtanen, C., Halfvarson, J., and Tysk, C. (2009). DNA methylation profiles in monozygotic and dizygotic twins. *Nature Genetics*, **41**(2), 240–245.

Kessler, R.C., Berglund, P., Demler, O., Jin, R., Merikangas, K.R., and Walters, E.E. (2005). Lifetime prevalence and age-of-onset distributions of DSM-IV disorders in the National Comorbidity Survey Replication. *Archives of General Psychiatry*, **62**(6), 593–602.

Klengel, T., Pape, J., Binder, E.B., and Mehta, D. (2014). The role of DNA methylation in stress-related psychiatric disorders. *Neuropharmacology*, **80**, 115–132.

Knafo, A. and Jaffee, S.R. (2013). Gene–environment correlation in developmental psychopathology. *Development and Psychopathology*, **25**(1), 1–6.

Lacourse, E., Boivin, M., Brendgen, M., Petitclerc, A., Girard, A., Vitaro, F., Paquin, S., Ouellet-Morin, I., Dionne, G., and Tremblay, R. (2014). A longitudinal twin study of physical aggression during early childhood: evidence for a developmentally dynamic genome. *Psychological Medicine*, **44**(12), 2617–2627.

Liang, L. and Cookson, W.O.C. (2014). Grasping nettles: cellular heterogeneity and other confounders in epigenome-wide association studies. *Human Molecular Genetics*, **23**(R1), R83–R88.

Lutz, P.E. and Turecki, G. (2016). DNA methylation and childhood maltreatment: from animal models to human studies. *Neuroscience*, **264**, 142–156.

Manuck, S.B. and Mccaffery, J.M. (2014). Gene-environment interaction. *Annual Review of Psychology*, **65**, 41–70.

McCrory, E.J. and **Viding**, E. (2015). The theory of latent vulnerability: reconceptualizing the link between childhood maltreatment and psychiatric disorder. *Development and Psychopathology*, **27**(2), 493–505.

McCutcheon, V.V. (2006). Toward an integration of social and biological research. *Social Service Review*, **80**(1), 159–178.

McGowan, P.O., Sasaki, A., D'alessio, A.C., Dymov, S., Labonté, B., Szyf, M., Turecki, G., and Meaney, M.J. (2009). Epigenetic regulation of the glucocorticoid receptor in human brain associates with childhood abuse. *Nature Neuroscience*, **12**, 342–348.

Meaney, M.J. (2010). Epigenetics and the biological definition of gene × environment interactions. *Child Development*, **81**(1), 41–79.

Morris, T.J., and **Beck**, S. (2015). Analysis pipelines and packages for Infinium humanmethylation450 beadchip (450k) data. *Methods*, **72**, 3–8.

Naumova, O.Y., Lee, M., Koposov, R., Szyf, M., Dozier, M., and Grigorenko, E.L. (2012). Differential patterns of whole-genome DNA methylation in institutionalized children and children raised by their biological parents. *Development and Psychopathology*, **24**(1), 143–155.

Nestler, E.J., Peña, C.J., Kundakovic, M., Mitchell, A., and Akbarian, S. (2016). Epigenetic basis of mental illness. *The Neuroscientist*, **22**, 447–463.

Nicolaides, N.C., Kyratzi, E., Lamprokostopoulou, A., Chrousos, G.P., and Charmandari, E. (2014). Stress, the stress system and the role of glucocorticoids. *Neuroimmunomodulation*, **22**(1–2), 6–19.

Non, A.L. and **Thayer**, Z.M. (2015). Epigenetics for anthropologists: an introduction to methods. *American Journal of Human Biology*, **27**(3), 295–303.

Peschansky, V.J. and **Wahlestedt**, C. (2014). Non-coding RNAs as direct and indirect modulators of epigenetic regulation. *Epigenetics*, **9**(1), 3–12.

Peter, C.J., Fischer, L.K., Kundakovic, M., Garg, P., Jakovcevski, M., Dincer, A., Amaral, A.C., Ginns, E.I., Galdzicka, M., and Bryce, C.P. (2016). DNA methylation signatures of early childhood malnutrition associated with impairments in attention and cognition. *Biological Psychiatry*, **80**(10), 765–774.

Relton, C.L. and **Davey Smith**, G. (2012). Two-step epigenetic Mendelian randomization: a strategy for establishing the causal role of epigenetic processes in pathways to disease. *International Journal of Epidemiology*, **41**(1), 161–176.

Richardson, T.G., Shihab, H.A., Hemani, G., Zheng, J., Hannon, E., Mill, J., Carnero-Montoro, E., Bell, J.T., Lyttleton, O., and McArdle, W.L. (2016). Collapsed methylation quantitative trait loci analysis for low frequency and rare variants. *Human Molecular Genetics*, **25**(19), 4339–4349.

Richmond, R.C., Simpkin, A.J., Woodward, G., Gaunt, T.R., Lyttleton, O., McArdle, W.L., Ring, S.M., Smith, A.D., Timpson, N.J., and Tilling, K. (2015). Prenatal exposure to maternal smoking and offspring DNA methylation across the lifecourse: findings from the Avon Longitudinal Study of Parents and Children (ALSPAC). *Human Molecular Genetics*, **24**(8), 2201–2217.

Roberts, S., Lester, K., Hudson, J., Rapee, R., Creswell, C., Cooper, P., Thirlwall, K., Coleman, J., Breen, G., and Wong, C. (2014). Serotonin transporter methylation and response to cognitive behaviour therapy in children with anxiety disorders. *Translational Psychiatry*, **4**, e444.

Rutter, M., Moffitt, T.E., and Caspi, A. (2006). Gene–environment interplay and psychopathology: multiple varieties but real effects. *Journal of Child Psychology and Psychiatry*, **47**(3–4), 226–261.

Schilling, E.A., Aseltine, R.H., and Gore, S. (2007). Adverse childhood experiences and mental health in young adults: a longitudinal survey. *BMC Public Health*, **7**, 30.

Shakya, K., O'Connell, M.J., and Ruskin, H.J. (2012). The landscape for epigenetic/epigenomic biomedical resources. *Epigenetics*, **7**(9), 982–986.

Spiers, H., Hannon, E., Schalkwyk, L.C., Smith, R., Wong, C.C., O'Donovan, M.C., Bray, N.J., and Mill, J. (2015). Methylomic trajectories across human fetal brain development. *Genome Research*, **25**(3), 338–352.

Suárez-Álvarez, B., Baragaño Raneros, A., Ortega, F., and López-Larrea, C. (2013). Epigenetic modulation of the immune function: a potential target for tolerance. *Epigenetics*, **8**(7), 694–702.

Sullivan, E.L., Nousen, E.K., and Chamlou, K.A. (2014). Maternal high fat diet consumption during the perinatal period programs offspring behaviour. *Physiology & Behaviour*, **123**, 236–242.

Sullivan, P.F., Daly, M.J., and O'Donovan, M. (2012). Genetic architectures of psychiatric disorders: the emerging picture and its implications. *Nature Reviews Genetics*, **13**(8), 537–551.

Teschendorff, A.E., West, J., and Beck, S. (2013). Age-associated epigenetic drift: implications, and a case of epigenetic thrift? *Human Molecular Genetics*, **22**(R1), R7–R15.

Turecki, G. and Meaney, M.J. (2014). Effects of the social environment and stress on glucocorticoid receptor gene methylation: a systematic review. *Biological Psychiatry*, **79**(2), 87–96.

van der Knaap, L.J., Oldehinkel, A.J., Verhulst, F.C., Van Oort, F.V., and Riese, H. (2015). Glucocorticoid receptor gene methylation and HPA-axis regulation in adolescents. The TRAILS study. *Psychoneuroendocrinology*, **58**, 46–50.

Wagner, J.R., Busche, S., Ge, B., Kwan, T., Pastinen, T., and Blanchette, M. (2014). The relationship between DNA methylation, genetic and expression inter-individual variation in untransformed human fibroblasts. *Genome Biology*, **15**(2), R37.

Walton, E., Pingault, J.-B., Cecil, C., Gaunt, T., Relton, C., Mill, J., and Barker, E. (2017). Epigenetic profiling of ADHD symptoms trajectories: a prospective, methylome-wide study. *Molecular Psychiatry*, **22**(2), 250–256.

Weaver, I.C., Cervoni, N., Champagne, F.A., D'alessio, A.C., Sharma, S., Seckl, J.R., Dymov, S., Szyf, M., and Meaney, M.J. (2004). Epigenetic programming by maternal behaviour. *Nature Neuroscience*, **7**(8), 847–854.

Weaver, I.C., Champagne, F.A., Brown, S.E., Dymov, S., Sharma, S., Meaney, M.J., and Szyf, M. (2005). Reversal of maternal programming of stress responses in adult offspring through methyl supplementation: altering epigenetic marking later in life. *Journal of Neuroscience*, **25**(47), 11045–11054.

Yehuda, R., Flory, J.D., Bierer, L.M., Henn-Haase, C., Lehrner, A., Desarnaud, F., Makotkine, I., Daskalakis, N.P., Marmar, C.R., and Meaney, M.J. (2015). Lower methylation of glucocorticoid receptor gene promoter 1 F in peripheral blood of veterans with posttraumatic stress disorder. *Biological Psychiatry*, **77**(4), 356–364.

Zannas, A.S. and West, A.E. (2014). Epigenetics and the regulation of stress vulnerability and resilience. *Neuroscience*, **264**, 157–170.

Ziller, M.J., Gu, H., Müller, F., Donaghey, J., Tsai, L.T.-Y., Kohlbacher, O., De Jager, P.L., Rosen, E.D., Bennett, D.A., and Bernstein, B.E. (2013). Charting a dynamic DNA methylation landscape of the human genome. *Nature*, **500**(7463), 477–481.

Chapter 13

Reacting to abuse

Richard Holton

Introduction

The findings of Essi Viding and her colleagues on the effects of childhood abuse and neglect are striking and sobering. Let me recap in broad strokes what I see as the main points of her Loebel Lectures: (1) among the children who show serious antisocial behaviour, there is good reason to distinguish two very different groups, characterized by those who exhibit callousness and those who don't; (2) the callous group show a large genetic component in their antisocial behaviour; (3) the uncallous group show a smaller genetic component, instead exhibiting an over-sensitization to possible threat, an over-sensitization that is probably caused by the abuse, and that is one of the factors in the antisocial behaviour.

In these brief comments I'll focus on the second group, on the children whose antisocial behaviour, together, no doubt, with much else, is affected by the abuse they have suffered. I want to discuss two things. The first concerns an idea that runs through much of Viding's work, the idea that characteristics that might be helpful in avoiding a threat in one environment might be damaging elsewhere. In pursuing this I will start with one particular phenomenon that Viding discusses, the 'overgeneral memory effect'. This is the finding that abused children tend to forget many of the specific happenings in their childhoods. Reflection on it can perhaps help to shed some light how memory, and its suppression, works. I will draw some parallels with the findings on delayed gratification that Viding also discusses. It is striking that in both cases we find a need to shut down certain sorts of thought; the therapeutic interest is in how and when we might get it going again.

My second focus is more general. I want to pose a question about how much the effects of childhood abuse are mediated by the expectations of the subjects. Many have claimed, with some plausibility, that we find such mediation in various psychological illnesses: that the way that subjects understand their own condition affects the symptoms that they display. I wonder whether here it could help explain the equifinality and multifinality that Viding discusses.

The overgeneral memory effect and delayed gratification

Children who have been maltreated tend to maintain only very general memories. (Valentino et al., 2009).[1] They may remember where they lived, where they went to

---

[1] Of course there are many other claims about the effects of abuse on children's memory which have been the subject of huge debate; I shan't get into them.

school, and so on, but will lose—or at least will lose access to—memories of specific events. It is plausible to see this as a defence mechanism: failing to remember specific events means failing to remember instances of abuse or other mistreatment. But a priori that seems surprising: wouldn't it be better to remember the good things while forgetting the bad? We might expect maltreated children to have selective specific memories rather than to lose them altogether.

I take it that the explanation of why this isn't the case is grounded in what is psychologically possible. It may be optimal to remember good things and forget the bad, but plausibly there is no way of doing that. Once the gates are open to some, the others will come crowding in. Reflecting on a good happening will jog a memory of the dreadful thing that followed. Better to keep the whole lot out.

If that explanation is right, then the overgeneral memory effect is another example of the class of phenomena that McCrory and Viding call 'latent vulnerability': a trait which is adaptive in some circumstances, but that remains latent, ready to be harmfully expressed in others (McCrory and Viding, 2015). They have shown that abused children are highly sensitive to facial expressions of emotion. For a child living with irascible and violent parents it is easy to see that this may be highly adaptive; they need to be responsive to the first sign of welling anger. But applied to other social settings it may be deeply harmful, leading to an over-readiness to perceive threat, and a tendency to display aggression in response. Viding's second example of latent vulnerability concerned delayed gratification. Walter Mischel famously showed that the ability as a child to refrain from eating one marshmallow in order to be rewarded with two—to delay one's gratification—is predictive of many good outcomes later, including academic, financial, and social success (Mischel, 1996). This can make it seem like an unalloyed good. However, he noticed early on that the ability to delay gratification is class marked: children from more affluent homes show it more markedly than those from poorer homes. And this has led more recent researchers to question whether it might be disadvantageous to delay gratification if one lives in an environment in which delay is typically not rewarded: perhaps someone will steal the marshmallows in the meanwhile, or the promise of more later will never be honoured. As evidence that this is indeed what is happening, note that children who have previously encountered unreliable adults will be less inclined to wait in a marshmallow test than those who have encountered trustworthy adults (Kidd et al., 2012). Again a trait that may be useful in an aggressive home environment may be harmful when applied elsewhere.

There are, moreover, further parallels between this example and the case of overgeneral memory, and it is useful to think about them. Other work on delayed gratification has shown that much of what happens when subjects yield to temptation is that they open up for reconsideration the question of whether they should resist; and that when they do so they revise downwards their judgements of the worth of what they were holding out for (Karniol and Miller, 1983). In effect, they rationalize succumbing. So a good strategy in resisting temptation is simply not to open the question: form a resolution and then stick to it without reconsidering. And an effective way of doing that is to make what Peter Gollwitzer calls 'implementation intentions': intentions that are triggered by features of the world and so do not require one to open the question (Gollwitzer, 1999). If one wants to diet, simply resolving to eat less is unlikely to do much good: the question of how much less will always come up, and once one starts thinking about it, it will be easy to come up with justifications for eating heartily this once—justifications that can then be used time and again. A better approach is to lock in prior intentions that are triggered by the environment: 'I will serve myself one plateful of food and if there are any leftovers I will freeze them immediately'; 'When I get to the dessert counter I will walk straight by'; and so on. Gollwitzer finds that such implementation intentions work much better than simple intentions to eat less. But he finds that if he gets his subjects to add a because-clause to them—'I will freeze the leftover immediately because this is the best way of losing weight'—all of the effectiveness is undone (Wieber et al., unpublished). The suggestion is that the because-clause brings them to reopen the question, and once that happens, the rationalizations come flooding in. As with the over-generalized memory, to keep out what one wants, one has to keep out everything.

Now of course these implementation intentions can also give rise to a 'latent vulnerability'. Perhaps there are times when we see that happening; perhaps anorexia is an example where a prior intention remains active even though it is clearly harmful. But it strikes me that this is unusual in the absence of other underlying problems. In general it seems that people manage to keep to their implementation intentions fairly flexibly. Even young children know that it is right to break a promise if that is a way of avoiding significant harm. Is there something that we can learn here about how latent vulnerability might be overcome—about how traits that are advantageous in one context can be constrained so that they do not spill into others where they are not?

Part of the difficulty in answering this question is that we do not really know how people succeed in having flexible intentions. If the secret to having an effective intention is not to reconsider it, then it surely cannot be the case that to have a flexible intention one would constantly need to consider whether to reconsider it: the higher-level consideration would surely spill into the lower, and the effectiveness of the intention would be lost. It may be that the key is to use a separate system, outside of consciousness, to monitor when to reconsider, in particular a system that works through affective rather than cognitive channels. That has some plausibility in the case of when to break a promise. Here the conscious thought may be 'I promised, so I have to do it, and I mustn't even contemplate not doing so'. But that block on reconsideration could be disrupted by a more visceral emotional jolt once the agent realizes that significant harm would be done by maintaining the promise.

If this is right about how we maintain flexible intentions, then it might explain why it is so hard to have flexibility when it comes to the kinds of tendency with which Viding is concerned. Return to the case of a hypersensitivity to the expression of emotion. The ideal there would be to have an ability to switch the sensitivity off in a non-threatening environment. How might that work? In the case of intentions, the idea was that an input from the affective system might tell us to reconsider a possibility that we had been excluding. But it is hard to see how anything like that could work here, since the problem is the other way around. Viding shows that the sensitivity to facial expressions of emotion is itself coming through the amygdala, and various subcortical pathways, that is, through an affective response. So the subject would be faced with the need to do the opposite to the intention case: to shut down an affective response using more cognitive methods. And that, as the increasing evidence on the ineffectiveness of cognitive behaviour therapy shows, is something that we are not good at doing.

If that is right, then it may be that developing a flexible response to expression of emotion is not possible. Once the oversensitivity has been acquired, an effective intervention would either have to involve a process of desensitization, or would involve helping the child to control their behaviour despite their alarm. But perhaps I have overlooked something and flexibility is possible. Clearly Viding's findings here have taken us into an area that is rich in possibilities for future research.

the role of expectations

There is evidence for many psychological illnesses that the symptoms presented are influenced by the patient's expectations. One extreme of this comes with psychosomatic illness: here it may be that the entire nature of the symptoms is determined by the patient's expectations. We need not venture into cases as extreme as these, but can focus on those where the expectations have some impact on the symptoms. Here are two examples, which vary in the degree of controversy they will elicit.

*Shell-shock.*First World War shell-shock produced a wide range of symptoms, some of which have been much less noticeable in other conflicts: witness the many kinds of odd gait that were remarked on by doctors at the time.[2] There is good evidence that at least some of these were affected by the attitudes of the patients. For instance, in their comparison of patients in Berlin and London, Linden and Jones found that functional seizures were over three times more common in the former group than the latter. Various factors could explain this, but they concluded that the most likely were cultural; more crudely put, that the German patients were more likely to expect to suffer seizures (Linden and Jones, 2014, pp. 542–4).[3]

*Eating disorders.*This is a more controversial case, but there is some reason to think that the particular form that eating disorders take is affected by the expectations of those who suffer from them. First, there is the issue of change over time. For many years it was thought that rates of anorexia nervosa increased dramatically from the 1960s until at least the 1990s. More careful studies called that into question, and rates from around 1990 look to be fairly steady.[4] But there does seem to have been a strong increase in the incidence of bulimia nervosa: that rose threefold in the period from the early 1980s to the end of the century (Currin et al., 2005; Hudson et al., 2007). Second, there is the issue of cross-cultural change. The best documented here is a set of studies by Lee Sing concerning anorexia in Hong Kong. Lee contends that a form of anorexia existed in the Chinese population but that it was very different to that seen in the West—it wasn't characterized by unhappiness about being overweight, nor

---

[2] They are discussed by Mott in the third of his Lettsomian Lectures (Mott, 1916).

[3] For a general history of psychological responses to twentieth-century war, one which emphasizes the complex interactions of expectations with other facts, see Shephard (2000).

[4] See van't Hof and Nicolson (1996) for summary and discussion of the earlier period; and Currin et al. (2005), and Hudson et al. (2007) for the more recent period.

was it connected with an unrealistic body image. This changed, he thinks, in the mid 1990s when a Western idea of anorexia was introduced (partly by journalists and by well-meaning public health official alarmed at the lack of preventative programmes), so that now most sufferers conform much more closely to those in the West. If eating disorders change across time and culture, an obvious explanation is that this is mediated by the attitudes of those involved.[5]

Other examples could be given—the increased prevalence of cutting among Western adolescents[6]; the rise, and decline, of multiple personality disorder[7]; the presentation of depression in cultures like Japan (Kitanaka, 2012). And there are many historical cases. All are somewhat controversial but all seem to show some evidence of an impact on the symptoms of the expectations of the subjects. This is not to say that the expectations change in a vacuum: they change in response to social pressures, which are equally causally important. Nor is it to say that there would be no such illnesses if it were not for the expectations of the sufferers. But psychological illness is typically a reflective phenomenon: people behave partly on the basis of their understanding of what is happening to them (it is thus 'model based' to use a currently fashionable notion); and as we know from the literature on self-efficacy, this can be important to how things turn out.

My question then for Viding is this: how much is the kind of antisocial behaviour that she is concerned with itself influenced by the expectations of those who engage in it: their expectations of how, given their upbringing, they will act, or of how it is appropriate for them to act? The answer may be: not at all. But Viding has stressed two phenomena that make her research more difficult. The first is multifinality: given the same exposures, different subjects will often react in different ways. The second is equifinality: given different exposures, different subjects will often react in the same way. I wonder whether the role of expectations can help explain this. For if they do have an important role, then if subjects from different backgrounds think that they have a great deal in common, then they might come to behave in rather similar ways; and likewise if subjects from similar backgrounds think that they are very different, they might come to behave in rather different ways.

All this is, of course, highly speculative. And even if there is an important role for expectations, there are, once again, no immediate lessons for how interventions should be designed. But thanks to Viding we are much closer to seeing what the questions are.

---

[5] For a popular summary of Lee's work see Watters (2010, chapter 1), and the references given there. Subsequent chapters give a similarly cultural relativist take on post-traumatic stress disorder, schizophrenia, and depression.

[6] The consensus among therapists and the like seems to be that this has increased rapidly, although the studies are not all bearing this out; see, for instance, Muehlenkamp et al. (2012).

[7] For an extensive but sympathetic discussion see Hacking (1995). Much recent work has been much more sceptical that it, or its successor, dissociative identity disorder, really exists; for a representative example see Piper and Merskey (2004a, 2004b).

References

Currin, L., Schmidt, U., Treasure, J., and Hick, H. (2005). Time trends in eating disorder incidence. *The British Journal of Psychiatry*, **186**, 132–135.

Gollwitzer, P. (1999). Implementation intentions: the strong effect of simple goals. *American Psychologist*, **54**(7), 493–503.

Hacking, I. (1995). *Rewriting the Soul: Multiple Personality and the Sciences of Memory*. Princeton, NJ: Princeton University Press.

Hudson, J., Hiripi, E., Pope, H., and Kessler, R. (2007). The prevalence and correlates of eating disorders in the National Comorbidity Survey Replication. *Biological Psychiatry* **61**(3), 348–358.

Karniol, R. and Miller, D. (1983). Why not wait? A cognitive model of self-imposed delay termination. *Journal of Personality and Social Psychology* **45**(4), 935–942.

Kidd, C., Palmieri, H., and Aslin, R. (2012). Rational snacking: young children's decision-making on the marshmallow task is moderated by beliefs about environmental reliability. *Cognition*, **126**(1), 109–114.

Kitanaka, J. (2012). *Depression in Japan: Psychiatric Cures for a Society in Distress*. Princeton, NJ: Princeton University Press.

Linden, S. and Jones, E. (2014). 'Shell shock' revisited: an examination of the case records of the National Hospital in London. *Medical History*, **58**(4), 519–545.

McCrory, E. and Viding, E. (2015). The theory of latent vulnerability: Reconceptualizing the link between childhood maltreatment and psychiatric disorder. *Development and Psychopathology*, **27**(2), 493–505.

Mischel, W. (1996). From good intentions to willpower. In: P. Gollwitzer and J. Bargh (Eds.), *The Psychology of Action* (pp. 197–218.). New York: The Guildford Press.

Mott, F.W. (1916). The Lettsonian Lectures on the effects of high explosives on the central nervous system, Lecture III. *The Lancet*, **187**(4828), 545–553.

Muehlenkamp, J., Claes, L., Havertape, L., and Plener, P. (2012). International prevalence of adolescent non-suicidal self-injury and deliberate self-harm. *Child and Adolescent Psychiatry and Mental Health*, **6**, 10.

Piper, A. and Merskey, H. (2004a). The persistence of folly: a critical examination of dissociative identity disorder. Part I. The excesses of an improbable concept. *Canadian Journal of Psychiatry*, **49**(9), 592–600.

Piper, A. and Merskey, H. (2004b). The persistence of folly: a critical examination of dissociative identity disorder. Part II. The defence and decline of multiple personality or dissociative identity disorder. *Canadian Journal of Psychiatry*, **49**(10), 678–683.

Shephard, B. (2000). *A War of Nerves: Soldiers and Psychiatrists in the Twentieth Century*. London: Jonathan Cape.

Valentino, K., Toth, S.L., and Cicchetti, D. (2009). Autobiographical memory functioning among abused, neglected, and nonmaltreated children: the overgeneral memory effect. *Journal of Child Psychology and Psychiatry*, **50**(8), 1029–1038.

van't Hof, S. and Nicolson, M. (1996). The rise and fall of a fact: the increase of anorexia nervosa. *Sociology of Health and Illness*, **18**(5), 581–608.

Watters, E. (2010). *Crazy Like Us*. New York: Simon and Schuster.

Wieber, F., Gollwitzer, P., Gawrilow, C., and Oettingen, G. Unpublished. Intending to lose weight: benefits of why reasoning and implementation intentions.

Chapter 14

The first steps on long marches: The costs of active observation

Peter Dayan, Jonathan P. Roiser, and Essi Viding

Introduction

One of the most important options on any of our multitudinous electronic devices is the 'factory reset', offering us the opportunity to wipe away all the catastrophes of past interactions and start afresh. We, the users of these devices, are of course not so forgetting of their past failures or our past frustrations. Furthermore, we frequently interact with other people and artefacts in the world that learn about us from these interactions. They will also typically not forget, and so may do back to us amplified or distorted versions of what we do to them, be this good or bad.

In this chapter, we examine these issues through the medium of Bayesian decision theory (BDT), which offers a crisp characterization of optimal choice in temporally extended, valenced, domains in which there can be various sorts of uncertainty (Berger, 1985; Körding, 2007; Ferguson, 2014). BDT, and in particular approximations to BDT that are sensitive to the typically insurmountable computational challenges it poses for humans and other animals, allow neurobiological, psychological, and environmental aspects of healthy and psychopathological performance to be tied together (Huys et al., 2015a). Much of the previous work on decision-theoretic psychiatry has focused on neurobiological and psychological facets, for instance, concentrating on individual differences and mechanistic flaws in various sorts of algorithms that learn to predict future rewards and punishments and hard-wired or plastic ways of choosing actions (known as policies) in the light of these predictions (Gillan et al., 2016; Huys et al., 2016a). Here, we concentrate on environmental factors—considering how early experience, and in particular actions provoked by that early experience, can colour later beliefs and actions.

In particular, we focus on the issue of partial observability—that there are aspects of the environment that we do not completely know. Ignorance needs to be reduced in order to determine appropriate actions; however, the optimal nature, extent, and effects of this reduction turn out to be subtle. Importantly, as we will show, it is not always optimal to remove ignorance entirely (Gittins 1989), in particular when it may be expensive or formally fruitless to do so. Furthermore, in environments containing other adaptive agents—think, for instance, of the interaction between a child and their caregiver—our actions can teach them unfortunate lessons about us, even when those actions are intended only to reduce our ignorance about those agents (Ray et al., 2009; Hula et al., 2015) or even are noise. The potential links to mis-attachment or escalating aggression are evident.

To put this another way, BDT specifies a way to choose actions that perfectly balances the costs and benefits of the reduction of ignorance. This equipoise is exquisitely sensitive to prior knowledge and assumptions. For instance, given the prior expectation that the current environment affords no worthwhile opportunity, it is adaptive not to attempt to explore, since nothing worth exploiting is anticipated (Huys et al., 2015a). However, the consequence of not exploring is never finding out that this prior is not (or perhaps is no longer) correct. Thus the unduly negative conclusion will persist.

There are two main sources of prior knowledge, both of which can lead to problems. One is history fossilized in terms of our genetic endowment. Many aspects of this are highly beneficial—for instance, we would not want to have to discover for ourselves what to do in the face of mortal threat (Bolles, 1970; Keay and Bandler, 2001). However, when evolutionary and current environments are mis-matched, oversensitivity to unfortunate aspects of the former could lead to the persistent problems in our interaction with the latter. The second source of prior knowledge is earlier individual experience. This can be conceptualized through the lens of filtering (Anderson and Moore, 1979), in which the posterior distribution at one step, after making some early observations, becomes the prior distribution for the next step, ready to absorb new data. Again, the circumstances that pertained in one's youth that determined the values of these priors could since have changed. This mismatch would nevertheless persist if exploration to discover it is not indicated. Genes and early environment are not, of course, entirely independent of each other (Jaffee and Price, 2007; Viding and McCrory, 2012).

That past evolutionary or personal experience can influence current interactions with the environment is known as path dependency—with early steps along one's individual path exerting significant influence at later points in time. The sorts of path dependency we have discussed are reminiscent of active gene–environment correlations (Jaffee and Price 2007)—albeit best conceived instead in terms of prior–environment correlations, to accommodate the different possible genetic and environmental routes to unfortunate priors that we mentioned previously. Subjects actively create their own environments—in the case discussed earlier, by refusing to explore—implying that the effective arrow of causality can be from subject to environment rather than vice versa.

A form of evocative prior–environment correlation (Jaffee and Price, 2007) is also readily possible in environments which contain other people or any other form of intentionally acting decision-making agent, rather than just the disinterested stochasticity of nature. In responding to our actions in such a way as to optimize their own goals, either mutually harmful competition or mutually beneficial cooperation (or both) can be stabilized (as in Axelrod's (2006) 'tit for tat' strategy for the prisoner's dilemma), again enshrining path dependence.

We start by briefly describing the elements of BDT to formalize the relevant sources of path dependency. We then discuss a classical example known as a Bayesian bandit problem (Berry and Fristedt, 1985; Gittins, 1989). This formalizes the widespread notion that subjects might have a menu of possible actions ('arms' of a bandit machine in the fanciful context of a casino), but incomplete knowledge about their relative merits. Reducing this ignorance is exactly what must be carefully managed because of the potential attendant costs of doing so. We use such a bandit to illustrate the issues that arise in active prior–environment correlations. We complement this with a more elaborate example from approximate Bayesian microeconomics (Harsanyi, 1967; Gmytrasiewicz and Doshi, 2005) which illustrates evocative prior–environment correlations. We end by discussing some of the other possible generators of path dependency in BDT, and by drawing out translational consequences of our argument in the context of vulnerability and resilience, using early caregiving as an example.

Bayesian decision theory

BDT is described in detail by Berger (1985) and Ferguson (2014); and some applications to behavioural and psychiatric modelling are considered by Dayan and Daw (2008) and Huys and colleagues (2015b). It has played a substantial part in helping to systematize thinking in the nascent field of computational psychiatry (Montague et al., 2012; Stephan and Mathys, 2014; Huys et al., 2016b); example applications to conditions such as psychosis and depression are discussed, for instance, by Adams and colleagues (2013), Huys and colleagues (2015a), Jardri and Denve (2013), and Moutoussis and colleagues (2011).

In brief, BDT comprises several elements. The first is a state of the world $x \in \mathcal{X}$, where X is the set of all possible states. The state need not be static, but could change. Where necessary, we will use subscripts to indicate the time t. There is also a possible observation $o \in \mathcal{O}$, from a set $\mathcal{O}$, a choice of action $a \in \mathcal{A}$, from a menu A, and a utility function $u(x, a)$, which determines the merit of doing action a if the state is actually x. Critically, subjects may be ignorant about the current state x_t, and so build and maintain probabilistic beliefs about it $p(x_t|\mathcal{D}_t)$, where $\mathcal{D}_t = \{o_0, a_0, o_1, a_1, \ldots, a_{t-1}, o_t\}$ represents all the information collected (and produced) up to time t. This posterior is also influenced by initial priors $p(x_0)$, and information about how the state itself changes over time (which is often simplified to be Markovian ($p(x_{t+1}|x_t, a_t)$), depending only on the current state and action). Subjects can then be assumed to have a goal such as choosing actions to maximize the long-run sum $V(\mathcal{D}_t)$ of expected future discounted utilities starting from every time t:

$$V(\mathcal{D}_t) = \mathbb{E}_{p(x_t|\mathcal{D}_t)}\left[\sum_{\tau=t}^{\infty} \gamma^{\tau-t}u(\mathrm{x}_\tau, a_\tau)\right]$$

The discount factor $0 \leq \gamma \leq 1$ downweights future utilities as a function of their temporal distance.[1] The expectation is over the subject's probabilistic uncertainty about all unknown quantities. Formally, this probabilistic structure is known as a partially observable Markov decision process (POMDP; Kaelbling et al., 1998).

One of the most important implications of optimizing choices over the long run is a trade-off between exploitation and exploration (Hills et al., 2015). For an example, consider the choice between staying at home with indifferent television (call this option φ) versus going to a new pub (option ψ) which could be either good (if the state $x = x^a$) or bad (if the state is $x = x^b$). Option φ is moderately good, no matter whether the pub is good or bad $u(x^a, \varphi) \simeq u(x^b, \varphi) \simeq 0$, and so is low risk. However, it obviously provides no information about whether or not the pub is good. The worth of option ψ depends on the state of the pub, $u(x^a, \psi) \gg 0 \gg u(x^b, \psi)$, and so it is more risky, since it could be that the pub is bad. However, crucially, by performing ψ, that is, by exploring, the quality of the pub will be discovered. If it is bad (if $x = x^b$), then one can watch television forever more. However, if it is good (if $x = x^a$), then it will be safe to take ψ in the *future*. The magnitude of the future benefit of this current exploration depends on the various utilities and the discount factor γ, which has to be large enough that the future matters sufficiently. It also depends crucially on the prior expectations about the relative initial probabilities that the pub is good.

In general, calculating optimal actions in the long run in the face of uncertainty is extremely taxing—for computers and humans alike. People therefore employ heuristics and approximations, which can themselves have psychiatric consequences. We have elaborated on the nature and effect of these approximations in previous work (Huys et al., 2015b). However, properties of the solution that is optimal according to BDT are at least indicative, and suffice to illustrate path dependence.

Most manifestations of BDT concern stochastic environments, with people playing games against an unnoticing nature. However, many psychiatrically important cases concern interactions with other sentient beings who have their own utility functions. In this case, game theoretic considerations become important (von Neumann and Morgenstern, 1955; Camerer, 2003)—and are particularly

---

[1] Behavioural results show that discounting is usually better described as being hyperbolic rather than exponential (Ainslie, 2001), but the distinction is immaterial for the present purposes.

rich when those utility functions quantify psychological factors such as guilt, envy, or intention that are associated with the joint choices and outcomes (Fehr and Schmidt, 1999; McCabe et al., 2003) but whose magnitude may be incompletely known to other participants. In this case, the standard game theoretic concept of a Nash equilibrium (roughly a collection of strategies for the players that none has an individual incentive to change) becomes a Bayes–Nash equilibrium (Harsanyi, 1967). The Bayesian aspect of this equilibrium involves each player performing inference about the characteristics of the other player that they do not know for certain. The equilibrium aspect includes the fact that the players know that their partners are learning about them. Players can thereby take account appropriately of the actions that their partners take in the light of their ignorance.

In practice, people do not play equilibrium strategies. Rather, it appears that they build and use more or less deep and recursive models of each other (player A's model of player B, which might include player B's model of themselves, and so forth, but for only a limited number of cycles of recursion; Costa-Gomes et al., 2001; Camerer et al., 2004). Mismatches between the complexity of the models of the players can lead to complex patterns of intended and unintentional cooperation and competition. In the case of imperfect knowledge, this has been captured in BDT terms using a construct known as an interactive POMDP (IPOMDP; Gmytrasiewicz and Doshi, 2005), and applied to problems such as trust games that have been used to probe interpersonal interaction in health and disease (King-Casas et al., 2005, 2008; Ray et al., 2009; Xiang et al., 2012; Hula et al., 2015, 2018).

In the next sections, we use two simple examples to examine facets of path dependence.

A Bayesian bandit and active prior–environment correlations

One of the simplest non-trivial instances of BDT is the so-called two-armed bandit—a task involving choosing between two actions based on partial knowledge of their returns. The actions $a = \{\varphi, \psi\}$ are often called 'arms', and provide a utility of £1 with probabilities θ^φ, θ^ψ respectively, where $0 \leq \theta^\varphi, \theta^\psi \leq 1$, and otherwise cost –£1. The state of the world $x = (\theta^\varphi, \theta^\psi)$ exactly comprises the probabilities of getting a positive reward; here, the observations o are just the rewards themselves. Subjects start not knowing the true value of x, just having a prior. They update this prior as they collect rewards (and observations).

In the most straightforward version of a two-armed bandit problem, the prior takes the form of a pair of independent beta distributions, $\theta^\varphi \sim \text{Beta}(\alpha^\varphi, \beta^\varphi)$; $\theta^\psi \sim \text{Beta}(\alpha^\psi, \beta^\psi)$. Here α_0, β_0 can be interpreted as pseudo-counts for the options, that is, just like a pool of pre-existing observations of £1 (for α) and of –£1 (for β). Bayesian inference amounts to nothing more than adding the number of actual £1s that are obtained to α for the arm concerned, and the number of actual –£1s that are obtained to β.

Inferences about the arms then become straightforward—for instance, the mean value is $£(\alpha - \beta)/(\alpha + \beta)$ and the variance $\alpha\beta/((\alpha + \beta)^2(\alpha + \beta + 1))$.

In this version, the exploration–exploitation trade-off was famously solved by Gittins (1989). This two-dimensional problem (since there are two arms) turns into two one-dimensional problems—each involving calculating a so-called Gittins index for an arm based on that arm's values of α and β. The Gittins index combines the benefits of exploitation and exploration—acknowledging the possibility of stopping choosing an arm when it is no longer worthwhile. The overall optimal policy is to choose the arm with the largest Gittins index. Calculating Gittins indices is computationally challenging; however, approximations (and tables) are available.

The relevance to path dependence is as follows—using an extension of the very simple previous example to make the point. Option φ involves 'staying-at-home', for which $\alpha_0^\varphi = \beta_0^\varphi \simeq \infty$, implying that it surely provides £0 on average (and so has a Gittins index of £0 too). The other option ψ ('going to the pub') is unknown, starting from prior values of $\alpha_0^\psi, \beta_0^\psi$.[2] The question is the circumstances under which it is *not* optimal to choose arm ψ. If it is indeed not, then since arm φ is pegged at its neutral value, and never changes, it will therefore be permanently the case that ψ is never chosen. Thus, even if it is *better* than φ, this fact will never be found—the subject will metaphorically stay at home forever more.

Figure 14.1 shows the resulting conclusions. The upper plots show approximate (Brezzi and Lai, 2002) Gittins indices for going to the pub, ψ, for the case in point for short-term ($\gamma = 0.25$) and long-term ($\gamma = 0.999$) horizons, and for various prior values of $\{\alpha_0^\psi, \beta_0^\psi\}$. The white dashed line separates those prior values from which it is worth exploring the pub (above) from those in which it is not (below). For values that are below, the subject will *optimally* fail to explore the pub, and so never discover whether it is better than staying at home. The lower plots show the distributions over θ^ψ for sample priors on either side of the separatrix (the asterisk shows a distribution that would not inspire sampling; the cross shows a distribution that would). For the more impulsive case (short-term horizon; left), even if the prior is actually correct, there is a substantial chance (31%) that the pub is better on average than staying at home, and yet will not be sampled. For the longer horizon (right), exploring is much more promising; however, there remains a non-zero probability of failing to discover that the pub is worthwhile.

In sum, this example shows that because of an unfortunate prior distribution, which could be set by a genetic endowment or some earlier interactions with the environment, or because of a short-term outlook (i.e. a low discount factor, γ), or both, it may be optimal not to sample an available option and so never to find out that it is, in fact, advantageous. This can be seen as an example of prior–environment correlation. The subject shapes the portion of the environment that she occupies (by refusing to explore one key option, thus restricting their choices); and thereby suffers negative potential consequences.

---

[2] The extension being that the unknown state x is not just binary ($x \in \{x^a, x^b\}$), but rather is the probability θ^ψ that the pub will stochastically be good on any occasion it is visited.

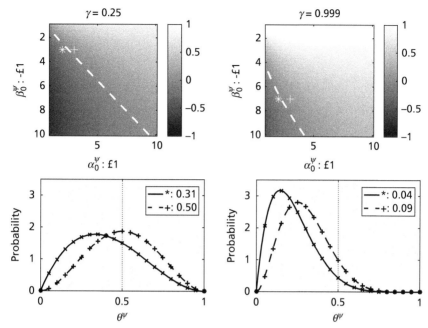

Figure 14.1 Gittins indices. The upper plots show approximate Gittins indices (using an expression from Brezzi and Lai 2002) for arm ψ given prior observations $\{\alpha^\psi, \beta^\psi\}$ associated with outcomes £$\{1, -1\}$ and for discount factors $\gamma = 0.25$ (short-term horizon; left) and $\gamma = 0.999$ (long-term horizon; right). The white dashed line shows the separatrix between prior values that favour sampling ψ (above) or ignoring it (below) when there is an alternative choice φ which is surely worth £0. The lower plots show the prior distributions over θ^ψ in the two cases for the values of $\{\alpha^\psi, \beta^\psi\}$ marked on the upper plots by the asterisk (solid) and cross (dashed), together with the total probability mass $p(\theta^\psi > \theta^\varphi)$ for the distributions.

Interactive POMDPs and evocative prior–environment correlations

In the bandit case, the environment is just defined by being stochastic. However, when the subject is involved in strategic interactions with other intentional agents, many additional complexities come to the fore. To illustrate this, we give a very brief description of a series of studies and analyses conducted by Montague and colleagues (King-Casas et al., 2005, 2008; Ray et al., 2009; Xiang et al., 2012; Hula et al., 2015, 2018) of a game designed to examine how two players can form and break trust in their mutual interactions (McCabe et al., 2003).

The game involves two players: an investor (we sometimes distinguish by sex as 'he') and a trustee ('she')—who normally do not know each other. On each of ten rounds, the investor receives a (sometimes notional) endowment of £20 from the experimenter; he can choose to keep or invest as much as he likes. The amount that he invests is trebled by the experimenter and given to the trustee. The trustee then plays a dictator game, choosing arbitrarily how much to return to the investor, and how much to keep for herself. It is called a trust game, since the investor has to trust that the trustee will return some money in order to make investing worthwhile, as otherwise he could choose to invest nothing, and walk away with £200 over the ten trials of the experiment.

Indeed, this null investment solution is the Nash equilibrium given standard notions of utility: on the *last* round, the trustee has no incentive to return any money at all; thus the investor has no incentive to invest anything; hence the last round can be discounted—but then the same argument applies to the penultimate round, and so on. However, this is neither economically efficient (since the experimenter is willing in principle to give out £600); nor is it socially appropriate. In practice, investments and returns generally happen, and indeed exhibit a rich dynamical interaction. However, players suffering from psychiatric conditions such as borderline personality disorder or antisocial personality disorder suffer worse outcomes, and indeed inspire less economically efficient choices from healthy control players with whom they interact. For instance, cooperation between healthy volunteer investors and trustees more frequently breaks down in early and middle rounds when those trustees suffer from borderline personality disorder than when they are healthy (King-Casas et al., 2008).

We originally modelled (Ray et al., 2009; Xiang et al., 2012; Hula et al., 2015) the interaction as a form of IPOMDP (Gmytrasiewicz and Doshi, 2005) in which players have other-regarding preferences—namely guilt (Fehr and Schmidt, 1999). What makes it a POMDP is that they do not know each other's preferences, but learn from their patterns of investment and return—this is rather like the case for the bandit. What makes it interactive is the way they model each other in making inferences. This structure admits substantial intricacy—particularly when the models have different degrees of complexity (e.g. the investor just models the trustee, but the trustee also models the investor's model of herself). This is known as a cognitive hierarchy (Costa-Gomes et al., 2001; Camerer et al., 2004), and is a psychologically plausible replacement for the radically computationally intractable Bayes–Nash equilibrium (Harsanyi, 1967). The equivalent of exploration here is trying investing or returning a little less or a little more to be able to learn from the other player's response. The problem is that doing so can make the other player think something different about oneself, and thereby interact in a potentially less favourable manner. This then can lead to a negative spiral.

Figure 14.2 shows an example of the sort of interactions that can result in models of this class. Here, we have included an additional unknown interactive parameter (called ζ^I, for the investor) that governs *irritation* (Hula et al., 2018). That is, when one's partner defects, by investing or returning less than expected it is possible to be become irritated. The more irritated a player, the more narrowly and myopically self-serving they play, even at their own longer-term expense. Conversely, larger-than-expected investments and returns reduce irritation, favouring normal interactions. The extent to which an individual is irritable (or in the way we formalize it, susceptible to both irritation and calming) is a random quantity that players need to infer about each other as they play. As before, prior beliefs about how irritable a player might be can interact with unfortunate early experience to cause irreparable breakdown in cooperation. We write $b^T(\zeta^I)$ for the trustee's prior belief about the investor's irritability. In the figure,

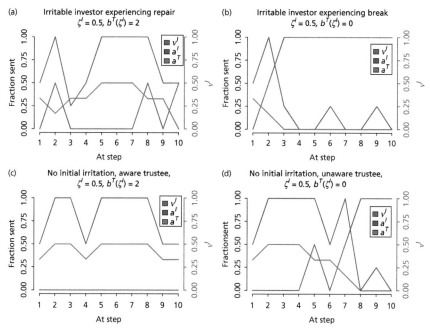

Figure 14.2 Evocative prior–environment correlations. These plots show the dynamics of the fractional investments (a^I; blue), returns (a^T; red), and the fractional irritation of the investor (v^I; brown) over ten rounds of the trust task. In all cases, the investor is moderately irritable ($\zeta^I = 0.5$); we then have a factorial arrangement of a trustee that is ($b^T(\zeta^I) = 2$; A;C) or is not ($b^T(\zeta^I) = 0$; B;D) aware of the potential for this irritability; and first two starting investments and returns that are malign (A;B) or benign (C;D).

This figure was generated by Andreas Hula as part of a collaboration with Read Montague.

this is either $b^T(\zeta^I) = 0$, for a trustee who is sure that the investor is *not* irritable (i.e., is *unaware*), or $b^T(\zeta^I) = 2$, for a trustee who instead allows for this possibility (is *aware*).

Figure 14.2 illustrates this by showing four different interactions between two different dyads. In all cases, the investor is the same; being mildly irritable. We consider two types of trustee: one who is aware (A;C); and the other who is unaware (B;D) of the investor's potential irritability. We also preprogram the first two interactions to be either malign (A;B), with the investor *increasing* his investment on step 2 and the trustee *reducing* her return; or benign (C;D), with the trustee also *increasing* her return. The figures show the path of simulated investments (blue) and returns (red) over the ten rounds as fractions of the amount that is available to each on a round. The brown line shows how irritated the investor is (v^I).

The figures show the range of possibilities. Consider first the malign case with the trustee being preprogrammed to defect in step 2 (by returning less) despite the investor's (pre-programmed) increased investment (A;B). If the trustee is aware that the investor might be irritable (A), then she responds beneficently in step 3 to the investor's decreased investment, and repairs cooperation. If she is unaware (B), then she responds poorly, and cooperation is minimal for the remaining trials.

If, however, the trustee's preprogrammed return on trial 2 is more benign (C;D), then the investor's irritation is not initially triggered, and so there is no immediate rupture to repair. However, even in this case, there remains some benefit for the trustee to be aware of the investor's potential irritability, to prevent the cooperation from disintegrating later.

In this case, we are seeing what could be thought of as an evocative prior–environment interaction, from the perspective of the trustee. The trustee's behaviour in Figure 14.2b has elicited a behavioural pattern in the investor that is substantially deleterious, in fact to both parties. The circumstances leading to this are a little more delicate than for the case of the bandit, notably with a requirement for a degree of irritability in the investor—but have been shown to characterize aspects of actual interactions (Hula et al., 2018).

Discussion

In this chapter, we used two highly simplified examples to study the consequences of ignorance for active observers in statistical and intentional environments. Observers are active in a decision-theoretic sense when they control their own sources of information, rather than being merely passive observers. This control is important when observers are ignorant. However, it poses the problem of trading off exploitation, in which existing knowledge is used, with exploration, which reduces ignorance, potentially enabling better future exploitation, but typically at some real or opportunity cost. We saw the consequences of this in terms of evolutionary- or experience-driven path dependence—that is, that active observers might get to the point at which they choose not to acquire information that would seemingly be useful—and related this to active prior–environment correlations. We also saw how problems from path dependency can arise when interacting with intentional, rather than merely stochastic others, related to evocative prior–environment correlations.

Both of the cases we studied were highly abstracted and simplified to make rather narrow points. For instance, for the case of the bandits, the expected benefit of exploration is critically dependent on generalization: experience gained from exploration is more valuable if it provides information that can be used to judge multiple actions (e.g. multiple pubs) based on their similarity. The expected scope of generalization is determined by an aspect of the prior over the environment (Huys et al., 2015b)—with many psychiatric consequences. For example, environments are not unitary, containing little more than just a single pair of arms. Rather they have hierarchical components, with multiple tasks of varying qualities, difficulties, and affordances. Success or failure in solving one task has implications for the chance of solving future tasks. However, those implications depend both on how one conceives of the first task (Kaney and Bentall, 1989), for instance, whether the outcome is attributed to one's own competence or rather that the task was easy or difficult, and the expected similarity structure between the tasks. Both of these are facets of prior expectations.

Indeed, such higher-order structures are important for considering exploration at another scale—how useful it is to explore and learn to gain competence in one task, even if this is not currently very rewarding, because it is expected to help in future tasks. The case we considered of a single uncertain choice is thoroughly anaemic in this respect; however, BDT can extend to provide an appropriate grounding for what is often known as intrinsic motivation (Oudeyer et al., 2007; Dayan, 2013). The quantitative benefits depend sensitively on subtle aspects of prior expectations—reinforcing the narrow separatices associated with path dependence.

We have so far mostly pretended that subjects are capable of performing optimal inference according to BDT to work out what to do to turn (potentially genetically based) prior distributions into appropriate actions. However, we also noted that the calculations are often radically intractable, implying that various shortcuts and heuristics are necessary (Huys et al., 2015b). One set of shortcuts is a system of Pavlovian or reflexive actions that are automatically elicited (Breland and Breland, 1961) by biologically significant outcomes or predictions thereof. In the case of negative outcomes, these include passive and active defensive actions (e.g. Bolles, 1970), which can also significantly affect the possibilities of learning about partially known environments. Both human and animal studies indicate that individual differences in the responsiveness of this system are partly due to genetic differences (e.g. Hettema et al., 2003; Shumake et al., 2014). This indicates that Pavlovian actions elicit a different repertoire of behaviours in different individuals, which in turn has consequences for that individual's subsequent environmental inputs and canalization of behaviours over time.

Along with externally directed Pavlovian actions that can influence choices, there may be internally directed ones that influence computations concerning appropriate actions (Dayan, 2012), and so can cause or exacerbate path dependencies. For instance, one standard method for estimating the future worth of present actions in the face of state uncertainty is to build a tree of future possibilities (Silver and Veness, 2010). There is evidence for a calculational shortcut in which branches of the tree associated with initial losses are (potentially maladaptively) 'pruned' (Dayan and Huys, 2008; Huys et al., 2012). Aspects of this pruning have been ascribed to the subgenual cingulate cortex (Lally et al., 2017), a region implicated in affective disorders and aversive processing (Amemori and Graybiel, 2012; Dunlop and Mayberg, 2014). Equally, serotonin, a neuromodulator of great importance in depression, anxiety, and other psychiatric conditions, has been suggested as being involved in determining the degree of discounting (Schweighofer et al., 2007, 2008). We saw that this latter effect helped determine path dependence in exploration. Individual, and indeed significantly heritable, differences in the operation of serotonergic neuromodulation are often described (Pinborg et al., 2008; Clauss et al., 2015).

Conversely, an unwillingness to build extensive and deep trees of possible futures can also be protective. For instance, it may take substantial chains of reasoning to work out the true extent to which one is being exploited in complex game-theoretic contexts such as the trust task described previously. Ignorance, or at least a refusal to calculate how, might sometimes be bliss—one need never appreciate one's vulnerability, and therefore not expect the worst in the future.

These various routes to potential problems can be seen in terms of equi- and multifinality (Cicchetti and Rogosch, 1996; Luyten, et al., 2008). Equifinality arises when there are many different routes to the same apparent set of symptoms or behaviours. In our previous psychiatric analyses of BDT, we have considered maladaptive characterizations of the problem—that is, priors, likelihoods (which tie observations to underlying states), and utilities; or maladaptive calculations—that is, heuristic evaluation or choice of options (Huys et al., 2015b). We have already seen that an equifinal outcome of a refusal to explore to find a good option that is actually available can have roots in both priors and calculations.

However, other issues can also be important leading to the same, equifinal outcome. For instance, there is some evidence that forms of depression in which anhedonia is particularly significant (i.e. formerly rewarding outcomes lose their positive subjective quality) are associated with issues concerning at least secondary utilities (Eshel and Roiser, 2010; Huys et al., 2013, 2015a). Equally, approximations in calculating and maintaining uncertainty about the quantities about which there is ignorance can themselves lead to path dependency. One worked example is the case of highlighting (Kruschke, 2006; Daw et al., 2008; see also Shteingart et al., 2013). Here, path dependency is apparent as a form of primacy, with information that the subjects learn at the beginning of a set of trials expressing itself more strongly at later points in learning, than information in the middle of the set. One explanation of this is that subjects do not model the entire distribution of their uncertainty correctly—and by thereby throwing away information, the earliest examples can unfairly dominate (Kruschke, 2006; Daw et al., 2008).

One of the most important clinical consequences of equifinality is that similar symptomatic presentations may be associated with different possible causes, and therefore very different prognoses and treatment efficacies. One of the most important directions in computational psychiatry is trying to use computational models of decision-making tasks to interrogate the underlying causes of equifinal outcomes in order to make steps towards this outcome.

Multifinality is complementary to equifinality, considering instead cases in which individuals who have *similar* histories nevertheless exhibit very *different* (e.g. developmental) outcomes. The sorts of path dependency that we have been examining can have the effect of amplifying small differences in individual endowments—including the degree of discounting, the propensity to prune, and prior expectations about the chance of reward. This can then lead to substantially different, multifinal, outcomes based on what start off as the same actions and observations. One notion of multifinality is that it arises from the interaction between multiple separate systems responsible for behaviour, with only a subset of those systems being different. The differences engendered by these are then amplified. One can well imagine this in the architecture of choice that we have described, with responsibility for some facets of decision-making being ascribed to discrete systems, for instance, with pruning coming as a form of internal behavioural inhibition. Note the consequence of active observation, however, that the progressive divergence in the conclusions drawn from experience will lead to a further divergence in the future experience that is sought, and so forth.

Finally, we should consider the implications for latent and overt vulnerability and resilience (McCrory and Viding, 2015). Since our discussion has so far been rather abstract, we would like to illustrate these issues by painting an outline picture of its implications for these most important facets. Consider, therefore, the interaction between a child and their caregiver. If the caregiver suffers from a substance use disorder, their interactions with the child may be impoverished in terms of the range of emotions expressed, and unpredictable in terms of meeting the child's needs for safety, comfort, and physical well-being. The child may, over time, learn that any emotional expression on behalf of the caregiver can (though does not always) lead to extreme physical danger. As a result, the child learns to be particularly vigilant for any perceived change in affect, which can serve a purpose in the home, but translates less well to social interactions outside the home. For example, routinely attributing hostile intent to teachers or school friends is likely to colour the child's social exchanges negatively and curtail their opportunities to develop positive, trusting relationships.

It is unfortunately rather easier to see routes to vulnerability than resilience, since in many of the cases we have described, maladaptive path dependencies are actually optimal solutions according to BDT—and so are, in a particular sense, ideal. One main defence against optimizing forms of path dependency is a commitment to the possibility of continual change—a belief that things are never fixed (and so constantly need revisiting; i.e. a factory reset). Of course, this is not cost-free itself.

Acknowledgements

We are very grateful to Julian Savulescu and the Oxford Uehiro Centre for Practical Ethics for organizing the Loebel Lectures that led to this chapter, and also to Will Davies and Hannah Maslen for comments. We particularly thank Andreas Hula for producing Figure 14.2, stemming from a collaboration between him, Read Montague, and PD. Funding was from the Gatsby Charitable Foundation (PD).

References

Adams, R.A., Stephan, K.E., Brown, H.R., Frith, C.D., and Friston, K.J. (2013). The computational anatomy of psychosis. *Frontiers in Psychiatry*, **4**, 47.

Ainslie, G. (2001). *Breakdown of Will*. New York: Cambridge University Press.

Amemori, K.-I. and Graybiel, A.M. (2012). Localized microstimulation of primate pregenual cingulate cortex induces negative decision-making. *Nature Neuroscience*, **15**(5), 776–785.

Anderson, B.D. and Moore, J.B. (1979). *Optimal Filtering*. Englewood Cliffs, NJ: Prentice-Hall.

Axelrod, R.M. (2006). *The Evolution of Cooperation*. New York: Basic Books.

Berger, J. (1985). *Statistical Decision Theory and Bayesian Analysis*. New York: Springer.

Berry, D.A. and Fristedt, B. (1985). *Bandit Problems: Sequential Allocation of Experiments* (Monographs on Statistics and Applied Probability). Dordrecht: Springer.

Bolles, R.C. (1970). Species-specific defense reactions and avoidance learning. *Psychological Review* **77**(1), 32–48.

Breland, K. and Breland, M. (1961). The misbehavior of organisms. *American Psychologist* **16**(9), 681–684.

Brezzi, M. and Lai, T.L. (2002). Optimal learning and experimentation in bandit problems. *Journal of Economic Dynamics and Control*, **27**(1), 87–108.

Camerer, C. (2003). *Behavioral Game Theory: Experiments in Strategic Interaction*. Princeton, NJ: Princeton University Press.

Camerer, C., Ho, T., and Chong, J. (2004). A cognitive hierarchy model of games. *The Quarterly Journal of Economics*, **119**(3), 861–898.

Cicchetti, D. and **Rogosch, F.A.** (1996). Equifinality and multifinality in developmental psychopathology. *Development and Psychopathology*, **8**, 597–600.

Clauss, J.A., Avery, S.N., and **Blackford, J.U.** (2015). The nature of individual differences in inhibited temperament and risk for psychiatric disease: a review and meta-analysis. *Progress in Neurobiology*, **127–128**, 23–45.

Costa-Gomes, M., Crawford, V., and **Broseta, B.** (2001). Cognition and behavior in normal-form games: an experimental study. *Econometrica*, **69**(5), 1193–1235.

Daw, N.D., Courville, A.C., and **Dayan, P.** (2008). Semi-rational models of conditioning: the case of trial order. In: N. Chater and M. Oaksford (Eds.), *The Probabilistic Mind: Prospects for Bayesian Cognitive Science* (pp. 431–452). Oxford: Oxford University Press.

Dayan, P. (2012). How to set the switches on this thing. *Current Opinion in Neurobiology*, **22**(6), 1068–1074.

Dayan, P. (2013). Exploration from generalization mediated by multiple controllers. In: G. Baldassarre and M. Mirolli (Eds.), *Intrinsically Motivated Learning in Natural and Artificial Systems* (pp. 73–81). New York: Springer.

Dayan, P. and **Daw, N.D.** (2008). Decision theory, reinforcement learning, and the brain. *Cognitive, Affective & Behavioral Neuroscience*, **8**(4), 429–453.

Dayan, P. and **Huys, Q.J.** (2008). Serotonin, inhibition, and negative mood. *PLoS Computational Biology*, **4**(2), e4.

Dunlop, B.W. and **Mayberg, H.S.** (2014). Neuroimaging-based biomarkers for treatment selection in major depressive disorder. *Dialogues in Clinical Neuroscience*, **16**(4), 479.

Eshel, N. and **Roiser, J.P.** (2010). Reward and punishment processing in depression. *Biological Psychiatry*, **68**(2), 118–124.

Fehr, E. and **Schmidt, K.** (1999). A theory of fairness, competition, and cooperation. *The Quarterly Journal of Economics*, **114**(3), 817–868.

Ferguson, T.S. (2014). *Mathematical Statistics: A Decision Theoretic Approach*, Vol. **1**. New York: Academic Press.

Gillan, C.M., Kosinski, M., Whelan, R., Phelps, E.A., and **Daw, N.D.** (2016). Characterizing a psychiatric symptom dimension related to deficits in goal-directed control. *Elife*, **5**, e11305.

Gittins, J.C. (1989). *Multi-Armed Bandit Allocation Indices* (Wiley Interscience Series in Systems and Optimization). Chichester: John Wiley & Sons Inc.

Gmytrasiewicz, P. and **Doshi, P.** (2005). A framework for sequential planning in multi-agent settings. *Journal of Artificial Intelligence Research*, **24**, 49–79.

Harsanyi, J. (1967). Games with incomplete information played by 'Bayesian' players. *Management Science*, **14**(5), 159–182.

Hettema, J.M., Annas, P., Neale, M.C., Kendler, K.S., and **Fredrikson, M.** (2003). A twin study of the genetics of fear conditioning. *Archives of General Psychiatry*, **60**(7), 702–708.

Hills, T.T., Todd, P.M., Lazer, D., Redish, A.D., Couzin, I.D., and **Cognitive Search Research Group** (2015). Exploration versus exploitation in space, mind, and society. *Trends in Cognitive Sciences*, **19**(1), 46–54.

Hula, A., Montague, P., and **Dayan, P.** (2015). Monte Carlo planning method estimates planning horizons during interactive social exchange. *PLoS Computational Biology*, **11**(6), e1004254.

Hula, A., Vilares, I., Dayan, P., and **Montague, P.** (2018). A model of risk and mental state shifts during social interaction. *PLoS Computational Biology*, **14**(2), e1005935.

Huys, Q.J., Daw, N.D., and **Dayan, P.** (2015a). Depression: a decision-theoretic analysis. *Annual Review of Neuroscience*, **38**, 1–23.

Huys, Q.J., Eshel, N., O'Nions, E., Sheridan, L., Dayan, P., and **Roiser, J.P.** (2012). Bonsai trees in your head: how the Pavlovian system sculpts goal-directed choices by pruning decision trees. *PLoS Computational Biology* **8**, e1002410.

Huys, Q.J., Goölzer, M., Friedel, E., Heinz, A., Cools, R., Dayan, P., and **Dolan, R.** (2016a). The specificity of Pavlovian regulation is associated with recovery from depression. *Psychological Medicine* **46**(5), 1027–1035.

Huys, Q.J., Guitart-Masip, M., Dolan, R.J., and **Dayan, P.** (2015b). Decision-theoretic psychiatry. *Clinical Psychological Science*, **3**(3), 400–421.

Huys, Q.J., Maia, T.V., and **Frank, M.J.** (2016b). Computational psychiatry as a bridge from neuroscience to clinical applications. *Nature Neuroscience*, **19**(3), 404–413.

Huys, Q.J., Pizzagalli, D.A., Bogdan, R., and **Dayan, P.** (2013). Mapping anhedonia onto reinforcement learning: a behavioural meta-analysis. *Biology of Mood & Anxiety Disorders*, **3**(1), 12.

Jaffee, S.R. and **Price, T.S.** (2007). Gene-environment correlations: a review of the evidence and implications for prevention of mental illness. *Molecular Psychiatry*, **12**(5), 432–442.

Jardri, R. and **Denve, S.** (2013). Circular inferences in schizophrenia. *Brain*, **136**(Pt 11), 3227–3241.

Kaelbling, L.P., Littman, M.L., and **Cassandra, A.R.** (1998). Planning and acting in partially observable stochastic domains. *Artificial Intelligence*, **101**(1), 99–134.

Kaney, S. and **Bentall, R.P.** (1989). Persecutory delusions and attributional style. *The British Journal of Medical Psychology*, **62**(Pt 2), 191–198.

Keay, K.A. and **Bandler, R.** (2001). Parallel circuits mediating distinct emotional coping reactions to different types of stress. *Neuroscience and Biobehavioral Reviews*, **25**(7–8), 669–678.

King-Casas, B., Sharp, C., Lomax, L., Lohrenz, T., Fonagy, P., and **Montague, P.** (2008). The rupture and repair of cooperation in borderline personality disorder. *Science*, 321(5890), 806–810.

King-Casas, B., Tomlin, D., Anen, C., Camerer, C., Quartz, S., and **Montague, P.** (2005). Getting to know you: reputation and trust in a two-person economic exchange. *Science*, **308**(5718), 78–83.

Körding, K. (2007). Decision theory: what "should" the nervous system do? *Science*, **318**(5850), 606–610.

Kruschke, J.K. (2006). Locally Bayesian learning with applications to retrospective revaluation and highlighting. *Psychological Review*, **113**, 677–699.

Lally, N., Huys, Q.J., Eshel, N., Faulkner, P., Dayan, P., and **Roiser, J.P.** (2017). The neural basis of aversive Pavlovian guidance during planning. *The Journal of Neuroscience*, **37**(42), 10215–10229.

Luyten, P., Vliegen, N., Van Houdenhove, B., and **Blatt, S.J.** (2008). Equifinality, multifinality, and the rediscovery of the importance of early experiences: pathways from early adversity to psychiatric and (functional) somatic disorders. *The Psychoanalytic Study of the Child*, **63**, 27–60.

McCabe, K., Rigdon, M., and **Smith, V.** (2003). Positive reciprocity and intentions in trust games. *Journal of Economic Behavior & Organization*, **52**(2), 267–275.

McCrory, E.J. and Viding, E. (2015). The theory of latent vulnerability: reconceptualizing the link between childhood maltreatment and psychiatric disorder. *Development and Psychopathology*, **27**, 493–505.

Montague, P.R., Dolan, R.J., Friston, K.J., and Dayan, P. (2012). Computational psychiatry. *Trends in Cognitive Sciences*, **16**, 72–80.

Moutoussis, M., Bentall, R.P., El-Deredy, W., and Dayan, P. (2011). Bayesian modelling of jumping-to-conclusions bias in delusional patients. *Cognitive Neuropsychiatry*, **16**(5), 422–447.

Oudeyer, P., Kaplan, F., and Hafner, V. (2007). Intrinsic motivation systems for autonomous mental development. *IEEE Transactions on Evolutionary Computation*, **11**(2), 265–286.

Pinborg, L.H., Arfan, H., Haugbol, S., Kyvik, K.O., Hjelmborg, J.V.B., Svarer, C., Frokjaer, V.G., Paulson, O.B., Holm, S., and Knudsen, G.M. (2008). The 5-HT2A receptor binding pattern in the human brain is strongly genetically determined. *NeuroImage*, **40**(3), 1175–1180.

Ray, D., King-Casas, B., Montague, P.R., and Dayan, P. (2009). Bayesian model of behaviour in economic games. In: D. Koller (Ed.), *Advances in Neural Information Processing Systems 21* (pp. 1345–1352). Cambridge, MA: MIT Press.

Schweighofer, N., Bertin, M., Shishida, K., Okamoto, Y., Tanaka, S.C., Yamawaki, S., and Doya, K. (2008). Low-serotonin levels increase delayed reward discounting in humans. *The Journal of Neuroscience*, **28**(17), 4528–4532.

Schweighofer, N., Tanaka, S.C., and Doya, K. (2007). Serotonin and the evaluation of future rewards: theory, experiments, and possible neural mechanisms. *Annals of the New York Academy of Sciences*, 1104, 289–300.

Shteingart, H., Neiman, T., and Loewenstein, Y. (2013). The role of first impression in operant learning. *Journal of Experimental Psychology: General*, **142**(2), 476.

Shumake, J., Furgeson-Moreira, S., and Monfils, M.H. (2014). Predictability and heritability of individual differences in fear learning. *Animal Cognition*, **17**(5), 1207–1221.

Silver, D. and Veness, J. (2010). Monte-Carlo planning in large POMDPs. In: J.D. Lafferty and C.K.I. Williams and J. Shawe-Taylor and R.S. Zemel and A. Culotta (Eds.), *Advances in Neural Information Processing Systems 23* (pp. 2164–2172). Cambridge, MA: MIT Press.

Stephan, K.E. and Mathys, C. (2014). Computational approaches to psychiatry. *Current Opinion in Neurobiology*, **25**, 85–92.

Viding, E. and McCrory, E.J. (2012). Genetic and neurocognitive contributions to the development of psychopathy. *Development and Psychopathology*, **24**(3), 969–983.

von Neumann, J. and Morgenstern, O. (1955). *Theory of Games and Economic Behavior*. Princeton, NJ: Princeton University Press.

Xiang, T., Debajyoti, R., Lohrenz, T., Dayan, P., and Montague, P. (2012). Computational phenotyping of two-person interactions reveals differential neural response to depth-of-thought. *PLoS Compututational Biology*, **8**(12), e1002841.

Chapter 15

Psychiatry's inchoate wish for a paradigm shift and the biopsychosocial model of mental illness

Tim Thornton

Overview

In recent years, there have been repeated calls for a 'paradigm shift' in psychiatry. In this chapter, I take this idea seriously and explore its consequences. Having illustrated calls for a paradigm shift, I sketch the Kuhnian account of science from which the idea is taken and highlight the connection to incommensurability. I then outline a distinction drawn from Winch between putative sciences where the self-understanding of subjects plays no role and those where it is fundamental. I argue that psychiatry falls into the latter kind. This suggests that the wish for a paradigm shift in psychiatry is either incoherent or a wish for a radical but unpredictable overhaul of a significant aspect of our self-understanding as subjects and agents. The biopsychosocial model of mental illness is thus a helpful reminder of the cost of a paradigm shift in psychiatry.

Introduction: the inchoate desire for a psychiatric paradigm shift

During preliminary discussions of the development of the fifth edition of the *Diagnostic and Statistical Manual of Mental Disorders* (*DSM-5*, then referred to as '*DSM-V*') there was a widespread assumption expressed that psychiatry needed a 'paradigm shift'. For example, in the introduction to *A Research Agenda for DSM-V* (Kupfer et al., 2002), the editors, including the *DSM-5* Task Force Chair Dr David Kupfer, claimed that:

> limitations in the current diagnostic *paradigm* suggest that research exclusively focused on refining the DSM-defined syndromes may never be successful in uncovering their underlying etiologies. For that to happen, an as yet unknown *paradigm shift* may need to occur. Therefore, another important goal of this volume is to transcend the limitations of the current DSM *paradigm*. (Kupfer et al., 2002, p. ix, emphasis added)

In an article published 8 years later (but before *DSM-5*) called 'Paradigm shifts and the development of the Diagnostic and Statistical Manual of Mental Disorders: past experiences and future aspirations', one of those editors, Michael First, expressed pessimism about such a possible radical change:

> Work is currently under way on the preparation of DSM-5, which is due in May 2013. From the outset of the DSM-5 revision process in 1999, its developers were hopeful that the changes would be so significant so as to constitute a *paradigm shift* in psychiatric diagnosis. (First, 2010, p. 691, emphasis added)

> Despite hopes that DSM-5 may be able to move beyond its current descriptive categorical *paradigm* as a result of the fruits of the past 16 years of scientific research, based on *A Research Agenda for DSM-V*, the DSM-5 research planning conference presentations, and the initial drafts of the DSM-5 proposals, it seems evident that DSM-5 will continue to follow the DSM-IV *paradigm*, namely, a descriptive categorical system augmented by dimensions. Any future *paradigm shift* will have to await significant advances in our understanding of the etiology and pathophysiology of mental disorders. (First, 2010, p. 698, emphasis added)

Allan Frances, the Task Force Chair of the previous *DSM-IV* (American Psychiatric Association, 1994), later described the initial optimism about the possibility of such a change as 'absurdly premature':

> The *DSM-V* goal to effect a '*paradigm shift*' in psychiatric diagnosis is absurdly premature. Simply stated, descriptive psychiatric diagnosis does not now need and cannot support a *paradigm shift*. There can be no dramatic improvements in psychiatric diagnosis until we make a fundamental leap in our understanding of what causes mental disorders. The incredible recent advances in neuroscience, molecular biology, and brain imaging that have taught us so much about normal brain functioning are still not relevant to the clinical practicalities of everyday psychiatric diagnosis. The clearest evidence supporting this disappointing fact is that not even 1 biological test is ready for inclusion in the criteria sets for *DSM-V*. (Frances, 2009a, p. 2, emphasis added)

Elsewhere, in 'Whither DSM-V?' he wrote:

> Not surprisingly, the disappointing conclusion of all this effort was that there are no biological markers even remotely ready for inclusion in DSM-V. The good news is that the remarkable revolutions in neuroscience, molecular biology, and genetics of the past three decades have given us great insights into the functioning of the normal brain. The bad news is that our understanding of psychopathology is fairly primitive and may remain so for some time … Thus, it is obvious that our field lacks the fundamental understanding of pathogenesis that will be required before we can take the next meaningful step forward towards a *paradigm-shifting* aetiological model of diagnosis. (Frances, 2009b, p. 391, emphasis added)

Such passages imply that the nature of the radical shift envisaged was a turn towards a biological disease model for psychiatry and that this was undermined by the lack of biological markers for psychiatric diagnostic categories. But even those who rejected a disease model still appealed for a 'paradigm shift'. In a position paper written in the same year as *DSM-5* was published (American Psychiatric Association, 2013), the British Psychological Society wrote:

> The DCP [Division of Clinical Psychology] is of the view that it is timely and appropriate to affirm publicly that the current classification system as outlined in DSM and ICD, in

respect of the functional psychiatric diagnoses, has significant conceptual and empirical limitations. Consequently, there is a need for a *paradigm shift* in relation to the experiences that these diagnoses refer to, towards a conceptual system which is no longer based on a 'disease' model. (British Psychological Society, 2013, p. 1, emphasis added)

Since the publication of *DSM-5*, hope for a biological disease model for psychiatry has been placed, instead, on the National Institute of Mental Health's (NIMH's) Research Domain Criteria (RDoC). It is not a rival taxonomy but rather a research framework to underpin new approaches to investigating mental disorders:

RDoC itself does not propose an alternative nosology, but rather seeks to unfetter research from clinical definitions and provide an initial framework and set of constructs for reconceptualizing psychiatric research directions in line with basic neuroscience concepts … The RDoC framework seeks to reorient conceptions of psychopathology by encouraging infusion of neuroscientific thinking and data into such conceptions. (Hettema, 2016, p. 349)

NIMH gave emphasis to RDoC as a *paradigm* with the hypothesis that research based on already defined behavioral constructs with known neural circuits will accelerate the development of fundamental knowledge applicable to psychopathology while reducing problems associated with heterogeneous clinical syndromes. (Carpenter, 2016, p. 562, emphasis added)

In 'Research domain criteria: a final paradigm for psychiatry?', the philosopher of psychiatry, Walter Glannon, sums up an assessment with the claim that:

Despite its limitations, RDoC offers the most conceptually coherent and scientifically sound *paradigm* for explaining psychiatric disorders. (Glannon, 2015, p. 3, emphasis added)

As I will explain (briefly) later in this chapter, the fact that RDoC is not a rival taxonomy to *DSM-5* but a framework and set of constructs for research provides some rationale for the use of the label 'paradigm'. Putting that specific feature of RDoC aside, the earlier quotations suggest a more general point. There is a widespread assumption that psychiatry is in need of a paradigm shift whether towards or away from a more biomedical approach. But this prompts the question: for what does one hope if one hopes for such a thing?

'Paradigm' is the great term of art of the historian of science, Thomas Kuhn. In the next section, I will draw out some of the consequences of the call for a paradigm shift for psychiatry on a broadly Kuhnian picture of science. Central to this picture is the connection between paradigms and the meanings of theoretical terms and hence the connection between changing paradigms and the consequent incommensurability of the meanings of terms across time. It is this that helps to support Kuhn's theoretical scepticism about whether sciences can be said to progress. And this in turn calls into question whether the wish for a paradigm shift could be rational.

In the third section, I address a related but more substantial point. While the wish for a paradigm shift typically reflects optimism about the developments of neuroscience, psychiatry aims to use its technical innovations to relieve human distress. An improved psychiatry should thus be better able to address those issues. But if so, its understanding of mental illness and distress—which guides diagnosis, treatment, management, and shared plans for recovery—had better remain closely wedded to the self-understanding of those it is supposed to help. And if so, any plans for a paradigm shift threaten either to disconnect medical psychiatry from the understanding of human agents which should guide it or to revise radically and in unpredictable ways much of every day human self-understanding.

Paradigms, paradigm shifts, and incommensurability

The widespread and sometimes indiscriminate use of the word 'paradigm' in the description of scientific change is the result of the popularity of Kuhn's *Structure of Scientific Revolutions* in which it is a key term (Kuhn, 1962/1996). Margaret Masterman (a pupil of Wittgenstein and founder of the Cambridge Language Research Laboratory) identified 21 different ways in which Kuhn used the word but suggested that there were three main ideas (Masterman, 1970, p. 61). These are paradigm as a metaphysical worldview, a sociologically describable body of activity, and a particular concrete instance such as a textbook. To shed light on these, it will be helpful to offer a thumbnail sketch of his account of scientific practice.

Kuhn argues that scientific activity falls into two sorts. In the main, scientists are engaged in 'normal science'. This comprises the articulation and application of stable dominant theories and meta-theoretical assumptions to new areas. Kuhn uses the word 'paradigm' to refer to both the background worldview and agreed forms of activities (the first and second of Masterman's uses). The paradigm offers a way of seeing the world and one such tool is a paradigmatic worked example, or classic solution (Masterman's third sense). The business of normal science is puzzle solving: using familiar methods to arrive at solutions to problems against a background assumption that the paradigm provides the resources for such solutions.

As I advertised earlier, these characteristics suggest a rationale for calling RDoC a 'paradigm'. Rather than being merely a new taxonomy to rival the *DSM-5*, RDoC is intended to encourage a characteristic approach to explaining mental illness emphasizing biological and neurological causes. It offers a way of seeing mental illness as a biological disease.

During periods of normal science, no serious attempt is made to refute or even defend the theoretical background and shared practices, which are instead simply presupposed. But these stable periods of normal science are punctuated by brief periods of revolutionary theory change. Sparked both by the accumulation of anomalous results—such as 'puzzles' that resist solution—and by the development of rival theories or even rival meta-theoretical assumptions, the dominant orthodoxy is cast aside and a new theory or set of theories put in its place. Only during these revolutionary periods is the truth of both the previous and the new orthodoxies called into question. Afterwards, the previous paradigm is rejected and the new one taken for granted.

Thus, while during periods of normal science some measure of progress can be based on an increasing ability to solve recognized puzzles against the background of a stable paradigm, that measure does not apply over periods of revolutionary change:

> In the first place, the proponents of competing paradigms will often disagree about the list of problems that any candidate for paradigm must resolve. Their standards or their definitions of science are not the same. (Kuhn, 1962/1996, p. 148)

This reason for a lack of a common measure—the claim that standards of assessment are internal, and hence relative, to a paradigm—is called 'the incommensurability of standards'. But it is not the only reason to think that different paradigms are incommensurable:

> More is involved, however, than the incommensurability of standards. Since new paradigms are born from old ones, they ordinarily incorporate much of the vocabulary and apparatus, both conceptual and manipulative, that the traditional paradigm had previously employed. But they seldom employ these borrowed elements in quite the traditional way. Within the new paradigm, old terms, concepts, and experiments fall into new relationships one with the other. The inevitable result is what we must call, though the term is not quite right, a misunderstanding between the two competing schools. (Kuhn, 1962/1996, p. 149)

This source of incommensurability follows from his view, influential at the time, of the meaning of theoretical terms. Like other philosophers and historians of science, Kuhn reacted against an influential view of the meaning of theoretical terms taken from the logical empiricists of the 1930s (Feigl, 1970). On that older view, theories could be judged against the standard of theoretically neutral observations and that neutrality was supposedly maintained by the independence of observation from theoretical language. Although theoretical terms were grounded in the observational predictions that they collectively inferentially warranted, observational terms were thought to be definable antecedently.

A group of arguments towards the end of the twentieth century undermined that distinction between theory and observation (establishing instead the 'theory dependence of observation') (e.g. Hanson, 1958; Kuhn, 1962/1996; Churchland, 1979). Kuhn concludes that the holism that had been thought to apply to theoretical terms—albeit a holism constrained from the outside by their implications for observation claims—must apply to theoretical and observational terms collectively. But without a stable set of neutral observation claims against which to judge theoretical claims, the new holism seems to imply that a change of overall theory would change the context and hence the meaning of all now hybrid theory-observation terms. This seems to suggest that there is no standard by which to compare overall theories across a paradigm change, since different paradigms defined different scientific languages leaving no resources for an objective translation manual. Translation depends instead on difficult judgements about the best way to render one description into another. And thus, paradigm change is *incommensurable*, undermining the very idea that science progresses.

Kuhn himself notoriously suggests that, after such a shift, scientists inhabit a different world:

> These examples point to the third and most fundamental aspect of the incommensurability of competing paradigms. In a sense that I am unable to explicate further, the proponents of competing paradigms practise their trades in different worlds. (Kuhn, 1962/1996, p. 150)

This is not the only way to view the meaning of theoretical terms and thus not the only view of the impact on the possibility of comparing theories of potential meaning change. One possible alternative, motivated by referential approaches to meaning influenced by Hilary Putnam, puts weight on the role of actual samples in fixing the extension of scientific terms (Putnam, 1975). But part of the force of the idea of a paradigm shift is that the change of worldview is radical and Kuhn's view of meaning incommensurability is part of the reason to think that such a change is radical. The use of the phrase 'paradigm shift' and commitment to meaning incommensurability go hand in hand. Any less radical account of the consequences of theory change, perhaps sustained by a non-Kuhnian account of the meaning of scientific terms, would undermine the point of deploying the suggestive phrase 'paradigm shift'.

This, however, suggests that, at the very least, there is something strange about psychiatry's frequently expressed wish to usher in a new paradigm. Without a standard by which to judge progress across such a change, what rational motive is there to wish in advance for such a change? By what pre-shift standard can a replacement be said to be rationally preferable? Afterwards, there might equally be no grounds for rational regret and perhaps even a parochial preference for the newly familiar, but that does not provide a rational argument to favour the change.

It may be that this is not what the authors of the many calls for a 'paradigm shift' in psychiatry have had in mind. Such calls may have been, and continue to be, made on the rational grounds that the existing categories do not mark genuine distinctions in kind, that they are not predictive, and do not help in designing treatments for mental illnesses, etc. And hence it is rational to think that *some* change to psychiatry is needed whatever precisely that is.[1] My reason for taking the use of the phrase 'paradigm shift' seriously and literally is that, whatever the intentions of such authors, it helps shed light on the connection between psychiatry and its therapeutic purposes. In the next section, I will suggest that a paradigm shift would come at a high price for psychiatry and that the apparent willingness to pay that price suggests a radical scepticism about solving psychiatry's current conceptual problems. At the very least, a call for a 'paradigm shift' is the wrong response to the challenges psychiatry faces.

Scientific and lay understanding of mental illness

In order to develop my main concern, I will return to (and requote) the passage from Frances I quoted earlier. The most obvious reason for thinking that psychiatry needs a paradigm shift is developments at the hard science end of psychiatry. Even Frances mentions 'incredible recent advances in neuroscience, molecular biology, and brain imaging' when discussing others' confidence in the possibility of a new paradigm.

---

[1] This reasonable point was suggested—in these words—by a referee. It also has structural parallels with a commonly proffered explanation of why, in the 2016 UK referendum, many voters voted to leave the European Union despite living in communities that would very probably be significantly disadvantaged by such a move. The explanation proposed is that, despite that likely consequence, their vote was a rational response to well-founded and legitimate political grievances. In this chapter, I am exploring the consequences of responding to the weaknesses of current psychiatric taxonomy by calling for a paradigm shift. This is not to deny that there are genuine problems with the conceptual foundations of psychiatry but is instead to deny that a fashionable slogan is a guide to the right solution to genuine needs (cf. 'Brexit'). In this case, the consequence of taking the slogan seriously also sheds light on the nature of psychiatry.

Frances himself argues that 'descriptive psychiatric diagnosis does not now need and cannot support a paradigm shift' but he goes on to say that there 'can be no dramatic improvements in psychiatric diagnosis until we make a fundamental leap in our understanding of what causes mental disorders' and that the absence of biological tests in diagnostic criteria suggests that this has not been reached. But that comment does not distance him from what might seem a plausible aspiration for a biomedical psychiatry. What is needed, on this assumption, is greater biological understanding of 'what causes mental disorders' and a sufficiently 'fundamental leap' in that understanding might give us the hoped-for paradigm shift.

I think there are two fundamental complexities that this view—a view from which Frances does not sufficiently distance himself—ignores. The first is that, within psychiatry, the focus of neuroscientific, biological, and brain imaging technology is, nevertheless, mental pathology. Progress has been recently made in these areas and more progress is needed but, additionally, progress is also needed in determining not just what *causes* mental disorders but what they *comprise*. What is it, in other words, for something to be a mental disorder? There is no reason to think that an answer to this question can be provided by neuroscience, molecular biology, and brain imaging. In so far as these can help shed light on psychopathology, one needs first to have decided the extension of that concept, then to study its neurological and biological underpinnings. Given the conceptual complexity of the very idea of mental disorder, and given that what is classed as such is so contested, any leap forward in knowledge of brain mechanisms needs to go hand in hand with answers to that question.

The second complexity follows from the first. Suppose that innovations in neuroscience, molecular biology, and brain imaging were to lead to discoveries concerning the neurological underpinnings of familiar psychiatric diagnostic classifications of psychopathology. Suppose, further, that a future neuroscience identified some neurologically very similar states, which caused (or were identical with) no mental distress or suffering but which, on the basis of the neurological similarity, were proposed as asymptomatic forms of the previous diagnostic categories. Assuming that these were not predictive of mental distress or suffering, such a proposal would not, I suggest, mark a triumph of neuroscientific psychiatry. Rather, it would amount to psychiatry losing its primary focus on *mental* illness (cf Muang, 2016, Pickard, 2009).

This point suggests a more general moral that derives from the Wittgensteinian philosopher Peter Winch's arguments in *The Idea of a Social Science and its Relation to Philosophy* (Winch, 1958). Winch argues that there can be no such thing as a social science. The argument for this conclusion starts from the assumption that a central element of understanding meaningful behaviour is an understanding of the nature of rules. For this he draws on Wittgenstein's lengthy discussion of rules, rule following and understanding in the *Philosophical Investigations* (Wittgenstein, 1953). Winch makes three claims:

1. Rules are central to so-called social science because actions are constituted *as* the actions that they are by the rules that govern them. Thus, to give one of his examples, putting a cross on a piece of paper is an act of voting given the right context of rules. Sound patterns, similarly, are constituted as meaningful assertions only given the rules of spoken language.

2. Explaining an action by citing a rule presupposes a grasp of the rule not just by the putative social scientist but also (to a first approximation) by the agent whose behaviour is being explained.

3. Rule following is grounded in implicit practical knowledge of what actions count as going on in the same way. Rule following cannot rest entirely on explicit linguistically codified knowledge because that explicit knowledge would require further implicit knowledge of how the written prescription is to be understood.

Rules have a further implicit but important feature. They are *normative*: they prescribe correct and incorrect moves. In the example mentioned previously, they prescribe the difference between a successful vote and a spoiled ballot paper. Only certain actions count as casting a vote. Thus, if understanding what type of action an event is involves relating it to a rule, this form of understanding involves a notion of correctness. It involves understanding what makes it correct or appropriate as a piece of voting behaviour. This is not the same as saying that most votes are cast at a particular time of day or night or by a particular socioeconomic proportion of the electorate. That may be discovered by empirical study. The normative rules that characterize an event as an act of voting are not provided by any such statistical generalizations.

With these claims in place, Winch goes on to argue that so-called social science is fundamentally dissimilar to natural science:

> [W]hereas in the case of the natural scientist we have to deal with only one set of rules, namely those governing the scientist's investigation itself, here *what the sociologist is studying*, as well as his study of it, is a human activity and is therefore carried on according to rules. And it is these rules, rather than those which govern the sociologist's investigation, which specify what is to count as 'doing the same kind of thing' in relation to that kind of activity. (Winch, 1958/1990, p. 87)

In understanding social phenomena, the understanding possessed by the objects of study (human subjects) of their own behaviour plays a key role and this is not reflected in, say, the physics of billiard ball motion. The putative social scientist has to understand social behaviour by understanding it, at least in part, through the understanding that the agents he or she studies have. This follows from the idea that social science studies subjects' actions and that those actions are constituted as the actions they are by reference to the rules that subjects follow. Consider a social science study of the differing use of setting an off-side trap in football by different teams with more or less defensive strategies. No such study would be possible in ignorance of the off-side rule as understood by the players. Ignoring those rules threatens to cut the social scientist off from his or her domain of study. That is not to say that the analysis of social phenomena can go no further than agents' self-understanding. But it is rooted in it:

> I do not wish to maintain that we must stop at the unreflective kind of understanding of which I gave as an instance the engineer's understanding of the activities of his colleagues. But I do want to say that any more reflective understanding must necessarily presuppose, if it is to count as genuine understanding at all, the participant's unreflective understanding. (Winch, 1958/1990, p. 89)

Winch himself uses these points to argue, contentiously, that there can be no such thing as social *science* and, even more contentiously, that the proper study of social phenomena is continuous with philosophical analysis. Neither of these conclusions is necessary, however, for the more modest point that there is an important distinction between cases where the understanding of phenomena by those who are being studied is important and those where, because there is no such self-understanding (in the realm of physics, for example), it plays no role.

Psychiatry is not merely a disinterested study of the brain. It is a branch of medicine concerned with the amelioration of human distress and suffering and specifically mental distress and suffering. In identifying that subject matter it has, according to the Winchean analysis set out previously, an essential connection to norms governing social dysfunction, emotional dysregulation, and so on, since these are the norms that constitute its subject matter. Thus, it has an essential connection to the concepts with which we, as subjects and agents, make sense of ourselves. This suggests the importance of a biopsychosocial model of psychiatry. It helps to highlight the central role of psychological and social norms in constituting its focus (Engel, 1977).

The implication from Winch's analysis is that norms, deviation from which constitute mental illnesses, have to be understood, at least initially, via agents' self-understanding of them. This suggests a distinction between psychiatry and at least some of the natural sciences. While there seems to be no constraint imposed by the subject matter of much of natural science on the limits of conceptual innovation (as long as the concepts arrived at can still be understood by at least some scientists), the concepts of psychiatry need to retain some connection to those concepts in terms of which we ordinarily make sense of ourselves. Only so can human experiences play at least some guiding role for psychiatric diagnosis, theorizing, and care.

Implications for psychiatric paradigm shifts and the biopsychosocial model

If the Winch-inspired argument described earlier is correct, then psychiatry, unlike, for example, quantum physics, has to keep one foot on the ground via a lay understanding of the norms governing mental illness, disorder, dysfunction, and distress. That in turn has implications for paradigm shifts in psychiatry, given their connection to incommensurability. If, on the one hand, a future psychiatry maintains its links to the ordinary understanding of mental illness that currently sets the agenda for mental healthcare, then that ordinary understanding provides a bridgehead for scientific understanding, undermining the very idea of there being a paradigm shift. If the Winchean argument is right, while psychiatry can go beyond ordinary agents' understanding of the norms deviations from which amount to illness, it must still be rooted in it. If, on the other hand, a radical change in psychiatry severs those links, that might amount to a genuine paradigm shift for medical psychiatry—because that would imply a lack of the commensurability—but it would lose its identity as a response to mental illness and distress. It would no longer be psychiatry.

Consistent with this basic framework, there is one other possibility. The call for a paradigm shift may be intended not just to cover scientific psychiatric theorizing about the causes of mental illnesses and distress—for example, a turn to more biological models and biomarkers—but also everyday conceptualizations of them. That is, it might be a kind of counsel of despair. On the assumption that everyday thinking about mental illness is essentially confused and raises insoluble conceptual questions of the sort expressed in the dilemma 'mad or bad?', it might be thought that the rational response is a kind of conceptual radical overhaul. But given the consequences of a Kuhnian paradigm shift, such a move risks putting into an unpredictable future not merely elements of medical science but also a significant element of our self-understanding as agents, the basic norms governing actions, emotions, responsibility, and free will.

If this working through of the combination of Kuhn and Winch is correct, then the wish for a paradigm shift in psychiatry seems doubly misplaced. First, the connection to incommensurability necessarily undermines the rationality of the wish, even when limited to an area of medical science. Second, a change which did *not* sever the connection to the concepts we use to make sense of ourselves would not be a paradigm shift. Anything leaving those connections in place would allow standards for rational assessment of the technical innovations, and hence would not count as a paradigm shift on the Kuhnian view. But a paradigm shift localized to psychiatry which rendered the pre- and the post-shift worldviews incommensurable would have to sever the connection to those grounding concepts and that could only be because psychiatry had lost its way. Finally, a paradigm shift of not only medical psychiatry but also of the everyday norms against which folk conceptions of illness, distress, and suffering are measured is such a radical view that there is no way now to conceptualize what it is for which one would be wishing.

Against this long-standing inchoate wish for a paradigm shift in psychiatry, the biopsychosocial model of psychiatry is a helpful reminder of its potential costs (Engel, 1977). Our understanding of mental illness is not merely rooted in biological natural science. It is much more broadly rooted in psychological and sociological basic norms and rules governing activity, thought and feeling. Genuine fundamental change in that whole conceptual package is not something to be lightly entertained.

References

American Psychiatric Association (1994). *Diagnostic and Statistical Manual of Mental Disorders* (4th ed.). Washington, DC: American Psychiatric Association.

American Psychiatric Association (2013). *Diagnostic and Statistical Manual of Mental Disorders* (5th ed.). Washington, DC: American Psychiatric Association.

British Psychological Society (2013). *Classification of Behaviour and Experience in Relation to Functional Psychiatric Diagnoses: Time for a Paradigm Shift* (DCP Position Statement). Leicester: The British Psychological Society.

Carpenter, W.T. (2016). The RDoC controversy: alternate paradigm or dominant Paradigm? *American Journal of Psychiatry*, **173**(6), 562–563.

Churchland, P. (1979). *Scientific Realism and the Plasticity of Mind*. Cambridge: Cambridge University Press.

Engel, G.L. (1977). The need for a new medical model: a challenge for biomedicine. *Science*, **196**(4286), 129–136.

Feigl, H. (1970). The 'orthodox' view of theories: remarks in defense as well as critique. In: M. Radner and S. Winokur (Eds.), *Analyses of Theories and Methods of Physics and Psychology*

(Minnesota Studies in the Philosophy of Science, Vol. IV) (pp. 3–16). Minneapolis, MN: University of Minnesota Press.

First, M. (2010). Paradigm shifts and the development of the Diagnostic and Statistical Manual of Mental Disorders: past experiences and future aspirations. *Canadian Journal of Psychiatry*, **55**(11), 692–700.

Frances, A. (2009a). A warning sign on the road to *DSM-V*: beware of its unintended consequences. *Psychiatric Times*, **26**(8), 1–9.

Frances, A. (2009b). Whither DSM-V? *The British Journal of Psychiatry*, **195**(5), 391–392.

Glannon, W. (2015). Research domain criteria: a final paradigm for psychiatry? *Frontiers in Human Neuroscience*, **9**, 488.

Hanson, N.R. (1958). *Patterns of Discovery*. Cambridge: Cambridge University Press.

Hettema, J.M. (2016). Psychophysiology of threat response, paradigm shifts in psychiatry, and RDoC: implications for genetic investigation of psychopathology. *Psychophysiology*, **53**(3), 348–350.

Kuhn, T.S. (1962/1996). *The Structure of Scientific Revolutions*. Chicago, IL: University of Chicago Press.

Kupfer, D.J., First, M.B., and Regier, D.A. (Eds.) (2002). *A Research Agenda for DSM-V*. Washington, DC: American Psychiatric Association.

Masterman, M. (1970). The nature of a paradigm. In: I. Lakatos and A. Musgrave (Eds.), *Criticism and the Growth of Knowledge* (pp. 59–90). Cambridge: Cambridge University Press.

Maung, H.H. (2016). To what do psychiatric diagnoses refer? A two-dimensional semantic analysis of diagnostic terms. *Studies in History and Philosophy of Biological and Biomedical Sciences*, 55, 1–10.

Pickard, H. (2009). Mental illness is indeed a myth. In: L. Bortolotti and M. Broome (eds.), *Psychiatry as Cognitive Science: Philosophical Perspectives* (pp. 83–101). Oxford: Oxford University Press.

Putnam, H. (1975). The meaning of meaning. In: *Mind Language and Reality* (pp. 215–271). Cambridge: Cambridge University Press.

Winch, P. (1958/1990). *The Idea of a Social Science and its Relation to Philosophy*. London: Routledge.

Wittgenstein, L. (1953). *Philosophical Investigations* (Trans. G.E.M. Anscombe). Oxford: Blackwell.

Chapter 16

Ignoring faces and making friends

Matthew Parrott

Introduction

A staggering amount of scientific evidence shows that individuals who are physically, sexually, or emotionally abused or neglected when they are infants or very young
children are at a much greater risk of developing psychiatric disorders later in life,
including anxiety, depression, and schizophrenia (for an overview, see Gilbert et al.
(2009) cf. McCrory and Viding (2015)). As one would expect, not everyone who suffers from childhood maltreatment goes on to develop psychiatric symptoms. Many
adult victims of child abuse or neglect lead well-adjusted, happy, and healthy lives.
However, the fact that childhood maltreatment is highly correlated with the manifestation of psychiatric symptoms later in life does suggest that something about being
abused in early life significantly alters one or more aspects of a person's psychological
or neurocognitive functioning, in ways that make the person more vulnerable to other
factors that might contribute to the eventual emergence of psychiatric symptoms.[1]

If we wish to understand precisely how childhood maltreatment might make a
person susceptible to developing psychiatric symptoms, we need to clarify two things.
First, we need to understand precisely how prolonged exposure to an abusive environment in early life changes an individual's psychological or neurocognitive systems.
How exactly are information-processing pathways within the mind adjusted in response to the extreme trauma of child abuse or neglect? Second, we need a much
clearer picture of how the identified maltreatment-induced alterations in these systems could put someone at higher risk than average for developing a psychiatric disorder later in life. How exactly might certain functional changes to psychological or
neurocognitive systems increase the probability that a person will develop anxiety,
depression, or some other kind of psychiatric condition? Answering these questions
will not only give us a substantive theory of how childhood maltreatment makes a

---

[1] Some might be reluctant to go so far as to say that childhood maltreatment is a *cause* of the
psychiatric disorders that emerge in adulthood. But if we think of a cause as 'something that
makes a difference', it would be hard to deny, given the data, that childhood maltreatment
makes a difference to whether or not one becomes depressed, anxious, or unusually aggressive.
Similarly, it is pretty clear that if we were interested in significantly decreasing the incidence of
psychiatric disorders in the adult population, we could do this by intervening upon the rates
of childhood maltreatment. The promise of such a social intervention suggests that there is a
type of causal relationship between theses variables (cf. Woodward 2005, 2008; Pearl, 2009).

person vulnerable to various psychiatric disorders, it would also go a long way towards helping us design effective medical interventions to target specific parameters implicated in the onset of those disorders.[2]

Childhood maltreatment is correlated with an astonishing number of psychiatric symptoms, not to mention other negative outcomes such as poverty and poor physical health. It is therefore very likely that more than one psychological or neurocognitive system is transformed by experiences of maltreatment in early childhood. In this chapter, I shall focus on only one system that looks to be rather significantly affected by sustained childhood maltreatment.

A number of studies have shown that individuals who experience childhood maltreatment exhibit significant differences in the way they process information associated with threat. More specifically, several studies have shown that individuals who are maltreated as young children respond differently to angry facial expressions, which are commonly thought of as 'threat-related cues' or 'threat-related stimuli' (McCrory and Viding, 2015). The experimental data seem to indicate that experiences of abuse makes a person more adept at identifying or recognizing visually presented stimuli of angry facial expressions.

Since sensitivity to actual threats in the environment is crucial to an organism's survival, one very plausible hypothesis is that an unusually hostile or abusive environment changes the neurocognitive systems responsible for processing information concerning angry faces precisely because, in a hostile environment, angry faces are extremely dangerous and threatening (Pollak and Sinha, 2002; Pollak et al., 2009; McCrory et al., 2013; 2017; McCrory and Viding, 2015). In an environment in which angry faces reliably indicate the presence of an immediate and significant physical or emotional threat to an organism, it would be important for the organism to be highly attuned to the presence of angry faces. Thus, heighted responsiveness to angry facial expressions can be seen as a kind of information-processing adaptation to an unusually hostile environment.

This naturally suggests a corollary hypothesis about how the same heightened responsiveness to angry faces may contribute to the eventual onset of psychiatric symptoms. The basic idea is that a specific calibration of an information-processing system can be adaptive or beneficial to an organism in one kind of environment but detrimental in another. As McCrory and colleagues claim, 'such adaptations are equally thought to incur a longer-term cost as they may mean that the individual is poorly optimized to negotiate the demands of other, more normative environments, thus increasing vulnerability to future stressors' (McCrory et al., 2017, p. 339, cf. McCrory et al., 2012). So, whether or not amplified responsiveness to angry faces is beneficial to an organism depends crucially on the type of environment in which the organism is embedded. Generally, this is a plausible idea, but we still need to understand precisely why heightened responsiveness to angry facial expressions becomes 'maladaptive' in a non-hostile environment. How exactly does an enhanced capacity to visually

---

[2] McCrory and Viding (2015) term a theory of how maltreatment makes one susceptible to developing psychiatric disorders a 'theory of latent vulnerability' (cf. McCrory et al., 2017).

recognize or identify angry facial expressions increase a person's vulnerability to developing psychiatric symptoms?

In this chapter, I shall focus on this last question. After reviewing some of the empirical evidence that shows how childhood maltreatment affects the ways in which a person responds to angry facial expressions, I shall briefly present three hypotheses suggested by McCrory and Viding (2015) to account for why an individual who manifests heightened responsiveness to angry facial expressions might thereby be more vulnerable than average to developing psychiatric symptoms. The aim of this chapter is to develop the second of these hypotheses, which claims that maltreatment-induced alterations to neurocognitive processing 'leads to behaviours that shape the child's environment over time in ways that increases the likelihood of stressor experiences and decreases the likelihood of protective experiences' (McCrory and Viding, 2015, p. 500). Although I shall agree with McCrory and Viding that maltreatment-induced alterations in neurocognitive systems ultimately contribute to a more aversive and distressing social environment, one in which a person is exposed to factors that contribute to developing psychiatric symptoms, I shall develop this proposal in a slightly different direction that the one they suggest.[3]

McCrory and Viding think that angry facial expressions are classified or coded by spectators as 'threat-related cues'. There are two senses in which a presented stimulus might be thought of or categorized as a 'threat-cue'. First, certain stimuli tend to elicit a range of proprietary responses in various physiological or neurocognitive systems that seem to prepare an organism for an encounter with something harmful or dangerous. For instance, they tend to generate defensive responses in the autonomic nervous system, such as an increase in heart rate and blood pressure, and the release of hormones such as adrenocorticotropic hormone and epinephrine. In this sense, a stimulus qualifies as a 'threat-cue' by virtue of the effects that it has on an organism. But, it is very natural to think that stimuli have these internal consequences precisely because they reliably indicate the proximity of actual environmental threats. Thus, a stimulus may also be a 'threat-cue' in the sense of being a reliable indicator of an environmental threat to an organism. These two senses of 'threat-cue' are not necessarily independent, since some types of autonomic responses, such as high blood pressure, are, if sustained, dangerous for an organism. So, any external stimulus which caused such a response would be a kind of environmental threat.

It seems clear that angry faces generally elicit defensive physiological and behavioural responses in a subject's threat-processing systems and therefore are 'threat-cues' in the first sense (McCrory et al., 2017; cf. LeDoux, 2000; Whalen et al., 2001; Öhman, 2002). But it is plausible to think that this is partly because angry faces reliably indicate the proximity of environmental threats and so are 'threat-cues' in the second sense (cf. Öhman et al., 2001; Fox et al., 2000; Öhman, 2009). The type of environmental threat one faces may vary; for example, an angry face may indicate the presence of a severe

---

[3] I think the proposal presented in this chapter is a plausible way of expanding upon McCrory and Viding's (2015) brief presentation of the second hypothesis (cf. McCrory et al., 2017). However, it is worth noting that since it is not something that they explicitly discuss, it is not clear whether or not it will be something which they find congenial.

physical danger in a hostile environment, but only the presence of some social threat in an ordinary environment. Nevertheless, one might naturally think that the visual system categorizes or codes angry facial expressions as threatening in the second sense precisely because angry faces reliably indicate the presence of some kind of environmental threat. This would explain why other neurocognitive threat-processing systems respond in ways which prepare the organism for aversive consequences.

In this chapter, I shall argue that this last idea is mistaken and propose instead that the reason heighted responsiveness to angry facial expressions can be detrimental to an organism in a non-hostile environment is because, in that kind of environment, angry faces do not reliably indicate the presence of threat, neither physical nor social. I shall also claim that for this reason engaging in friendly, mutually supportive, pro-social behaviour with others, including those who are most likely to actively contribute to our personal welfare and further our interests, requires a person to learn to attenuate behavioural responses to angry faces.

Experimental evidence

A number of studies show that individuals who have experienced childhood maltreatment respond differently to angry faces. In several experiments, Seth Pollak and colleagues have shown that victims of abuse perform better than controls in visual recognition tasks that involve stimuli of angry facial expressions. For example, in one study (Pollak et al., 2009), children were shown sequences of stimuli which correspond to what Pollak and colleagues call a 'naturalistic unfolding of emotional expressions' (2009, p. 245). They were asked to determine, for each image in a sequence, what emotion was being felt by the person in that image. In another study (Pollak and Sinha, 2002), children were presented with a sequence of images of a single emotional expression, for instance, anger, where the image quality gradually becomes less degraded as one progresses through the members of the sequence. Once again, for each image in the sequence, children were asked to identify the emotion depicted. In both experiments, children who have experienced child abuse were able to accurately identify angry facial expressions on the basis of less perceptual information (i.e. at an earlier stage in the sequence). In a related study (Pollak and Kistler, 2002), children were presented with a continuum of facial expressions ranging, for example, from definitely angry to definitely sad.[4] Maltreated children categorized a wider range of expressions on this continuum as 'angry' than controls. Furthermore, in all of these studies, there

---

[4] This is an interesting result, but it is difficult to say what it indicates. The continua of emotions that Pollak and Kistler present have something like an artificial borderline between two different types of expressions, which is simply the middle image on the continuum, an artificially created 50% blend of each emotion being compared. It isn't clear to me that this artificial image corresponds to anything like a natural border between facial expressions of, for instance, sadness and anger. So, rather than thinking that the experimental results show that abused children categorize too many facial expressions as angry, one may interpret the results as showing that controls categorize too few facial expressions as angry. It isn't clear that either interpretation is preferable. It is also notable that neither group set their subjective border near the artificial midpoint.

was no observed difference in the way maltreated children responded to facial expressions of emotions other than anger.

These experimental results seem to be confirmed by neurophysiological studies. Electroencephalography studies have shown that, when they are asked to search for or actively pay attention to angry faces, maltreated children manifest a comparative increase in brain activity, specifically a higher Pb3 amplitude, which is correlated with high levels of anxiety (Pollak et al., 1997; McCrory and Viding, 2015). In addition, a number of recent functional magnetic resonance imaging (fMRI) studies show neurofunctional differences in the way maltreated children respond to angry faces. For example, McCrory and colleagues (2013) used fMRI to measure pre-attentive neural responses to facial expressions of emotion and found that maltreated children exhibited greater activation in the right amygdala when processing information about angry faces.[5] A related fMRI study (McCrory et al., 2011a; cf. McCrory et al., 2017) also found that maltreated children exhibited greater activation in the right amygdala as well as in the anterior insula when processing angry facial expressions.

Among many developmental psychologists, these studies are taken to demonstrate that children who have been maltreated at a young age respond differently to angry faces. In what follows, I shall assume that this is the correct interpretation of the experimental results.

Explaining neurocognitive alterations

The notion that a neurocognitive system might develop in a manner that displays heightened responsiveness to angry faces is not difficult to grasp. As many theorists have remarked, it is quite plausible that abused children are exposed to an unusually high number of angry faces in early childhood (Pollak and Sinha, 2002; Pollak et al., 2009; McCrory et al., 2013, 2017; McCrory and Viding, 2015). More importantly, in an extremely hostile environment, the presence of an angry face is plausibly associated with immediate harmful outcomes. Since children in these environments need to protect themselves from various physical and emotional harms, angry facial expressions naturally acquire heightened salience. Therefore, it is plausible that learning to rapidly detect an angry face may be beneficial in such an environment. As Pollak and Sinha claim, 'physically abused children learn to make decisions about the signalling of anger using minimal visual information. The development of increased perceptual sensitivity for the fine-grained details of variation in affective expressions may provide a behavioural advantage for living in threatening contexts, allowing earlier identification of emotion' (Pollak and Sinha, 2002, p. 786; cf. McCrory et al., 2017).

Indeed, mere exposure to a greater frequency of angry faces may itself be sufficient for explaining why a subject acquires the ability to accurately identify or recognize angry

---

[5] A second interesting result of this study is that these children also showed greater right amygdala activation when processing happy faces. This is slightly at odds with the experimental results of Pollak and colleagues (Pollak and Kistler, 2002; Pollak and Sinha, 2002; Pollak et al., 2009) which showed no information-processing differences with respect to expressions of happiness.

facial expressions quickly, or on the basis of less perceptual information. According to standard theories of perceptual learning, perceptual systems can learn to identify and discriminate a type of visual stimulus more quickly after repeated exposure to that stimulus (Goldstone, 1998; Hagemann et al., 2010). We therefore have some basic grasp of why someone exposed to an unusually high number of angry faces, especially in early life, might become more proficient at visually recognizing them.

Let's assume that an explanation along these lines can account for why maltreated children exhibited augmented visual responsiveness to angry faces. It is still not obvious why this type of information-processing bias would increase the probability of developing a psychiatric disorder. A plausible idea is that alterations to the way a subject processes information about angry faces is only beneficial in a hostile environment. When subjects are removed from this type of environment, it is no longer adaptive, perhaps because the frequency of exposure to angry faces diminishes. But, although it may be correct to think that a superior capacity to visually recognize angry faces on the basis of less information is less beneficial in a non-hostile environment, it does not follow from this that it would thereby be maladaptive or somehow put one at risk for developing a psychiatric disorder.

Suppose that I am born and raised in an environment where the primary source of food is a certain type of berry, but that 30% of these berries are poisonous. It would not be an evolutionary surprise if I learned to become very good at picking out or identifying these poisonous berries. Maybe I could learn to do this on the basis of the way they look or smell. If so, I might also become more attentive to the way these berries look or smell, especially when compared to other visible or olfactible properties. My capacity to process information relevant to identifying and recognizing these berries would be a kind of adaptive response to my environment. But now suppose that I move to an environment where only 0.05% of the berries are poisonous and there is also a much wider variety of nourishing food. My capacity to visually recognize poisonous berries may no longer be a clear evolutionary advantage, but it does not thereby become a deficit or something that puts me at risk of developing psychiatric or social problems. By analogy, it is difficult to see why being especially adept at visually identifying angry faces would itself constitute a disadvantage to an organism.

So even though we have evidence linking childhood maltreatment to altered neurocognitive processing of angry facial expressions, we still need to understand how these processing alterations contribute to the onset of a psychiatric disorder. McCrory and Viding (2015) propose the following three candidate hypotheses. First, they suggest that having an enhanced capacity to visually recognize or identify angry faces is best accounted for in terms of a subject being hypervigilant to angry faces. The thought is that individuals who have experienced abuse are able to visually recognize angry faces on the basis of less perceptual information because they are more vigilant to the presence of angry faces. As a result of this hypervigilance, their attentional resources are diverted from other domains. Specifically, McCrory and Viding propose that less attention will be allocated to domains relevant to 'optimal development in nonthreat environments' (2015, p. 500; cf. McCrory et al., 2017).

The second hypothesis presented by McCrory and Viding is that heightened responsiveness to angry faces leads to propensities for certain types of behaviour that 'shape the child's environment over time in a way that increases the likelihood of stressor experiences and decreases the likelihood of protective experiences' (2015, p. 500). How might this happen? McCrory and Viding again appeal to hypervigilance. They think it is plausible that children who are hypervigilant to angry faces are more likely to *misattribute* threat to peers and then behave towards those peers as if they were threatening (cf. Pollak and Kistler, 2002). As a result, their peers are more likely to become reactively aggressive, which in turn gives rise to a much more stressful social environment, one in which prosocial relationships are difficult to create and sustain. It is not easy to form a mutually supportive relationship with someone whom one treats as a threat, and, without such relationships, one is at greater risk of developing psychiatric symptoms.

McCrory and Viding's final hypothesis is that greater sensitivity to angry faces recalibrates a person's affective systems such that they manifest amplified responses to future environmental stressors. For example, they may have generally higher levels of anxiety. Experiencing highly aversive affective responses may also lead an individual to develop negative coping strategies such as avoidance or repression, which would also increase one's chances of developing psychiatric symptoms.

For all three of these hypotheses, it is not the case that being adept at visually recognizing angry faces is itself what puts someone at risk of developing a psychiatric disorder. It is rather that changes to the neurocognitive systems underlying this discriminatory capacity have additional negative consequences, such as misattributing anger to non-angry people, or having generally high levels of anxiety. The three hypotheses are not mutually exclusive. It is possible that any or all of them could be true.[6] At this stage, they are highly speculative and in need of empirical confirmation (or disconfirmation). Nevertheless, in the following section, I would like to explore the second hypothesis more fully.

Anger and threat

McCrory and Viding's second hypothesis is that, by virtue of being hypervigilant to angry faces, individuals who have experienced childhood maltreatment develop a tendency to treat their peers as threats. Prima facie this sounds plausible. It does seem natural to think that an individual who has been exposed to a large number of angry faces would frequently be on the lookout for them. In that case, it would make sense if the individual had a greater propensity to miscategorize facial expressions as angry.

---

[6] These three hypotheses account for vulnerability to psychiatric disorder in terms of neurocognitive functioning. But they are not intended to exclude other explanations in terms of neurophysiology, genetics, or epigenetics. Indeed, there is evidence that many psychiatric symptoms associated with childhood maltreatment are heritable. For example, Caspi and colleagues have demonstrated that individuals who carry the low-activity variant *MAOA* allele are at greater risk for developing patterns of antisocial behaviour (Caspi et al., 2002; cf. McCrory et al., 2011b). Genotypes that predict a high risk of developing psychiatric disorder might also help to explain why certain subjects select high-stress or aggressive social environments, in which case a genetic account would also underlie a functional neurocognitive explanation (for further discussion, see McCrory et al. (2017)).

This would explain the results of the experiment conducted by Pollak and Kistler (2002) in which subjects of childhood maltreatment categorized a greater range of facial expressions as angry. Hypervigilance to angry faces would also plausibly explain why individuals exposed to maltreatment were more adept at recognizing actual angry faces on the basis of less perceptual information.

McCrory and Viding's presentation of this second hypothesis is extremely brief, so it will be useful to highlight its central claims. First, McCrory and Viding are in a position to claim that hypervigilance to angry faces puts one at greater risk of developing a psychiatric disorder because they assume that misattributing anger to someone is closely connected, or perhaps equivalent, to misattributing threat (cf. Öhman et al., 2001). Yet, it is really the latter that is more crucial to their explanation. The reason why they think individuals who have experienced childhood maltreatment become more vulnerable to psychiatric disorders is because they think these individuals are far more likely to treat non-threatening peers as if they were serious threats. The sort of treatment they have in mind consists in robustly exhibiting avoidance behaviour or antisocial behaviour such as acts of aggression. To exacerbate matters, in response to this type of behaviour, non-threatening peers are more likely to engage in reactive aggression.

This proposal makes sense but it is worth noting that the last step of McCrory and Viding's hypothesis has two stages. First, non-threatening peers are mistakenly categorized or identified as threats. For this to be at all relevant to experimental work on how individuals respond to facial expressions, there must be some connection between visually identifying a facial expression as angry and visually coding or classifying that same expression as threatening. As we have seen, McCrory and Viding follow a tradition of thinking of angry faces as 'threat-cues'. On the assumption that all angry faces are 'cues' or 'indicators' of some kind of environmental threat, identifying someone as expressing anger implies classifying them as a threat.

The second stage of McCrory and Viding's explanation claims that after someone identifies a person's facial expression as threatening, the subject will subsequently come to treat that person as a serious threat. According to McCrory and Viding, behaving towards one's peers in these ways directly contributes to a more stressful and detrimental social environment, which in turn increases one's chances of developing a psychiatric disorder. Notice that 'treating' one's peer as if they were threatening is not merely displaying a pattern of autonomic responses. As we have already seen, there is a sense in which an organism 'treats' a stimulus as a threat simply in so far as the stimulus activates certain processes in one's autonomic nervous system. But those responses are not sufficient to generate a detrimental social environment; rather, they need to be connected to sustained patterns of antisocial or avoidance behaviour. So even if a wider range of facial expressions cause autonomic arousal in children who have experienced childhood maltreatment, we still need to understand how this leads to the sort of antisocial or avoidance behaviour that put individuals at risk of developing psychiatric disorders, or at least understand why these sorts of responses are not regulated or attenuated (cf. Lyons et al., 2009; Sell et al., 2009).

With this in mind, there seem to be four steps to McCrory and Viding's proposed explanation:

1. People who have experienced childhood maltreatment become highly sensitive (hypervigilant) to angry facial expressions. For this reason, they tend to miscategorize facial expressions as angry.

2. Assuming that angry facial expressions are 'threat-cues', categorizing someone's face as angry means categorizing them as a threat.

3. Individuals who have been maltreated as children respond to the people that they have classified as threatening with antisocial behaviour such as aggression, or with avoidance.

4. Antisocial and avoidance behaviours undermine prosocial and potentially supportive relationships (in part by provoking reactive aggressive responses from one's peers).

According to McCrory and Viding's proposal, what primarily contributes to the greater risk of psychiatric disorder is the way an individual treats people who are not really expressing anger, rather than the way they react to angry peers (although it is consistent with their view that the latter may also be a contributing factor). This an attractive hypothesis, but it is worth reflecting on whether angry faces really are 'threat-cues' in the sense of reliably indicating the presence of an environmental threat. As we have already seen, in a hostile environment, angry faces reliably precede harmful outcomes, and so they are plausibly reliable indicators of immediate and serious physical or emotional threat. This partially explains why a high frequency of angry faces in such an environment recalibrates a child's information-processing systems such that the child becomes more responsive to them. It is natural to think that angry faces also reliably indicate the presence of a threat in non-hostile environments, even though the degree and nature of that threat may be different. Indeed, it is natural to think that basic emotional expressions generally have a function of reliably indicating properties in the environment relevant to an organism's interests (cf. Frijda and Mesquita, 1994). However, although this is a common way to think of emotional expressions such as anger, I would like to present an alternative conception of expressions of anger in the following two sections.

Looking angry

In the experiments presented earlier, we saw that subjects were presented with visual stimuli of angry faces for an extremely brief interval. So classifying or coding a facial expression as angry is a task carried out by the visual system, at least in the first instance. Let's assume this is true. The visual system responds to the way angry facial expressions look or appear, and it categorizes or identifies a person's face as angry because of how it looks or appears. The question is whether the visual system can also classify the person's face as threatening.

In what follows, I shall define a *distinctive look* as follows: the way something looks is a *distinctive look* of some property F if and only if most of the things in a spectator's environment that manifest that look really are F (Millar, 2000; Martin, 2010). So, for example, being round and yellow in a specific way is the distinctive look of *lemons*. Why? Because most of the things in our environment that look that way, most of the things that *look lemony*, really are lemons.

Of course, not all lemons look lemony; some of them have begun to rot and look rather different. An object can *be* F (it can be a lemon) without manifesting the distinctive look of F (without looking lemony). Moreover, not everything that looks lemony is a genuine lemon. My daughter has a plastic toy replica lemon that is a dead ringer for the real thing. But it isn't. So an object can manifest the distinctive look of F (it can look lemony) without in fact being F (it can be a plastic toy). Nevertheless, since most of the things in our environment that look lemony are lemons, a lemony look is the distinctive look of lemons.

This shows that whether or not a look or appearance is distinctive of some property depends on features of a spectator's environment. In my environment, the majority of the things that look lemony really are lemons. But if I took a lemon from my fruit bowl to a non-standard environment, such as one where there are a number of factories manufacturing plastic toy replicas, then the way my lemon looked would no longer be distinctive of *lemons*. That is because it would not be true in that environment that most of the things that manifest a lemony look are lemons; rather most would be plastic toys. That does not mean that my fruit's appearance has changed. It looks the same no matter where you take it. What changes is whether the way it looks is *distinctive* of some property F (being a lemon or being a certain type of plastic toy).

All visible things have looks or appearances. Yet subjects do not always have the appropriate visual capacities to be sensitive to every way that an object looks. For instance, my neighbour is an avid aviculturist and has the capacity to visually discriminate a female house finch from a female Cassin's finch. I don't. But even though the two of us have different visual recognitional capacities, the two birds manifest the same appearance to both of us. It is just that one of us has learned to be visually sensitive to the way a female house finch looks and the other one of us has not.

Thus, whether or not a spectator is able to visually recognize or identify objects to be lemons on the basis of how they look depends on two things. First, a spectator must have the appropriate type of visual capacities; they must have the ability to visually recognize lemony looks. Second, the way the object looks must be distinctive of lemons. In the imagined scenario with toy factories, I would not be able to visually recognize or identify a piece of fruit as a lemon on the basis of how it looks. This is not because I am not sufficiently visually sensitive to that look, but because, in that environment, the way it looks is distinctive of plastic toys, not lemons.

How does this relate to our discussion of facial expressions? Facial expressions are standardly identified or classified by the way they look. This makes it plausible that angry facial expressions have a distinctive look.[7] Given our definition, the way a face looks is distinctive of anger if and only if most of the faces in a spectator's environment that manifest that look really are angry. In such an environment, someone with the appropriate recognitional capacities will be able to visually recognize or identify faces as angry on the basis of how they look. It seems clear that human beings have this ability

---

[7] There is a further question of whether the ability to recognize angry facial expressions on the basis of how they look is sufficient to secure perceptual knowledge that a person is angry. This question is outside the topic of this chapter but is discussed at some length in Parrott (2017; cf. Gomes 2019; McNeill 2019).

from a very young age (Kestenbaum and Nelson, 1990; Kahana-Kalman and Walker-Andrews, 2001; Pollak et al., 2009).

Consider now a hostile environment in which a child is subjected to severe physical and emotional maltreatment. We have seen that in that type of environment angry faces immediately precede harmful outcomes and are therefore a reliable indicator of threat. It follows from this that, in a hostile environment, the way an angry face looks is also a distinctive look of threat. If most of the faces that manifest a particular type of facial expression (i.e. the ones that look angry) are in fact threatening, it follows that most of those faces *look* threatening. Generally, for any property G that is reliably correlated with F (if the way something looks is distinctive of F (if most of the things in the environment which manifest the look are F), then it will also be distinctive of G. So, in a hostile environment, angry facial expressions present a distinctive look of *both* anger and threat, and a subject with the appropriate recognitional capacities will be able to visually recognize or identify threats on the basis of how they look.

But what about a non-hostile environment? Is it the case that in this type of environment angry facial expressions present a distinctive look of threat? I would like to propose that they do not because, in this type of environment, it does not seem that angry faces are reliably correlated with the presence of threats. Most of the people that manifest anger towards me do not pose a threat to me and certainly do not harm me physically or emotionally. One group of people that I encounter with angry facial expressions are complete strangers—angry drivers, angry bystanders, angry commuters on the London Underground. Since these people are expressing anger, I'm able to visually recognize them as angry. But after our brief encounter, I never see them again. Partly for that reason, they are not threatening to me and, unlike in an abusive environment, their angry facial expression is not followed by harmful consequences. The other class of people that look angry are my family members and friends, people that tend to share my interests and wish to promote my well-being. These people are also not threatening. Rather than causing me serious harm, they tend to foster my health and happiness.[8] So, in an ordinary environment, it seems that most of the faces that look angry are not threatening.[9]

This last claim gains further support from the view that the emotion of anger evolved because of its social function. Many evolutionary psychologists believe that anger evolved in order to organize complex human behaviour into cooperative social relationships (Frijda and Mesquita, 1994; Keltner and Haidt, 1999; Haidt, 2003). As such, the primary function of anger is not to indicate the proximity of physical or social harm, but rather to signal to one's peers that there has been a perceived violation of a

---

[8] One might think that these people are threatening, it is just that the type of threat they present is different from the sort of physical or emotional threat once faces in an abusive environment. Thus, one might feel emotionally shaken by angry commuters or, especially if your loved ones are angry at you, their angry facial expressions might be thought to indicate a type of social threat, such as displeasure or the withdrawal of affection. This is an important line of objection to which we shall return in the following section.

[9] Angry faces may nevertheless be threatening in the sense of causing defensive autonomic responses. But if the argument in this section is right, then this causal relation is brute—it is not a response to the visual system having recognized or identified an environmental threat.

norm or expectation governing social cooperation. In this sense, expressions of anger function to facilitate cooperative behaviour. For instance, according to the model developed by Sell and colleagues, the function of anger is to 'recalibrate the target of the anger by showing the target that it will be worse off by continuing to behave in ways that place to little weight on the actor's interests' (Sell et al., 2009, p. 15074). Moreover, since the function of anger is to promote cooperation, it is normally diminished once the event which initially triggered the anger is appropriately redressed (Lerner et al., 1998; Keltner and Haidt, 1999). If this is right, then adults in non-hostile environments will normally have learned that expressions of anger pose no threat of physical or social harm to those who are appropriately engaging in cooperative behaviour. By contrast, children raised in a hostile or abusive environment experience unprovoked, random, or dysfunctional anger, which does not diminish in response to clear signals of cooperative behaviour. Thus, these children have not had an opportunity to learn how expressions of anger function to foster social bonds.

By contrast, in non-hostile environments, a spectator will likely encounter a fair number of faces that manifest the distinctive look of anger, but the majority of these will not be threatening. It follows from this that, in a non-hostile environment, angry facial expressions do not present a distinctive look of threat. So a spectator in this environment will not be able to visually recognize or identify *threats* on the basis of how someone's face looks, just as a spectator is not able to visually recognize lemons on the basis of a lemony look in the imagined toy-factory scenario. Of course, it is possible that threatening individuals manifest some kind of distinctive look, which is to say that there may be some way that people can look such that most of the people that look that way are actually threatening. But it is not the look of an angry face. For that reason, it is not clear whether this would be a look that an ordinary spectator has the ability to recognize, or whether it is more like the look of a female house finch, which can only be recognized after significant training.

This suggests an alternative way of developing the second hypothesis presented by McCrory and Viding. Recall that according to their proposed explanation the proximate factor contributing to the higher risk of developing a psychiatric disorder is that a more stressful environment shaped the fact that an individual treats non-threatening people as if they were threats. As we saw in the previous section, McCrory and Viding claim that this results from misidentifying the facial expressions of people who are not actually angry. However, we can now see that rather than misattributing anger to non-angry facial expressions, it is possible that individuals mistakenly attribute *threat* to people which their visual system correctly identifies as angry. If, as I have claimed, angry facial expressions do not present a distinctive look of threat, then it is possible for a spectator to correctly recognize an angry face on the basis of how it looks, but lack an adequate basis for visually identifying that face as threatening. Nevertheless, a spectator may take themselves to be recognizing a threat because they mistakenly think angry facial expressions present a distinctive look of threat.[10]

---

[10] Notice that this suggestion is compatible with McCrory and Viding's idea that the individuals are also misidentifying people as angry. Of course, if these people are also misidentifying people as angry then the problem will be amplified.

We actually should expect this sort of mistake whenever a spectator's environment is significantly changed. Suppose that I go to the environment dominated by lemon factories after having spent some time growing up on a lemon farm. I would naturally think that I am able to visually recognize *lemons* on the basis of how they look and I would take myself to be exploiting this capacity in the new environment. However, in that environment I am not in a position to visually discriminate lemons on the basis of how they look, only plastic toys. Nonetheless, since my behavioural responses are attuned to the lemon farm, I would naturally treat the plastic toys as if they were lemons, at least initially. Especially if I am not aware of the extent of environmental changes, I might not be in a position to know that I cannot visually identify genuine lemons on the basis of their lemony look. So, it would not be surprising if I responded to the plastic toys as if they were lemons because I take their look to be the distinctive look of lemons.

As we have seen, children who are abused in early life learn to visually discriminate facial expressions in a hostile environment wherein angry faces do present a distinctive look of immediate threat. This explains why they are predisposed to treat people with angry faces as threats. This predisposition would naturally continue after one is removed from a hostile environment. So, someone who has learned to associate angry faces with threating or harmful people will naturally respond to angry faces as threats, even after they have moved to a non-hostile environment. Moreover, they will not have had an opportunity to learn the appropriate responses to expressions of anger in a non-hostile environment in which the emotion functions to promote cooperative social relationships.

Let me note how the explanation proposed in this section differs from the one presented by McCrory and Viding. First, both explanations hold that people who have been severely maltreated as children develop heightened visual responsiveness to angry facial expressions. For this reason, they are especially adept at visually recognizing angry facial expressions. But whereas McCrory and Viding appeal to hypervigilance to account for this heightened responsiveness, the explanation proposed in this section does not. Instead, it claims that individuals are able to acquire a set of heightened recognitional capacities in a hostile environment where people who express anger are threatening, even though, in a non-hostile environment, they are not in a position to visually discriminate threats. This seems anodyne on McCrory and Viding's view because they assume that angry faces are correlated with some type of environmental threat.

This brings us to the second difference between the two proposals, namely that the proposal in this section rejects the notion that angry faces are reliable indicators of threat in all environments. Instead, it proposes that angry faces present a distinctive look of threat only in a hostile environment. In a non-hostile environment, it is more common for non-threatening people to look angry. This is partly why behaviourally responding to angry people as if they were threatening can be detrimental to an individual in a non-hostile environment. Thus, whereas McCrory and Viding's explanation focuses on problematic responses to peers who are not really angry, the explanation proposed in this section focuses on how certain kinds of responses to angry people might contribute to a higher risk of developing psychiatric disorders.

Despite these differences, the explanation I have sketched in this section is compatible with McCrory and Viding's suggestion that individuals who are exposed to childhood maltreatment misattribute anger to non-angry people. So it is not really a competing hypothesis. The explanation also accepts their claim that the most proximate factor contributing to an increased risk of developing a psychiatric disorder is the more stressful environment generated by treating one's peers as if they were threatening. As McCrory and Viding point out, responding to non-threating peers in this manner makes it much more difficult to create and sustain supportive and mutually beneficial relationships, which plausibly increases one's chances of developing psychiatric problems.

If your closest friends can be angry without being a threat to you, then so can your potential friends. Learning to dissociate expressions of anger from threat is one of the keys to forming lasting, mutually supportive social relationships. By taking angry facial expressions to be presenting a distinctive look of threat, subjects who have experienced childhood maltreatment risk missing out on these sorts of positive relationships.

Two types of emotion

The explanation I have just proposed relies on the notion that, in a non-hostile environment, expressions of anger are not reliably correlated with any kind of environmental threat. This might strike people as counterintuitive. The term 'expression' is factive—someone can *express* anger only if they are actually angry (cf. Green, 2007; Gomes, 2019). This means it is trivial that angry facial expressions are reliably correlated with actual anger. But we might naturally think that the emotion of anger is itself a kind of threat. Especially in cases where people are angry at *you*, another person's anger might directly cause strong feelings of displeasure, or other kinds of negative arousal. Along these lines, some theorists have claimed that part of what it is to *be angry* with someone is to be a potential source of physical, emotional, or psychological harm to that individual. For example, Martha Nussbaum claims that it is part of the very concept of anger that it consists of 'a wish for things to go badly somehow, for the offender' (2015, p. 46). Part of the reason Nussbaum thinks this is that she believes anger is a characteristic response to a perceived offence; it is a feeling that one has in response to being wronged by another. In that sense, even in cases where someone harms me accidentally, I feel angry in the sense of desiring some kind of retribution for the wrong done to me.[11] As we have already seen, in normal contexts, this anger will diminish so long as the offending party apologizes or redresses the wrongdoing. But even so, if part of what it is to be angry involves wishing for the object of one's anger to be harmed, then it might seem that all angry people are threatening, at least to the extent that they wish for some kind of negative outcome for the object of their anger. If this is right, then the emotion of anger may be reliably correlated with threat, even in non-hostile environments. It is just that the nature and degree of threat varies

---

[11] My anger might very well vanish once the offender apologizes. But, on Nussbaum's proposal, even in this case, my short-lived anger will constitutively involve a 'wish for things to go badly somehow'.

significantly from the sort that one faces in a heavily abusive environment. But if angry faces express anger and anger is reliably correlated with threat, then the explanation I have proposed in the previous section cannot work.

Before responding to this objection, it is important to note a distinction between the idea that angry facial expressions reliably indicate the presence of some type of environmental threat and the idea that angry facial expressions are harmful. Many of us might find that expressions of anger, even by strangers, cause unpleasant feelings. We want those who we love to have positive feelings towards us, and the manifestation of anger can easily hurt, or cause anxiety, or other forms of distress. We have also seen that angry facial expressions directly stimulate defensive responses in the autonomic nervous system, at least some of which might reasonably be considered to be harmful. Nothing that I have proposed in this chapter is inconsistent with the idea that angry facial expressions can themselves be emotionally, psychologically, or physiologically harmful. But this is not equivalent to them indicating the presence of some kind of environmental threat. Whether or not someone is a threat depends on what they are going to do, either in the immediate future or at some other future time. So, for example, seeing a family member express anger might immediately cause negative arousal, but it might also indicate to me that the person is going to withhold affection from me for some length of time. Similarly, seeing a potential friend express anger might cause a detrimental emotional response, but it might also be taken to indicate that the individual is someone who is likely to cause negative effects in the future. Harm is a matter of degree and it is the fact that individuals who have experienced significant childhood maltreatment expect their peers to cause them serious harm in the future that undermines positive social relationships. This is the sense in which they treat their peers as threats.

Let's return to the objection, which claims that angry faces are reliable indicators of some type of threat. There are two ways to avoid this objection. The first would deny that the emotion of anger reliably manifests itself in harmful behaviours. Like any emotion, being angry involves dispositions to act and react in certain ways. But, there appear to be a wide range of different behaviours associated with anger (Kuppens et al., 2004). So, although anger does give rise to aggressive or assertive behaviours, or to inhibition of them, there is evidence that anger also leads to prosocial behaviours (Rime et al., 1991; Kuppens et al., 2004). This should be expected if, as we saw previously, anger has a positive social function. So, it seems that anger does not invariably lead to harmful behaviours. Nevertheless, it may seem that the majority of cases of anger involve at least a *disposition* to treat the object of one's anger with some sort of aggression.

The second way to avoid the objection denies that expressions of anger are reliably connected to a disposition towards harmful or aggressive behaviour. To see how this could be true, it will be helpful to appeal to a distinction introduced by Richard Wollheim. According to Wollheim, our everyday vocabulary for speaking about the emotions is ambiguous. Sometimes we use words like 'anger' or 'happiness' to refer to psychological attitudes.[12] These are persisting, dispositional features of a person's psychology that manifest themselves in the person's behaviour. So, as we have seen,

---

[12] Wollheim classifies these as psychological dispositions.

part of what it is to have an emotional attitude is to have a corresponding disposition or dispositions to behave in certain ways. In Wollheim's terms, emotional attitudes provide a creature with 'an *orientation*' towards the world (1999, p. 15).

However, Wollheim also points out that we sometimes use the very same emotion-words to refer not to attitudes or dispositions, but to transitory mental *events* 'in which the emotions manifest themselves'[13] (1999, p. 9). That is, we sometimes use words like 'anger' or 'happiness' to refer not to a persisting attitude, but to refer to an episodic conscious event that momentarily occupies our thought (cf. Frijda and Mesquita, 1994).

We can avoid this ambiguity by describing conscious events as 'feelings'. For instance, when I am abruptly cut off by another driver on the motorway, I might naturally feel angry without also *being* angry in a more robust sense. That is, my conscious mental life might be occupied with a particular sort of conscious episode, which we might associate with anger. I might vent this feeling by yelling or cursing, but it would be natural for the conscious episode to be short-lived. Unless there is some underlying pathology, a conscious mental event is not something that tends to persist in my mental life.

Crucially, the fact that I have a conscious feeling of anger does not entail that I *am* angry, in the sense of having an underlying attitude which disposes me towards certain kinds of behaviour. Of course, someone who is angry in the attitude sense also tends to have corresponding conscious feelings of anger. That is part of what it is to have the emotional attitude of anger. But the converse is not true. One can simply experience a conscious feeling of anger without that meaning they are behaviourally oriented towards the world in any specific way.

If this is right, then conscious feelings need not be reliably connected with emotional attitudes. Even though attitudes like anger typically cause conscious feelings of anger, in ordinary environments those feelings are quite frequently caused by environmental conditions. It is because I was cut off by a driver on the motorway or because my favourite café is closed that I feel angry. Features of my environment directly cause the feeling; they cause a particular conscious event without having to also cause any persisting dispositional attitudes. If cases where conscious feelings such as anger are caused by environmental conditions, they do not reliably indicate the presence of any type of emotional attitude.

Let's assume that the attitude of anger is some kind of environmental threat. The account I proposed in the previous section is committed to the existence of an ontological gap between facial expressions of anger and the emotional attitude of anger. We can now see that there could be such a gap in cases where angry facial expressions are caused by conscious feelings, rather than by emotional attitudes. In such cases, a spectator would be in a position to visually discriminate people who *feel* angry on the basis of their facial expressions, but they would not thereby be able to visually discriminate

---

[13] Unlike many philosophers, Wollheim calls the transient events within a person's mind 'mental states'. But it is clear that he defines 'mental states' as events: 'mental states are those transient events which make up the lived part of the life of the mind, or to use William James's great phrase, 'the stream of consciousness' (James, 1890) (Wollheim, 1999, p. 1).

people with a persisting emotional attitude of anger. Yet it is only the latter that is plausibly a threat.

Facial expressions are transitory. One briefly vents a feeling of anger by grimacing or quickly expresses one's feeling of happiness by jumping for joy. Neither the grimace nor the jumping lasts for long. It seems to me that many facial expressions are directly caused by momentary conscious feelings. As such, the expressions are not a reliable indicator of any persisting attitudes or behavioural dispositions. For this reason, they have little evidential value in predicting how a person will be disposed to behave towards me, or whether the person's futures actions will be helpful or harmful. Thus, even though certain kinds of facial expressions such as anger may themselves be harmful in some sense, for instance, by causing momentary physiological distress, they indicate only what a person feels for a moment.

Of course, none of this is true in hostile environments. In that type of environment, conscious feelings are typically caused by underlying attitudes. The reason that an abusive parent tends to frequently experience conscious feelings of anger is that deep down he or she *is* extremely angry. The abusive parent has an underlying emotional attitude that orients them towards the world in a specific way and that attitude, rather than their surrounding environment, is directly responsible for their conscious feelings of anger. So, in a hostile environment, angry facial expressions are reliably connected to the emotional attitude of anger and since, especially in this type of environment, this attitude leads to extremely aggressive behaviour, it can reasonably be seen as a threat.

To make things worse, in an abusive environment, the emotional attitude of anger is itself dysfunctional. It occurs randomly or spontaneously and is therefore disconnected from the social function anger plays in non-abusive environments. Because the abusive parent's anger is clearly not a response to any offence or wrongdoing on the part of the child, and because it does not diminish in light of clear signals of cooperation, the maltreated child is unable to learn how to appropriately respond to anger, but responds instead with avoidance or aggression. There is simply no opportunity for the maltreated child to learn how anger serves to establish and regulate positive social relationships in non-abusive environments.

Conclusion

Correctly interpreting facial expressions is a complex problem. One needs not only to acquire the ability to visually discriminate the different ways a face can look, but one also needs to learn what these different expressive looks mean. For this reason, the environment in which one learns to visually recognize faces is crucial for determining precisely how one responds to different types of facial expressions.

As many psychologists have suggested, it is plausible that, in an abusive environment, angry facial expressions are indications of very serious threat. That is why it is beneficial for an individual's neurocognitive systems to develop to become highly sensitive to angry faces. When you are in a hostile environment, it is absolutely vital that you can recognize angry faces as quickly as possible.

Nevertheless, individuals whose neurocognitive systems manifest heightened responsiveness to angry faces seem to be at a much greater risk than average of developing psychiatric disorders later in life, once they are removed from an abusive environment. The main proposal of this chapter is that this risk can be explained as the direct result of the individual's behaviour shaping their environment to be more distressing and antisocial. Specifically, it is plausible that a person who has experienced childhood abuse will tend to treat non-threatening peers as if they were threats, which, significantly compromises the person's ability to develop supportive social relationships. This is the basic explanatory approach suggested by McCrory and Viding (2015).

However, I have also suggested that the way an individual who has experienced abuse responds to angry people may be inappropriate. This suggestion rests on the idea that in ordinary environments angry faces are not reliable indicators of threat, and so they are not a basis upon which a spectator can visually discriminate environmental threats. Indeed, in the previous section it was suggested that, in an ordinary environment, angry facial expressions are often not even caused by an underlying attitude of anger. Rather, in those environments, many of the people one encounters express anger because they have a momentary conscious feeling of anger.

In an ordinary environment, emotional expressions are often fleeting outbursts that serve to vent conscious feelings. They do not indicate any long-term disposition, or intention, or plans on the part of the person who looks angry, or sad, or happy. So, we do not need to fear, or take precautions against people that express anger. The majority of these people either have our best interests in mind, or are completely innocuous. This is why in order to maintain positive relationships with friends and family members, and to craft new positive social relationships, one must learn to respond appropriately to angry facial expressions. One can form a lasting friendship with someone who expresses their feeling of anger, but only if one does not respond to the person as if they are some kind of threat. In a sense, making new friends, and keeping old ones, means learning to overlook angry faces.

Acknowledgements

I would like to express my gratitude to Eamon McCrory and Essi Viding for offering many insightful comments on an earlier version of this chapter. I'm sure there are parts of this chapter with which they will disagree but I believe that my proposed explanation is in accordance with the spirit of their second hypothesis. Thanks also to Anil Gomes and Josh Shepherd for several helpful conversations on the topic of this chapter and to the participants of the London Mind Group.

References

Caspi, A., McClay, J., Moffitt, T.E., Mill, J., Martin, J., Craig, I.W., Taylor, A., and Poulton, R. (2002). Role of genotype in the cycle of violence in maltreated children. *Science*, **297**(5582), 851–854.

Fox, E., Lester, V., Russo, R., Bowles, R.J., Pichler, A., and Dutton, K. (2000). Facial expressions of emotion: are angry faces detected more efficiently? *Cognition & Emotion*, **14**(1), 61–92.

Frijda, N.H. and Mesquita, B. (1994). The social roles and functions of emotions. In S. Kitayama and H.R. Markus (Eds.), *Emotion and Culture: Empirical Studies of Mutual Influence* (pp. 51–87). Washington, DC: American Psychological Association.

Gilbert, R., Widom, C.S., Browne, K., Fergusson, D., Webb, E., and Janson, S. (2009). Burden and consequences of child maltreatment in high-income countries. *The Lancet*, **373**(9657), 68–81.

Goldstone, R.L. (1998). Perceptual learning. *Annual Review of Psychology*, **49**(1), 585–612.

Gomes, A. (2019). Perception, evidence, and our expressive knowledge of others' minds. In A. Avramides and M. Parrott (eds.), *Knowing Other Minds* (pp. 148–172). Oxford: Oxford University Press.

Green, M. (2007). *Self-Expression*. Oxford: Oxford University Press.

Haidt, J. (2003). The moral emotions. *Handbook of Affective Sciences*, **11**, 852–870.

Hagemann, N., Schorer, J., Cañal-Bruland, R., Lotz, S., and Strauss, B. (2010). Visual perception in fencing: do the eye movements of fencers represent their information pickup? *Attention, Perception, & Psychophysics*, **72**(8), 2204–2214.

James, W. (1890). *The Principles of Psychology*. New York: Henry Holt.

Kahana-Kalman, R. and Walker-Andrews, A.S. (2001). The role of person familiarity in young infants' perception of emotional expressions. *Child Development*, **72**(2), 352–369.

Keltner, D. and Haidt, J. (1999). Social functions of emotions at four levels of analysis. *Cognition & Emotion*, **13**(5), 505–521.

Kestenbaum, R. and Nelson, C.A. (1990). The recognition and categorization of upright and inverted emotional expressions by 7-month-old infants. *Infant Behavior and Development*, **13**(4), 497–511.

Kuppens, P., Van Mechelen, I., and Meulders, M. (2004). Every cloud has a silver lining: Interpersonal and individual differences determinants of anger-related behaviors. *Personality and Social Psychology Bulletin*, **30**(12), 1550–1564.

LeDoux, J.E. (2000). Emotion circuits in the brain. *Annual Review of Neuroscience*, **23**(1), 155–184.

Lerner, J.S., Goldberg, J.H., and Tetlock, P.E. (1998). Sober second thought: the effects of accountability, anger, and authoritarianism on attributions of responsibility. *Personality and Social Psychology Bulletin*, **24**(6), 563–574.

Lyons, D.M., Parker, K.J., Katz, M., and Schatzberg, A.F. (2009). Developmental cascades linking stress inoculation, arousal regulation, and resilience. *Frontiers in Behavioral Neuroscience*, **3**, 32.

Martin, M.G.F. (2010). What's in a look? In B. Nanay (Ed.), *Perceiving the World* (pp. 160–225). Oxford: Oxford University Press.

McCrory, E.J., De Brito, S.A., Kelly, P.A., Bird, G., Sebastian, C.L., Mechelli, A., Samuel, S., and Viding, E. (2013). Amygdala activation in maltreated children during pre-attentive emotional processing. *The British Journal of Psychiatry* **202**(4), 269–276.

McCrory, E.J., De Brito, S.A., Sebastian, C.L., Mechelli, A., Bird, G., Kelly, P.A., and Viding, E. (2011a). Heightened neural reactivity to threat in child victims of family violence. *Current Biology*, **21** (23), R947–R948.

McCrory, E.J. De Brito, S.A., and Viding E. (2011b). The impact of childhood maltreatment: a review of neurobiological and genetic factors. *Frontiers in Psychiatry*, **2**, 48.

McCrory, E., De Brito, S.A., and Viding, E. (2012). The link between child abuse and psychopathology: a review of neurobiological and genetic research. *Journal of the Royal Society of Medicine*, **105**(4), 151–156.

McCrory, E.J. and Viding, E. (2015). The theory of latent vulnerability: reconceptualizing the link between childhood maltreatment and psychiatric disorder. *Development and Psychopathology*, **27**(2), 493–505.

McCrory, E.J., Gerin, M.I., and Viding, E. (2017). Childhood maltreatment, latent vulnerability and the shift to preventative psychiatry—the contribution of functional brain imaging. *Journal of Child Psychology and Psychiatry*, **58**(4), 338–357.

McNeill, W.E.S. (2019). Expressions, looks, and others' minds. In A. Avramides and M. Parrott (Eds.), *Knowing Other Minds* (pp. 173–199). Oxford: Oxford University Press.

Millar, A. (2000). The scope of perceptual knowledge. *Philosophy*, **75**, 73–88.

Nussbaum, M.C. (2015). Transitional anger. *Journal of the American Philosophical Association*, **1**(1), 41–56.

Öhman, A. (2002). Automaticity and the amygdala: nonconscious responses to emotional faces. *Current Directions in Psychological Science*, **11**(2), 62–66.

Öhman, A. (2009). Of snakes and faces: an evolutionary perspective on the psychology of fear. *Scandinavian Journal of Psychology*, **50**(6), 543–552.

Öhman, A., Lundqvist, D., and Esteves, F. (2001). The face in the crowd revisited: a threat advantage with schematic stimuli. *Journal of Personality and Social Psychology*, **80**(3), 381.

Parrott, M. (2017). The look of another mind. *Mind*, **126**(504), 1023–1061.

Pearl, J. (2009). *Causality*. Cambridge: Cambridge University Press.

Pollak, S.D., Cicchetti, D., Klorman, R., and Brumaghim, J.T. (1997). Cognitive brain event-related potentials and emotion processing in maltreated children. *Child Development*, **68**(5), 773–787.

Pollak, S.D. and Kistler, D.J. (2002). Early experience is associated with the development of categorical representations for facial expressions of emotion. *Proceedings of the National Academy of Sciences*, **99**(13), 9072–9076.

Pollak, S.D., Messner, M., Kistler, D.J., and Cohn, J.F. (2009). Development of perceptual expertise in emotion recognition. *Cognition*, **110**(2), 242–247.

Pollak, S.D. and Sinha, P. (2002). Effects of early experience on children's recognition of facial displays of emotion. *Developmental Psychology*, **38**(5), 784–791.

Rime, B., Mesquita, B., Boca, S., and Philippot, P. (1991). Beyond the emotional event: six studies on the social sharing of emotion. *Cognition & Emotion*, **5**(5–6), 435–465.

Sell, A., Tooby, J., and Cosmides, L. (2009). Formidability and the logic of human anger. *Proceedings of the National Academy of Sciences*, **106**(35), 15073–15078.

Whalen, P.J., Shin, L.M., McInerney, S.C., Fischer, H., Wright, C.I., and Rauch, S.L. (2001). A functional MRI study of human amygdala responses to facial expressions of fear versus anger. *Emotion*, **1**(1), 70–83.

Wollheim, R. (1999). *On the Emotions*. New Haven, CT: Yale University Press.

Woodward, J. (2008). Mental causation and neural mechanisms. In J. Hohwy and J. Kallestrup (Eds.), *Being Reduced: New Essays on Reduction, Explanation, and Causation* (pp. 218–262). Oxford: Oxford University Press.

Woodward, J. (2005). *Making Things Happen: A Theory of Causal Explanation*. Oxford: Oxford University Press.

Part 4

Neurobiology and the Biopsychosocial Model

Chapter 17

Mental illness: The collision of meaning with mechanism

Steven E. Hyman and Doug McConnell

Note

The purpose of this chapter is to present the views SEH put forward in his Loebel Lectures. Therefore, in co-authoring this chapter, DM has set aside a couple of his disagreements with SEH. These disagreements are discussed in DM's commentary on this chapter (Chapter 18, this volume).

Introduction

The human brain gives rise to cognition, emotion, and behaviour, to social interactions and self-consciousness, and, importantly for the arguments to follow, it does so by mechanisms that are absolutely opaque to introspection. Mental disorders result from malfunctioning of this highly complex and subtle machine, and effective treatment should be conceptualized as repairing or mitigating those malfunctions.[1] Importantly, neurobiology like all mainstream science is explicitly non-Cartesian; thus, both the causes of mental illness and contributors to their repair may come from any source that affects the structure and function of the brain, including those taken on board by (partly) conscious mechanisms, including lived experience, social interactions, and ideas (including those learned in psychotherapy), as well as by genes, metabolic and other bodily factors, drugs, implanted electrodes, and so on. From what we might call the neurobiological perspective, clinicians examine the patient with an objectifying gaze that looks for diagnostic clues, evidence of improvement or worsening, and for beneficial or deleterious effects of treatment. The neurobiological view is, however, incomplete; notwithstanding its focus on descriptions of the patient's symptoms and functioning, it has no place for sufferers as human beings with subjective experience, their interpretations of their experiences in terms of meaning, and their

---

[1] At the risk of complicating the argument, some diagnosed mental disorders such as personality disorders might be better conceptualized in terms of maladaptive brain functioning rather than malfunctioning—and there is no bright line between the two. We know precious little about the neurobiology of these conditions, but there is little to suggest that the brains of people with personality disorders would have identifiable abnormalities of the sort founds in, for example, schizophrenia (discussed later).

narrative describing how, and perhaps why, they find themselves in their current predicaments. Patients' narratives of their experience living with mental disorder and its damaging effects on their lives and goals are invitations to the clinician to switch from the objectifying view, needed to diagnose and select treatment, to an interpersonal perspective that engages the patient as a subject. From this interpersonal perspective, it is the sufferer's subjective distress and sense of disruption in their life narrative that we care about, even while we recognize that their narratives and explanations are not objectively true. While damaging and counterproductive narratives, such as those that might be driven by depressed or psychotic states, must be appropriately confronted, a successful clinical encounter typically demands that patients experience the clinician as able to empathize with them, treat them respectfully whatever their symptoms or status in society, and grasp their perspective on the meaning of their symptoms.

There is a shaky truce within psychiatry and clinical psychology between those who predominantly favour what we might cell an objectifying or neurobiological perspective and those who favour an interpersonal perspective. In the extreme, the former believes the latter to be engaged in the non-scientific practice of folk psychology which accepts at face value people's intuitive sense of self and false explanations of illness.[2] Folk psychology, on this view, has led many psychotherapists and other clinicians astray by their putting too much stock in the meanings of patients' first-hand reports and causal theories, often leading them on wild goose chases, and at worst to false and damaging theories and interpretations illustrated by psychoanalytical explanations of autism or schizophrenia. From a purely neurobiological perspective, subjective reports are useful when their form and content provide clues to diagnosis, responses to treatment, treater, and setting, but have no further utility. Those who favour an interpersonal approach counter that, in fact, it is the neurobiologists who are blind to the central problem of a mental disorder—pathological mental content and intersubjective relations. On this view, although pathological mental content is instantiated in the brain, the brain-level description of events confuses what is best understood and treated discursively in terms of intentionality and meaning. By casting the patient as an object, a diagnostic and therapeutic problem to be solved, the neurobiological perspective has been seen by some as entirely missing the active ingredient of successful treatment, discourse that leads the patient to accept a new and healthier life narrative. Other critics argue that at a minimum, the neurobiological perspective risks subverting the treatment alliance thus discouraging adherence to treatment or even exacerbating symptoms by alienating and dehumanizing the suffering person. An insistence on biological causation alone might also instil some patients with a sense of fatalism that might undercut the motivation to participate in treatment.

This chapter, based on the Loebel Lectures given by one of us (SEH), reflects on the effects that neurobiological advances will have on psychiatry, not only in terms of hoped for advancements in diagnosis and treatment, but also in terms of the cognitive

---

[2] We follow the current practice of using the term 'folk psychology' to describe the unscientific, intuitive picture of how people perceive, think, feel, make decisions, and act. For reasons discussed later, we share Jonathan Glover's reluctance, expressed in his commentary, to use the term because it seems to have a denigrating connotation that is undeserved.

frameworks by which we understand the clinical encounter. In his view, the challenge for psychiatry is to embrace the advancing views provided by neurobiology (with due scepticism for the sometimes overhyped claims of a young science) while resisting the temptation to trivialize the role of human interpersonal engagement and an interpersonal perspective in the clinical encounter. The challenge in Hyman's view is that these perspectives are epistemologically incommensurate, yet both are essential to good and effective clinical care and thus that psychiatrists must use both according to the demands of the clinical situation. Indeed, the caricatured clinicians who are narrowly and blindly rooted in neurobiology or in interpersonal views of the patient's needs are growing fewer as the younger generation of psychiatrists and clinical psychologists are increasingly trained to be pragmatic and eclectic in their practice. What we will argue may, therefore, initially seem counterintuitive. The neurobiological view as we will develop it and the folk psychological or interpersonal view are deeply incompatible. The folk psychological view takes as true the potent, indeed ineluctable, human intuition of a self with effective agency and ascribes truth value to illness narratives based on a person's values, motivations, decisions, and actions. Neurobiology sees such narratives as 'just so' stories and understands pathogenic mechanisms to be unavailable to introspection.[3]

We contrast a mechanistic view of mental illness grounded in neurobiology with what we call an interpersonal perspective (not to be confused with interpersonal psychotherapy for depression) that is grounded in folk psychology. We point out ways in which folk psychological concepts and empathy for those aspects of the patient experience that are meaning-laden remain critical for effective clinical care even if we adopt a mechanistic view of the illness. We explain why the most effective treatment will usually require the clinician to address both perspectives, taking care to avoid the Cartesian dualism that surfaces all too often in psychiatry, where psychopathology is erroneously parsed into biologically caused conditions, best treated with medications or neuromodulation and conditions caused by lived experience, best treated with psychotherapies. In fact, the patient's lived experience and interpersonal interactions can be understood as mechanistic contributors to pathogenesis and healing from the neurobiological perspective that views the patient as object. At the same time, the patient's lived experience, values, beliefs, and feelings must also be addressed from the stance of engaging the patient as a subject. This requires attention to the meanings and interpretations that the patient attributes to his illness. We conclude the chapter with a review of the emerging mechanistic picture of schizophrenia pathogenesis, which raises questions of how advances in neurobiology may change the clinical encounter. These advances will often tip the treatment balance further towards neurobiological approaches but will never eliminate the need for interpersonal engagement.

---

[3] In this sense, modern neurobiology has something in common with psychoanalytic theory, which also saw pathogenic mechanisms as unconscious—however, any similarities end there. The putative mechanisms of psychopathology espoused by various psychoanalytic theories lack any serious empirical support and are often incoherent.

A very brief introduction to brain structure and function

Human brains are biological machines of staggering complexity. They are composed of about 90 billion neurons and an approximately equal number of glial cells. The precise number of distinct neuronal cell types, based on their molecular composition, morphology, location in the brain, and connectivity, is not yet known, but there may be several thousand. Neurons make connections with each other at specialized structures called synapses, across which they communicate with one or more chemical neurotransmitters that carry signals by binding to diverse receptors. Specific neuronal cells types differ in their characteristic number of synapses, and the neurotransmitters they release. The mature human brain likely has more than 100 trillion synapses in total. The processes that extend from the cell bodies of neurons (axons from which neurotransmitters are generally released and dendrites, which typically receive neurotransmitter signals) and their synaptic connections give rise to circuits that range from small, local circuits that refine information processing to long-range circuits that bind together distant brain regions. Patterns of activity in neural circuits are the computational basis of information processing in the brain and its outputs including signals that regulate bodily physiology and behaviour.

Central to the survival of free-living organisms is the ability to learn and to adapt their behaviour to changing circumstances and environments. Such capacities are rooted in a critical property of brains, synaptic plasticity, the experience-dependent strengthening or weakening of synaptic connections. When, for example, experience produces a memory, the memory is encoded and consolidated by alterations in patterns of synaptic connectivity and thus the functioning of neural circuits. By altering patterns of connectivity within circuits, experience alters the subsequent computations that underlie relevant cognition and behaviour. Memories are encoded in a distributed manner across different brain regions (e.g. visual components of a remembered event in occipital cortex, tactile components in parietal cortex, and associated emotions in the amygdala or other emotion-processing structures). These aspects must be bound together, typically across multiple synapses, both anatomically and physiologically. For memories accessible to consciousness the hippocampus plays an obligatory role in such binding. The binding of diverse brain regions permits a specific complex memory to be evoked by a cue or a chain of associations and experienced as an integral whole. Some such connectional patterns can remain latent for many years permitting some childhood memories to be activated in adult years by a relevant reminder. An implication of memory involving the binding of multiple local circuits is that it is constructed and can be updated by new information. In this sense, memory is nothing like a video recorder that produces archival records, but an adaptive mechanism tuned to successful negotiation of changing circumstance including social networks.

The acquisition of new memories or updating of old memories in the context of new information relies on experience-dependent synaptic plasticity. As first codified by Donald Hebb, strong, correlated activity in synapses produced by experience increases the strength of synaptic connections, while others might be weakened. This is accomplished by molecular alterations in existing synapses and also by the production of new synapses and the pruning away of weak or inefficient synapses. Neural circuits thus remodelled alter the information content stored in the brain, and its responses to future stimuli because the activity occurring in these new patterns of connectivity perforce yield new computations. Plasticity and thus altered patterns of synaptic connectivity can be produced not only by experience but also by stages of development, ageing, skill acquisition, social environments, immune mediators, drugs, illnesses, and other influences. The diversity of human interests, abilities, temperaments, and personalities reflect the rich diversity of genetic, developmental, and environmental influences—including lived experience—that shape synaptic connections and circuits and thus information processing in different human brains. Mental and neurological disorders occur when such processes are significantly disrupted by aetiologically highly diverse pathological processes.

Neurobiological explanations for psychopathology and treatment

The aspiration of neurobiologists for psychiatry and clinical psychology is to understand the molecular, cellular, and synaptic mechanisms of mental disorders. Most importantly, as has been illustrated in other fields of medicine, an understanding of disease mechanism permits rational hypotheses about the design of effective treatments., which for mental illness might include cognitive behavioural therapies, drugs, neuromodulation, and before long, at least for monogenic neurodevelopmental disorders, gene therapies. The better we understand the brain malfunctions that cause a constellation of symptoms and impairments, the better we can target an intervention to mitigate or repair those malfunctions or potentially prevent them in the first place. In addition, knowledge of disease mechanisms would likely facilitate the discovery of biomarkers, which might be useful not only in diagnosis and staging of illness, but also to follow the effects of treatment.

In mature fields of medicine, diagnoses are grounded in the aetiology or pathophysiology (abnormal anatomy and physiology) that produces the relevant symptoms. This contrasts with the *Diagnostic and Statistical Manual of Mental Disorders (DSM)* that, in the absence of other information, categorizes mental disorders according to the symptoms patients report and the behaviour they exhibit. The *DSM* approach is problematic because different underlying causes can have similar presentations and similar causes can have different presentations, therefore *DSM* diagnoses of mental disorder cannot accurately indicate disorder aetiology. If diagnosis with a disorder of a certain kind doesn't provide an accurate guide to the cause of a disorder, then neither can it provide an accurate guide to the effective treatment that alters the progression of the disorder as opposed to palliating symptoms. To the extent that a *DSM* diagnosis groups together patients with different conditions with different underlying causes, there no reason to think that what effectively treats one patient will effectively treat another. Thus, much treatment today depends on trial and error. If, on the other hand, disorders are classified according to their aetiologies and pathological processes, then diagnosis links the patient's problem with causation. Treatments can then be provided (or more relevant to mental illness, developed) that directly operate on the causes of the disorder. Medicine increasingly relies on objective tests and algorithms to make diagnoses and select treatments. Cancer medicine, for example, often matches patients with appropriate drugs based on molecular markers within their tumours. The hope is that objective measures will be developed to match patients who suffer mental illnesses with treatments that will prove effective for them.

Successful advance of the neurobiological vision for psychiatry will yield interventions that prevent or repair the disordered brain mechanisms that cause mental disorders (whether their aetiology lays in biology, lived experience, or both). Such disease-altering treatments contrast with our current treatments that palliate symptoms but do not repair underlying disease processes. Importantly, the neurobiological vision laid out here eschews Cartesian dualism entirely. Thus, brain repair can proceed from what we might describe as 'top-down' approaches such as psychotherapies, 'bottom-up' approaches such as drugs, or both. Top-down approaches such as psychotherapies engage with the patient's conscious cognitive processes, emotions, beliefs, and behaviour. Psychotherapies, like all forms of learning, rely on synaptic plasticity to alter patterns of synaptic connectivity and thus information processing in the brain and its outputs such as behaviour. When effective, top-down approaches 'rewire' the brain through words, cognitive processing, and instructed actions in a manner that diminishes symptoms, impairments, and suffering. For example, cognitive behavioural therapy can effectively treat anxiety and panic disorder by helping patients develop skills of relaxation, mental habits for interpreting situations in less frightening ways, and better problem-solving skills (Foa et al., 2002). As these mental skills and habits are internalized and become automatic, there is preliminary evidence from brain imaging that fear circuitry is less likely to be activated inappropriately (e.g. in response to innocuous stimuli), excessively, or to remain active after the appearance of safety signals (de Carvalho et al., 2007). Top-down treatments cannot always effectively treat a mental disorder because experience-dependent neural plasticity appears to have limits. Some brain malfunctions would require too much time and effort to shape or are simply beyond such shaping through psychotherapies. In those cases, brain repair can only proceed from the bottom-up (either alone or in combination with psychotherapies), by altering pathological aspects of brain structure and function that cannot effectively be influenced through the patient's conscious engagement alone. Such treatments might involve pharmacology or neuromodulation, which includes deep brain stimulation, repetitive transcranial magnetic stimulation, or electroconvulsive therapy.[4] Such interventions are presently relatively crude, but they don't

---

[4] Some may dispute whether top-down approaches should be thought of as 'brain repair'. It could be argued that if a mental disorder can be most efficiently treated through discourse such as cognitive behavioural therapy, then the brain-level description of what has happened may not be usefully explanatory because it focuses on the 'wrong' level of analysis (in analogy with trying to describe why a peg fits in a certain hole in terms of the constituent atoms.) A response to this challenge from a neurobiological point of view is that an explanation 'one level down' (e.g. from psychology to circuits) usefully constrains our understanding of what is happening. Treatment efficacy does not actually depend on the patient comprehending a new explanatory framework, but rather on altered input–output relationships in the brain established by the therapy. It could be hypothesized based on neuroimaging evidence that efficacy of cognitive behavioural therapy for some anxiety disorders depends on altered interactions

need to completely repair the brain on their own, if they create conditions in which the brain itself can begin processes of repair. For example, increases in synaptic norepinephrine or serotonin produced by certain antidepressant drugs are hypothesized to modify the chemical milieu of the brain, perhaps enhancing neuroplasticity in circuits that affect mood regulation. For example, the drugs might facilitate a reduction in attentional biases toward negative stimuli thus shifting cognition toward mood elevation. It has been further hypothesized that as the patient's mood improves sufficiently to re-engage in her normal activities, a virtuous cycle develops between synaptic reorganization and lifting of depressive symptoms that in turn permits further healthy thinking and healthy activities. Unfortunately, all current treatments for mental disorders, whether top-down or bottom-up, have limitations in efficacy, and for some serious symptoms clusters, such as the disabling cognitive impairments of schizophrenia, there are no significantly effective treatments at all.

Pathogenic mechanisms of mental disorders have remained stubbornly hidden

Lacking insight into disease mechanisms, progress in treatment development for mental disorders has been slow. Most current drug treatments originated with serendipitous observations made on prototype compounds in the 1950s; cognitive behavioural therapy, which originated in the 1960s, is, in contrast to the drugs, based on theoretical insights into the relationship of cognition to depression and anxiety. The hunt for mechanisms of disease has been stymied historically not only by the complexity of the human brain, but also because it is essentially inviolable in life for both ethical and medical reasons. Thus, unlike cancer research where a surgeon who performs an excisional biopsy can hand the diseased tissue to a scientist, brain researchers are, for the most part, limited to postmortem examinations or indirect approaches to the brain, such as non-invasive neuroimaging or electroencephalography, which fall well short of the temporal or spatial resolution needed to observe individual cells and synapses at work. To make matters worse, mental disorders are very poorly modelled in laboratory animals because they are separated from humans by significant evolutionary distance and by very different selective environments in which they evolved. The ubiquitous laboratory rodent models are largely nocturnal, depend on olfaction and whiskers to engage the world, and are only modestly social. Humans are diurnal and visual, with complex and pervasive social interactions that played a significant role in the evolution of our brains.

Implicit in the foregoing discussion is commitment to a scientific project to gain a wholly mechanistic view of how the brain undergirds normal and pathological thought, emotion, and behaviour. This scientific project depends tactically on many

---

among prefrontal cortical circuits, hippocampal circuits, and amygdala-based fear circuits even if this result was achieved through a therapy taken on board via conscious interactions with a therapist. In that sense, both top-down and bottom-up treatments depend on effectively altering patterns of synaptic connectivity and neural circuit function, can be monitored (at least in theory) by brain imaging, and can appropriately be construed as brain repair.

reductionist experiments, which are necessary to render aspects of brain complexity experimentally tractable and to isolate molecules, synapses, or circuits in order to consider them as therapeutic targets. However, the ultimate goals are not reductionist. A realistic and therapeutically beneficial model of brain function and dysfunction will not be achieved by maximizing reductionist explanations as at each level of analysis, whether genetic, molecular, cellular, circuit, or cognitive and behavioural, complex systems are at play. An important challenge is to be able to understand causality as it acts both from the bottom (genes and molecules) up and from the top (cognition and behaviour) down. Successful treatments might consist of one or a combination of alterations in environmental context (e.g. to reduce cues associated with relapses of drug use), psychotherapies, modulation of large-scale neural circuits, interactions of drugs with molecular targets, or targeted editing of genes by CRISPR-Cas systems. In contrast with this mechanistic view and its scientific goals, those who hold that mental content and meaning are the key to understanding mental illness and its treatment would have little use for brain human tissue or animal models as discussed previously; they would also consider the focus on psychiatric genetics in the section that follows quite wide of the mark.

Our genomes hold clues to understanding pathogenesis and treatment

Given the complexity and inaccessibility of the living human brain, the most direct and useful clues to molecular mechanisms of mental disorders lie in our genomes. It has long been recognized that mental disorders run in families. Based on family, twin, and adoption studies, family resemblance for risk of mental disorders has been shown to be highly, albeit not exclusively, influenced by genes. In short, genes play an important role, but do not, by themselves, determine a person's fate with respect to mental illness. That said, schizophrenia, bipolar disorder, autism spectrum disorders (ASDs), and attention deficit hyperactivity disorder are among the most genetically influenced of common human ills across all of medicine, far more than most cancers for which environmental exposures often play critical roles. (Indeed, in an early genome-wide association study (GWAS) of lung cancer, the strongest association was not with genes directly involved in carcinogenesis, but rather with genes encoding nicotinic acetylcholine receptors that influence a far more heritable trait, smoking behaviour.) Genes play lesser but still significant roles in many other mental disorders, such as unipolar depression and anxiety disorders, where lived experience, including early childhood experience, potently influences risk.

The significant role for genes in risk of mental illness does not mean that these conditions result from one or even a few genes of large effect. Rather, the significant influence of genes on mental disorders—as well as normal human and cognitive traits—is highly polygenic, that is, it results from the sum of the effects of many, usually small, variations in the linear sequence of 'letters' (the four types of nucleotide bases) that encode information within the three billion base pairs in our genomes. The most common DNA variants are differences in single bases from person to person, which occur in tens of millions of places throughout human genomes. Most family resemblance in traits results from the fact that family members share DNA sequences; first-degree relative share on average 50%, second-degree relatives 25%, and so on. Conversely, much human diversity in physical, cognitive, and behavioural characteristics and much disease risk results from differences in DNA sequences.

While damaging mutations occur, the vast majority of sequence differences are best understood as variation—there is no reference human genome or human being. Of the tens of millions of (mostly) small sequence differences that characterize human genomes, several thousand influence the risk of schizophrenia, bipolar disorder, and other mental disorders through small nudges that affect the biological processes underlying brain development, brain structure, brain function, and responses to environmental stimuli ranging from diet to infections to social stressors. Other small genetic nudges influence the shapes of our noses, adult height (assuming adequate nutrition), risk of obesity, cognitive abilities, and almost all other bodily and psychological traits. The genetic loading that produces risk for a mental disorder such as schizophrenia, results from a grab-bag of disorder-associated DNA variants, a small fraction of the total of disorder-associated variants found across the entire human population, representing a different fraction from other people with this illness. Such risk-associated genetic variants act together with pathogenic events during brain development and early life, specific environmental risk factors, and context to give rise to a mental illness. The genetic complexity of mental disorders contributes to their heterogeneity, for example, in timing of onset, symptom pattern, severity, and treatment responsiveness.

The development of powerful new genomic and computational tools during the first years of the twenty-first century spurred by the Human Genome Project made it possible to identify the specific DNA sequences involved in pathogenesis of mental disorders. While this is still a work in progress, hundreds of specific DNA sequence variants that increase the risk of psychiatric disorders have been identified with a high degree of statistical confidence for schizophrenia, bipolar disorder, ASDs, major depressive disorder, and others (Schizophrenia Working Group of the Psychiatric Genomics Consortium, 2014; Sanders et al., 2015; Singh et al., 2017; Wray et al., 2018). Epidemiologists are already successfully using this information in the form of polygenic risk scores to stratify individuals by genetic loading—although much remains to be done, especially extending this research beyond European populations (Martin et al., 2019). The challenge for neurobiology is to use the subtle molecular clues emerging from genetics to elucidate the mechanisms that underlie mental illness, which in turn can undergird the discovery of biomarkers and new treatments. Early success in this endeavour can be illustrated by schizophrenia research (Sekar et al., 2016), as discussed later in this chapter.

Another important new technology permits high throughput identification of the genes expressed in individual cells including neurons (Macosko et al., 2015). Cell types in the body differ from each other based on which genes are active in that cell. There is currently a global consortium working to identify the genes expressed in every cell type in the human body including those of the brain (Regev et al., 2017). It has become possible to use results from genetic studies of disease risk to interrogate particular cell types by asking whether that cell type disproportionately expresses disease-associated genes. For mental disorders, such approaches are beginning to make it possible to focus neurobiological studies on certain neural cell types (from among the many hundreds or perhaps thousands in the brain) and the circuits in which those cells participate. Even at this early stage it appears that many genes involved in schizophrenia are expressed by excitatory neurons of the cerebral cortex, and more than half of the genes involved in late-onset Alzheimer's disease are expressed in microglia, the brain's major immune cell type (Lambert et al., 2013; Sims et al., 2017).

Emerging interventions to treat brain disorders

Despite many exciting technological advances and scientific discoveries, serious challenges remain if genetics and neuroscience are to yield discoveries that will improve the lives of people with mental illness (Hyman, 2018). The goal is development of well-targeted, preventive or disease-altering treatments that can be selected based on highly predictive biomarkers. Medicine is entering a period in which drugs will no longer be limited to small molecules synthesized by chemists or antibodies, such as those now widely used to treat cancer and autoimmune diseases. New emerging therapies include some that are aimed at adding, silencing, or swapping out specific genes in specific cells in the brain. Such gene therapies are no longer science fiction; a gene-modifying therapy is now approved in the USA and Europe for the most severe form of spinal muscular atrophy, a recessive genetic disease that had previously been uniformly fatal in infancy. Children in clinical trials are not only surviving, but achieving developmental milestones (Finkel et al., 2017). Gene therapies that silence, repair, or replace genes are currently in clinical trials for several brain disorders including Huntington's disease (gene silencing) and advanced Parkinson's disease.

Treatments based on electrical or magnetic stimulation are also being studied in clinical trials and some are approved and in clinical use. Deep brain stimulation is effective for movement disorders such as essential tremor and Parkinson's disease, conditions in which the affected neural circuitry was well understood based on animal models. There have been reports of initial promise in treating severe obsessive–compulsive disorder and treatment-resistant major depressive disorder with deep brain stimulation, but outcomes are still highly variable (Greenberg et al., 2006; Naesström et al., 2016; Holtzheimer et al., 2017). Compared with movement disorders, neural circuitry relevant to psychiatric disorders is poorly understood, in part because evolutionary distance resulting in structural and functional differences in relevant brain circuits and regions has made animal models far less useful (Hyman, 2012, 2018). Repetitive transcranial magnetic stimulation has been approved to treat major depressive disorder in many countries despite the limitations in efficacy observed in clinical trials (Fox et al., 2012). Electroconvulsive therapy is limited in its use by the need for general anaesthesia and by the side effects of retrograde and anterograde amnesia. It remains, however, the most effective treatment for severe depression that has not improved with psychotherapy and medication (Slade et al., 2017). Treatments based on electrical and magnetic stimulations will likely improve as we gain the ability to more accurately identify the human brain circuits involved in pathogenesis. In the future, interventions with conventional drugs, antibodies, gene therapies or gene editing, electrical stimulation, and cognitive therapies may prevent certain mental disorders from developing in the first place.

Were psychiatry to become exclusively technologically and biologically focused, as has occurred to an increasing extent in some fields of medicine, the place for engaging patients as subjects, for example, addressing their fears, beliefs, values, and social networks, would inevitably shrink. What could be a rationale for movement in such a direction, for emphasizing the brain as a machine in which to intervene, and de-emphasizing the patient as subject? There is extensive evidence, which can only be touched on here, that the *neural mechanisms* underlying not only mental disorders but indeed all cognition, decision-making, and behavioural control are opaque to human introspection and to interpersonal observations and inferences made by others. The advent of validated, objective biological tests to make diagnoses and predict treatment response will likely reduce the role of patients' subjective reports and reports of their social milieu as key sources of diagnostic information, perhaps relegating them to making corroborative observations and to playing assigned roles in treatment adherence and programmes of rehabilitation. At present, the neurobiologically minded psychiatrist is forced to rely on the testimony and behaviour of patients and their social milieu for clues to what might be happening at the brain-level because limitations in our technology and neurobiological understanding prevent us from identifying relevant brain-level abnormalities directly and accurately—even if we knew what to look for. For example, a basic unit of cellular organization and brain function in the cerebral cortex, the cortical column, is approximately two orders of magnitude smaller than the resolution of the structural magnetic resonance imaging technology in clinical use and the temporal resolution of functional magnetic resonance imaging is on the order of seconds while the brain operates on a time scale of milliseconds. Thus today, information reported by the patient and other human observers remains necessary along with the observations and checklists of clinicians in making diagnoses and evaluating responses to treatment. However, this state of affairs may start to change as technology companies develop sensors and algorithms that can make and interpret continuous or periodic observations of patients (Insel, 2017) and as genetically informed biomarkers are developed—polygenic risk scores, which contribute probabilistic information, having been the first to emerge (Martin et al., 2019).

All human beings, which of course include those with mental disorders, lack direct introspective access to the functioning of their brains. Ideas, theories, and explanations of aetiology or causation grounded in introspection and subjective report or in the attributions and inferences of family members, clinicians, and others are at best hazy proxies for actual brain mechanisms and at worst outright false. Human beings are subject to cognitive distortions with a penchant for constructing self-serving explanations for their beliefs, emotional reactions, and actions (Kahneman, 2011). Moreover, careful observers have long recognized that human memory is not an accurate recorder of lived experience; indeed memories are regularly updated and thus altered in the service of adaptive function rather than accuracy (Schacter and Addis, 2007). The malleability of memory makes it a routine occurrence for patients not only to reinterpret the past in light of new narratives and theories gained from multiple sources including therapy, but also, like all of us, to update and edit their remembered experience, creating false tableaus and narratives that are believed with great conviction. At the turn of the twentieth century, Freud highlighted the distortion of consciously available memories and the disconnect between conscious introspection and the unconscious sources of emotion, motivation, and action—albeit in terms of now soundly rejected constructs such as ego, id, superego, libido, and certain powerful instincts. Modern cognitive neuroscience recognizes critical differences in the properties and functions of conscious information processing—which is slow, serial, capacity-limited, and effortful—compared with unconscious processing which is fast, effortless, massively parallel, and able to access enormous information stores (Dennett, 1991; Cisek and Kalaska, 2010; Custers and Aarts, 2010; Haggard and Lau, 2013). Given such considerations, it makes sense that a neurobiologically oriented psychiatrist would prefer to make diagnoses and follow treatment through objective measures and biomarkers when possible, and to use first-hand reports judiciously when necessary.

For 'bottom-up' brain repair to work, the patient's role is primarily to cooperate with receiving treatment, for example, to adhere to a regimen of medication or consent to surgery. More is required of the patient when the brain is repaired in top-down treatments, such as cognitive behavioural therapy or when these are combined with medication or surgical approaches. Here, the patient's conscious, cognitive activity is necessary but from a neurobiological stance, the patient's effortful, conscious participation is required as a conduit to other synapses and circuits in the brain. Ultimately what matters is that cognitive behavioural therapy produces alterations in synaptic networks that result in more adaptive responses to social stimuli, threats, or other salient stimuli. It is of no consequence whether the patient retains an accurate memory of the therapist or the sessions.

Evolution has played a trick on us

The mechanistic-neurobiological view goes even further in effacing the patient as subject when we consider that there is no evidence for circuits or regional specializations in the brain that might serve as a locus for a subjective self, for anything like Freud's ego, or any virtual homunculus that could make decisions and exert agency. What is observed instead is a brain characterized by activity in diverse neural circuits that act both in parallel and via complex interactions. Activity within circuits performs the computations that underlie brain function ranging from sensory processing, to the encoding of diverse forms of memory, to imagination, to decision-making and control of behaviour. As alluded to, diverse circuits presumably support the neural computations that underlie our powerful, but scientifically false intuition of a self that authors our actions (Kable and Glimcher, 2009; Shadlen and Kiani, 2013; Xie and Padoa-Schioppa, 2016). Based on strong neurobiological evidence, the potent, intuitive human experience of free will and agency does not reflect the true sources of decisions to act or of the actions themselves. Rather, the sense of agency is the product of the circuits inaccessible to consciousness that plan and initiate volitional actions (Haggard, 2008; Haggard and Lau 2013). The resulting intuition of agency is not a report on the true state of affairs as they occur in the brain but may represent an adaptive mechanism that usefully informs individuals of what they are about to do. Such experience of authoring actions is associated with the intuition of a self in the role of actor. In his pioneering, albeit still controversial work, Benjamin Libet (1983) observed that the conscious experience of willing an action occurs hundreds of milliseconds after the decision has been made by unconscious brain mechanisms. This work has been extended using electroencephalography as Libet did and by non-invasive neuroimaging to detect an unconscious brain-based signal that predicts the action. The basic design of these experiments remains the same, however, comparing the timing of the subject's report of a decision to act with the timing of the brain-based predictive signal, a design that remains open to methodological concerns. Some recent experiments report that decisions made by unconscious mechanisms can occur significantly (seconds) earlier with respect to the conscious experience of deciding to act than Libet had initially observed (Haggard, 2008; Soon et al., 2008). Reflecting on such experiments and many observations made by cognitive scientists it could be said (metaphorically, of course) that evolution has played a trick on us. Our powerful and ineluctable experience of being a self that wills and acts freely seems useful and adaptive as we (and presumably other animals) interact rapidly with our world and with other members of our species. Of course, we have no insight into the history of natural selection as it pertains to human cognition, but without committing the sin of teleological reasoning, we can reflect that natural selection is based on survival and reproductive success. In that sense, evolution would not have favoured our ability to experience truthfully our underlying neural and cognitive mechanisms in their vastly cumbersome complexity, if that ability would have detracted from our ability to react to our environments and act rapidly and adaptively.

In a sense that differs starkly from folk psychology, human beings actually do author their actions; it is just that decisions and behaviour do not originate with a conscious self that chooses freely and causes actions, but in unconscious, massively parallel circuit-based mechanisms that are embedded in webs of external causal influences and internally represented states ranging from metabolic and homeostatic states to diverse forms of memory. The simple motor act of reaching for a cup of coffee requires the brain to calculate the angle and distance needed to grasp the cup, to direct the firing of just the right opposing muscle groups with just the right amplitude and timing while stabilizing certain joints, and to process sensory feedback such as joint position and the changing place of one's hand in space as it approaches the cup. Exquisite error detection and feedback systems are needed to keep the trajectory of the arm on track and ensure the right grip, which must be adjusted on the fly if the cup is heavier or hotter than expected. The focus of this brief discussion has been on motor decisions and acts because there is an extensive experimental basis for understanding the disconnection between human intuitions about agency and the neural mechanisms that actually underlie motor behaviour. However, other beliefs about the self and the human social milieu and about one's ability to exert control over one's own thought, emotion, and behaviour are almost certainly just as false with respect to what really happens in the brain.

The intuitive experience of being a self that freely decides and causes the body to move is false when tested against what we know scientifically; nonetheless these untrue intuitions deserve to be taken seriously rather than dismissed as mere illusions of no scientific interest. In short, the goal of these reflections is not eliminativist; it is not to dismiss universal human intuitions as fantasies that should be relegated to the cognitive dustbin along with such concoctions as Freud's id and ego. The experience of being a self with agency is not only a universal human cognitive trait to which considerable brain circuitry is dedicated, but is also ineluctable in the sense that we cannot think our way out of them except in artificial circumstances for a limited period of time. These reflections raise a hypothesis already alluded to: despite being false as a mechanistic explanation these intuitions serve important adaptive functions. As a thought experiment, imagine gaining introspective access to the true neurobiological mechanisms that underlie the simple decision to reach for a cup of coffee. In that case, you would become aware of the millions of computations performed by synapses and circuits that led to the decision to reach for the cup and the additional and likely larger number of computations needed to initiate and control the reaching and grasping action. These computations and their ultimate integration—even for a very simple motor act like reaching for a cup of coffee—would overwhelm the limited capacity of conscious cognition and even if they could be managed, would crowd out other important information that is constantly impinging on us from the world. The astonishing complexity of what brains must actually do to process and integrate diverse sources of information in order to make decisions, select actions, and cause the relevant behaviour—and to do so rapidly in the service of goals and ultimately survival—would seem to make introspective access to the actual computational mechanisms incredibly maladaptive. If to actually reach for a cup of coffee we had to engage seriously with the kind computational complexity previously suggested, it is doubtful that we would ever lift the cup or obtain a sip. The price of really knowing what we are doing in a manner that truly captures, let alone directs our neural machinery even in some abbreviated form, would have highly adverse consequences—probably lethal—for functioning and for survival in a fast moving, competitive, and often dangerous world.

There is another strand of evidence that argues for the functional importance of our false intuitive sense of self, will, and agency: circumstances and conditions that subvert our folk psychological expectations are associated with significant psychopathology and stress. For example, a pervasive sense of external control of one's self or one's actions is a symptom of psychosis. Diminished ability to attribute mental states and intentions to other people is a cardinal and disabling impairment of ASDs that can make navigation of the social world extremely difficult. Automatic attributions of moral responsibility to others (in the Aristotelian sense) do not capture the truth of the brain mechanisms by which people perform good or bad acts, but these attributions are often necessary for survival in a complex, rapidly changing social world. Finally, the experience of being unable to exert volitional control over one's actions or to act effectively in certain environments is highly stressful, accompanied by stress hormone release, activation of the sympathetic nervous system, and in animal models over repeat episodes, the maladaptive state of learned helplessness (Seligman, 1972; Peterson et al., 1995). The importance of such experiences of folk psychological intuitions to healthy functioning does not imply that they offer insight into mechanistic truth, but is evidence, worth understanding, of how our brains evolved to function effectively.

Folk psychology and the interpersonal perspective will likely always have an important role in the practise of psychiatry and clinical psychology

Some writers have speculated that ever more compelling mechanistic explanations of thought, emotion, and behaviour might push aspects of our intuitively experienced selves and our automatic attributions of intentionality and agency off centre stage (Greene and Cohen, 2004; Kong et al., 2017). This seems entirely unlikely. Recognizing the imperfections of science and a historical litany of false conclusions about the aetiology and treatment of mental illness, scientific investigation nonetheless eventually brings us closer to the true state of affairs and to practical technological applications, while folk psychology lacks such truth value. Despite the fact that they do not withstand scientific scrutiny, folk psychological understandings dominate human experience because they capture automatic and powerful intuitions about ourselves and others. Previously, we have laid out the odd case that universally held intuitions that purport to capture realities of human functioning, but that are nonetheless scientifically false, have an inescapably important role for healthy and adaptive engagement in the world and for interactions with other people. This assertion is made from a perspective inspired by evolutionary thinking about adaptiveness for reproductive success and survival. It is not meant as a value judgement as to whether such automatic cognitive mechanisms are beneficent. For example automatic attributions of intentions and moral attributes to others, while adaptive in the broad sense of helping a person make decisions rapidly in a potentially dangerous world, can be suffused with inaccurate and harmful implicit biases or can promote false and damaging attributions in legal proceedings.

From the foregoing discussion it can be concluded that the neurobiological view and folk psychology are completely incommensurate as explanations for human thought, emotion, and behaviour. These two views make competing claims and have an entirely different status based on the scientific evidence. From a scientific vantage, the intuitions captured by folk psychology are false even if adaptive; with further neurobiological research it will likely be possible to identify the circuit mechanisms that underlie the ineluctable, but false intuitions captured by folk psychology. Having starkly claimed that these epistemological stances are incompatible, we now face the difficult task of showing how psychiatry and clinical psychology can incorporate both views into clinical practice, as they must do in order to treat people with mental illness effectively.

Looking at healthcare as a whole, patients, families, and payers likely prioritize good treatment outcomes over such matters as whether the patient experiences a good rapport with the clinicians caring for him or her. Although good rapport and the feeling of being respected and understood may influence patients' acceptance of treatment recommendations and adherence to the prescribed regimen, many excellent procedure-oriented clinicians may be experienced as cold or uninterested by patients, while charlatans trade on their ability to create a rapport with patients rather than on scientific knowledge or technical skill. Psychiatry and clinical psychology represent areas of healthcare that perhaps uniquely rely for their success not only on successful diagnosis and treatment conducted skilfully from an objectifying cognitive stance, but also on the interpersonal perspective, the ability to engage the suffering person as a subject. Just as it is entirely unlikely that immersion in the study of cognitive neuroscience could supplant one's intuitive experience of selfhood and agency—or that it would be adaptive to do so—it is unlikely that scientific explanations of mental illness will drive out the experience of mental illness as intimate and as affecting the nature of the person's experienced self. In so far as mental illness is experienced as damaging to the person's concept of self and experience of relating to others including clinicians, the engagement of the person as subject may not only advance the acceptance of prescribed treatment, but may itself be therapeutic. We do not believe that this latter assertion is an appeal to mysticism or placebo responses. Rather for some people with mental illness, the experience of empathy, caring, and being listened to can initiate new learning, best taken in by such interpersonal channels both conscious and unconsicous, signifying that they are not outcasts, but deserving of empathy and respect, even in their current state.

Jonathan Glover (2014 and Chapter 19, this volume) argues that it is not only possible but desirable to *synthesize* what we have referred to as the neurobiological and the interpersonal perspectives, permitting the clinician to see the patient with what he calls 'binocular vision'. We entirely agree with Glover that both perspectives are critically important to good care. However, attempts to synthesize these incommensurate perspectives represent an epistemological error that is more than academic: it can adversely affect clinical care. From the point of view of the clinician, conflation of the intuitive language of a Cartesian self with the language of neurobiology risks confusion and misunderstanding. One problem arises when clinicians engage in a kind of scientism and unnecessarily efface the patient by discussing the patient's experience in objective terms. For example, when trying to reassure a patient who suffers from anxiety, it usually won't help to discuss the anxiety only in neurobiological terms, such as the sensitivity of their amygdala-based fear circuits, if the neurobiology doesn't connect with anything the patient experiences. While it is often beneficial to educate patients about relevant current scientific opinion, the clinician would do well to also find meaningful connections from the interpersonal realm the patient will understand. For example, it might prove more reassuring to know that other patients, ideally in well conducted clinical trials, receiving the same treatment have reported fewer panic attacks and a renewed ability to achieve their goals. Likewise, scientific discussions are muddied by blending them with folk psychological terms. This can be relatively benign, such as when saying that a receptor antagonist binds to its target receptor because it 'wants' or 'tries' to, when really it does so because of its chemical and physical properties. But it is more misleading if attempts at shorthand scientific explanations become teleological, reductive, or deterministic. The clinician may know better, but many people hear oversimplified discussions of genes or brain mechanisms as forms of causality against which they cannot effectively struggle. What matters when scientific explanations are given is to glean what the patient has taken in both cognitively and emotionally and to ensure that there is good agreement on the value of treatment, adherence, and follow-up. By arguing for a synthesis of neurobiological and folk psychological perspectives Glover's advice might give the clinician a case of disorienting double vision rather than beneficial binocular vision.

Eschewing a facile and incoherent synthesis: switching cognitive frames

Given that the neurobiological perspective and the interpersonal perspective are epistemologically incompatible but are both important for the clinical encounter, what can the clinician do? Clinicians must learn to switch cognitive frames between the neurobiological and objectifying perspective and the interpersonal perspective that treats the patient as a subject. Indeed, we believe that this is what good clinicians already do within the encounter. With experience, switching of cognitive frames becomes unconscious and automatic, guided by implicit social cues exchanged between the clinician and patient. The clinician may gain proxy information from engaging with patients in the interpersonal mode but should not muddle objective information needed for diagnosis and treatment with folk psychology or intuition of emotional states that may be been gleaned implicitly from the patient. If information obtained from the two different frames clash, the clinician is in a position to deliberate—a challenging position that would be obviated in some cases if psychiatry had objective biomarkers. Interpersonal intuitions may raise scepticism about information obtained from structured interviews or checklists—after all, not all information obtained in this manner is truthful—but that is one reason that it is valuable to keep the neurobiological and interpersonal perspectives distinct.

It is important for the clinician to recognize the meaning that illness and its consequences have for patients' self-concepts and social milieus without attributing meaning to the illness or its pathogenic mechanisms per se. The Scylla and Charybdis between which clinicians must steer are folk psychology's invitation to accept inappropriate self-blaming or other distorted views on the part of the patient or stigmatization of the patient by others as weak or deserving of illness versus the risk conferred by the biological perspective of instilling a sense of isolation and irretrievable difference from healthy people or producing inappropriate fatalism. The clinician has the task of empathetically acknowledging the patient's beliefs and feelings, but gently (and given our state of knowledge, humbly) correcting distortions about how the patient became ill and remains ill. At the same time, the clinician must be careful that the patient does not interpret mechanistic explanations as signifying that their condition is inevitably hopeless and beyond the reach of prescribed medications or psychotherapies.

The distinction between the neurobiological and interpersonal aspects of treatment often feels slippery because psychiatrists, psychologists, and patients, like all human beings, are intuitive Cartesians. Humans have the experience of being a self that is intuitively different from the body including the brain. People may recognize that their intuited self is embodied, but rarely do they experience their cognitive experience as body. Similarly, people have learned that their brains are necessary for cognitive processing, but do not have direct experience of their brains at work. As a result, it can feel counterintuitive to think that the conscious discourse of interpersonal therapies doesn't work through adjusting one's Cartesian self (i.e. the self that one takes to be the speaking and listening) but rather by influencing the unconscious brain processes underpinning both that discourse and the disorder from which the person is suffering. As suggested previously, cognitive psychotherapy for depression works by altering synaptic networks in our brains in a manner that diminishes attentional biases toward negative percepts and threats and reduces the tendency toward automatic negative interpretations of interpersonal interactions (DeRubeis et al., 2008; Garland et al., 2010; Challis and Berton, 2015). In parallel, the experience of engaging in and benefitting from cognitive therapy (or not) has meaning to the patient, enhancing the experience of agency or perhaps, if the therapy fails, exacerbating a sense of failure or incompetence. As described, a positive sense of agency is adaptive and healthy even if not a true description of neural mechanisms that underlie decision-making and action. A good rapport and strong alliance with the clinician also has meaning and there is evidence that the quality of the relationship can be a significant factor in whether the patient benefits from psychotherapy (Thompson and McCabe, 2012). The distinction between neurobiological and interpersonal frames in the clinical encounter represents the distinction between mechanism and meaning, not between pills and psychotherapies.

An emerging mechanistic picture of schizophrenia

In this final section we explore the advancing, and increasingly useful, mechanistic picture of schizophrenia as a basis for discussing how increasingly compelling neurobiological understandings may influence psychiatric treatment and affect clinical encounters. Schizophrenia has long been seen as a paradigmatic disorder for psychiatry. Its aetiology and treatment have attracted highly divergent theorizing, which, over time, has shifted from psychogenic models to neurobiological models.

Only a few decades ago most psychiatrists considered schizophrenia to be psychogenic, attributing its aetiology to maladaptive family interactions. In the 1930s and 1940s it was thought that schizophrenia was caused by mothers who were both rejecting and at the same time, controlling and overprotective, creating a psychological 'double bind'. The psychoanalyst Frieda Fromm-Reichmann (1948) crystallized a version of this theory of pathogenesis in the concept of the schizophrenogenic mother. According to such theories, families, and especially mothers, literally drove their children mad. The idea that schizophrenia was psychogenic in origin was very much alive when SEH began his medical training at Harvard Medical School in 1976. The junior psychiatrists who were the main instructors in his first psychiatry course believed that intensely negative, meaning-laden expressions of emotion by family members likely caused schizophrenia and undoubtedly exacerbated it. The patients on their wards did receive antipsychotic medication, but the drugs were seen as no more than adjunctive treatments to enhance participation in insight-oriented (not cognitive behavioural) psychotherapy. These young psychiatrists made inferences about the aetiologies of their patients' symptoms from the rambling, sometimes incoherent verbal productions of their chronically ill patients who they occasionally interviewed in front of us to demonstrate their symptoms. Their clinical practice reflected the now seemingly odd belief, but pervasive at the time, that the brain had essentially nothing to do with mental illness. The brain was treated as mere hardware that could, as this computer metaphor went, run any software program. What mattered was first-person experience and human meaning: this was the software. On this assumption, it made sense to think that insight-oriented forms of psychotherapy in the psychoanalytic tradition would be the best treatments because they addressed mental content directly; they could reload the computer with better software. During the 1990s, enthusiasm for psychoanalytically influenced treatment of schizophrenia waned not, it would seem, because these practitioners recognized its disutility, but because payers of insurance would no longer countenance costly, long-term treatments that lacked evidence of efficacy.

The psychiatrists observed by SEH during his medical training, both these junior clinicians and the professors, were riveted and seduced by the content-rich verbal productions of their psychotic patients—hallucinations that might involve multiple, often denigrating voices, bizarre and paranoid delusions, ideas of reference (belief that ordinary experiences contained hidden messages), the experience of thoughts being inserted into or extracted from their minds, and disorganization of speech, which at its extreme was described as 'word salad'. These psychiatrists relied on theoretical frameworks from diverse offshoots of psychoanalytic theory to guide their case formulations, which invariably pointed to family conflicts as the cause of their patients' schizophrenia, mediated by unconscious conflicts. They taught that the patients' verbal productions harboured clues to important unconscious processes, while focusing for the most part on what they perceived to be the meanings of the patients' speech. At times, after interviewing a patient in front of us, the junior psychiatrists would decode what seemed incoherent. They treated the language of their patients as distorted by psychosis, but still laden with meaning worth understanding. They did not imagine that these verbal outputs might reflect the outputs of a significantly malfunctioning brain rather than clues to what had caused the psychosis. Instead, these clinicians relied on patient verbal outputs as their major sources of information, presuming them to be interpretable in light of various psychoanalytic theories. Their preferred mode of treatment, intensive insight-oriented psychotherapy, relied on the idea that the verbal outputs, even of patients suffering with psychosis, provided clues to unconscious pathogenic processes.

Psychoanalytic theory and practice dominated American academic psychiatry for most of the mid-twentieth century, extending its purview from what was called neurosis, even to schizophrenia and bipolar disorder. In contrast, the late nineteenth-century psychiatrist Emil Kraepelin had recognized the importance of early onset and progressively worsening cognitive deterioration as a central feature of the condition that he called dementia praecox (early dementia), which was later renamed schizophrenia by Bleuler. Based on his careful observations, Kraepelin considered unremitting cognitive impairment to distinguish dementia praecox from manic-depressive illness (now bipolar disorder) in which patients might experience episodic psychosis without severe or progressive cognitive deterioration. Modern observations confirm Kraepelin's observation that the first symptoms of schizophrenia, appearing in adolescence are cognitive impairments affecting diverse aspects of cognitive function. These are accompanied by the onset of deficit symptoms such as impoverishment of thought, blunting of affect, and loss of motivation. Psychotic symptoms develop later in the course of the illness, often in the patient's late teens or twenties, beginning with attenuated symptoms such as hearing odd noises that other people do not hear, and then a first episode of florid psychosis followed by waxing and waning psychotic relapses thereafter. Antipsychotic medications shorten the duration of psychotic relapses and lengthen remissions, but at the cost of serious side effects. Moreover, after the first acute psychotic episode or two, medications generally fail to suppress psychotic symptoms fully.

Beginning in the late 1970s, non-invasive neuroimaging studies and postmortem studies began to identify anatomic abnormalities in schizophrenia, notably loss of grey matter, the component of brain tissue that contains neurons, accompanied by compensatory enlargement of the fluid-filled ventricles within the brain. As structural magnetic resonance imaging technology improved, it was observed that abnormal grey matter loss was most severe in the prefrontal and temporal regions of the cerebral cortex. Moreover, these deficits could be observed prior to treatment with antipsychotic drugs ruling out drug toxicity as a cause. It was later established that abnormal thinning of the cerebral cortex begins prior to the first episode of acute psychosis (Cannon, 2015; Satterthwaite et al., 2016). Postmortem studies of the brains of people with schizophrenia found that the grey matter loss did not result from cell death, as it does in Alzheimer's disease; instead, neurons in specific cellular layers in prefrontal and temporal regions of the cerebral cortex lose dendrites and the dendritic spines, the region of the neuron that receives synaptic connections. The conclusion is that people suffering from schizophrenia have synaptic loss that is most severe in prefrontal and temporal cerebral cortex, with the result that their brains would have a diminished ability to process information and generate outputs from these brain areas.

By carefully correlating the anatomic locations of grey matter loss with the results of cognitive testing, it could be concluded that the patterns of synaptic loss could explain the impairments observed in patients with schizophrenia (Walton et al., 2018). For example, the dorsolateral prefrontal cortex is typically the region most severely affected by grey matter loss in schizophrenia. This brain region plays a critical role in working memory, a capacity required for cognitive control of emotion and behaviour. Working memory and cognitive control are typically impaired in schizophrenia; thus, even when psychotic symptoms are under control, people with schizophrenia are rarely able to regulate their actions in accordance with their goals—and thus remain unable to participate effectively in school or to work.

Despite these findings, what was still missing at the turn of the twenty-first century was a likely mechanism of pathogenesis. During the last decade, new genomic and computational tools made it possible to obtain important information from genetic analyses, specifically the identification of DNA variants in human genomes that increase the risk of schizophrenia. The risk of schizophrenia, bipolar disorder, and ASDs is highly influenced by genes although developmental and environmental factors also influence disease risk. For schizophrenia, genes explain approximately 80% of the variance in the populations that have been studied (Sullivan et al., 2012; Hilker et al., 2018). Genes play a lesser but still significant role in major depressive disorder and anxiety disorders, explaining about 35% of the variance (Sullivan et al., 2012).

At the time of writing, nearly 100,000 individuals with schizophrenia and a larger number of matched comparison subjects have had their DNA subjected to GWASs and another 35,000 patients have had all of their DNA regions that encode proteins sequenced. GWASs have found more than 250 locations in the genome that influence schizophrenia risk. Many of these risk-associated variants affect genes that encode some of the many protein components of synapses, especially excitatory synapses in the cerebral cortex. Another risk-associated gene influences the level of expression in the brain of a protein called complement factor 4A (C4A), which had been known outside the brain for its role in the innate immune system where it is involved in marking bacteria or damaged cells for engulfment by immune cells (Sekar et al., 2016). In the brain, however, C4A has the role of marking weak synapses for removal by microglia, the brain's phagocytic cells (Salter and Stevens, 2017).

During infancy and childhood, the brain elaborates large numbers of synapses. As developing children experience their environments, synapses that get used for information processing are strengthened and those that go unused get weaker and are ultimately pruned away by microglia. These large-scale developmental processes follow the same principles that underlie memory formation where salient experiences lead to the strengthening of synaptic networks that encode a memory. As memories are updated and altered, new connections are made and strengthened while others are weakened and pruned away. During development, different brain regions mature at different rates, beginning with the visual cortex at the back of the brain, and finishing during adolescence and young adulthood with the prefrontal and temporal regions of the cerebral cortex that support high-level associations and cognitive control. The normal maturation of the prefrontal cortex is associated with a decrease in impulsivity that occurs as young people enter their third decade of life.

The elaboration of large numbers of synapses in early life is good preparation for information processing in an unpredictable world. (If animals, including humans, were born rigidly hardwired, they could not adapt to the very diverse circumstances they find themselves in.) As the maturing human brain reaches adolescent years, the person has accrued many years of learning and the person's brain has had many years of intense synaptic plasticity. In these years, a process of synaptic refinement occurs that produces an adult brain that has fewer synaptic connections than that of a child, but synapses that are on average far more efficient. A key step in adolescent synaptic refinement is the pruning of many weak and inefficient synapses by microglia. Weak synapses are thought to display complement factor C4 on their surface. C4 recruits another complement protein, C3, which provides a signal to microglia that the synapse is to be engulfed and thus eliminated (Stephan et al., 2012). The discovery that the variants of the *C4* gene that increase risk of schizophrenia increase levels of C4 protein expression in the brain, and the association of many genes that encode synaptic proteins tied together several observations leading to a mechanistic hypothesis of pathogenesis (Sekar et al., 2016).[5]

The age of onset of the first symptoms of schizophrenia is precisely during the time, adolescence, when wholesale synaptic refinement begins to occur in the prefrontal and temporal regions of the cerebral cortex. Given that people with schizophrenia have excessive loss of dendritic spines and synapses, it is now hypothesized that schizophrenia results from abnormal and excessive removal of synapses that is in large part

---

[5] Because many of the genes that influence the risk of schizophrenia affect synaptic structure and function, it has been speculated that they affect synaptic strength and other properties of synapses that influence plasticity and susceptibility to pruning.

influenced genetically by variants in genes that encode the protein building blocks of synapses and the *C4A* gene and other genes that affect complement and thus microglial activity. Given the heterogeneity of schizophrenia and indeed all common human traits, different genes, including C4A, play greater or lesser roles in different people. The anatomic locations of excessive synaptic loss observed by imaging and postmortem examination is consistent with the cognitive impairments and deficit symptoms that emerge as the illness develops. It has been further speculated that psychotic symptoms result from misprocessing of information that occurs as a result of synapse loss in schizophrenia as it does in late-onset neurodegenerative diseases such as Alzheimer's disease, Huntington's disease, and Parkinson's disease.

This emerging mechanistic picture is certainly incomplete and requires further corroboration. Risk-associated genetic variants are still being discovered at a rapid pace that may point in different directions from those discussed here (McCarroll et al., 2014; Hyman, 2018). That said, the picture of schizophrenia as a genetically influenced, developmentally triggered disorder of synapse loss provides a useful platform for further hypothesis testing. As in all of medicine, genetic findings also provide useful tools to refine our understanding of environmental risk factors. Epidemiology has implicated season of birth, urban birth, and migration as risk factors for schizophrenia (Schmidt, 2007). However, to date, these associations identify proxies rather than causal factors. As epidemiological study cohorts are stratified by the levels of genetic risk of their participants they will gain greater statistical power, and as the genes that influence schizophrenia risk are identified, scientists will be better able to refine epidemiological hypotheses. If, for example, season of birth is a proxy for prenatal viral infections which in turn produce immune activation, one could test whether this altered the behaviour of microglia, perhaps increasing their avidity. Notwithstanding such speculation, much remains to be discovered.

We have selected schizophrenia as an example because at present, more is known about its genetics and pathogenic mechanisms than is known for other mental disorders. More importantly for our purposes, the emerging mechanistic picture of schizophrenia confronts us with the need to rethink the clinical encounter in psychiatry. This picture, even if it must be significantly revised in coming years, is a potent reminder of the dangers of making inferences about the basis of mental illness based on folk psychological assumptions, for example, that human beings have insights into the aetiology of their conditions on which they can report—even when these reports are supplemented by elaborate psychological theories such as those derived from psychoanalysis. It must be acknowledged that schizophrenia typically produces more pervasive and devastating effects on thought, emotion, and behaviour than typical cases of depression or anxiety disorders. However, depression and anxiety disorders, no less than schizophrenia, result from altered functioning of the brain that is inaccessible to introspection, even if, relative to schizophrenia, verbal communication and empathy are often easier and the causal theories of patients and family members more plausible and cogent. Conversely, there is a risk that viewing the brain as a machine, which in mental illness is in need of repair, could undercut engagement with the patient as subject, which we have argued, remains a critical component of a successful clinical encounter and formation of a therapeutic alliance. Interactions with the patient as subject should not be taken to illuminate disease pathogenesis but, ideally, will address the patient's self-concept and jointly help explore their attribution of meanings to diagnosis, patient status, and treatment—making it possible to address potentially harmful misconceptions that could undercut treatment and damage life functioning.

As we gain understanding of the pathogenesis of mental disorders, it will be increasingly useful for clinicians to understand the relevant neuroscience and to educate patients and families about these illnesses—just as one might educate patients and families about diabetes mellitus or a particular cancer. When it comes to mental illness, education is trickier than it is for most other illnesses, however, because it invites erroneous Cartesian thinking, based on the deeply ingrained human folk psychological experience of being a self with agency and responsibility, and thus potentially morally at fault for being ill. In describing the brain as the basis of the person's mental illness, it will be important to communicate that, through their cells, synapses, and circuits, brains integrate genetic risk and other biological risk factors endogenous to the body, with environmental risk factors including inputs communicated through language and social interactions. Effective treatment may take the form of medication, neuromodulation, psychotherapy, management of the person's environment, or some combination. Clinical trials will ultimately reveal, as an empirical matter, which treatments are most effective whatever we believe the aetiology of the person's illness to be. Patient education about aetiology and treatment of mental illness requires a nuanced discussion that clinicians can best provide by engaging with patients and families not only in an objectifying scientific context, but also as subjects, maintaining curiosity about what models of illness patients and families are internalizing and what meanings they are attributing to illness and treatment. Ideally, the result is a new self-narrative for the patient and family that reduces stigma and blaming, and that enhances the motivation for appropriate self-care in the context of the best current understandings. Even for a severe condition such as schizophrenia, the interpersonal perspective remains critical to successful clinical encounters and to the development of constructive alliances that respect the patients' values in the service of treatment over time. This last statement deserves an important caveat, however. At times, schizophrenia and other illnesses that affect the brain are so severe that the interpersonal model loses relevance—the patient might have lost the ability to process information with any semblance of normalcy or may incorporate the clinician into the content of delusions. In such cases, with due care, there may be no alternative to an objectifying interaction to permit interventions that avoid harm.

We expect the advancing mechanistic understanding of schizophrenia to be mirrored over time in our understandings of other mental disorders, each with its particular mixture of risk factors, mechanisms, biomarkers, and treatment. Clinical practice needs to make the most effective use of this new information for the benefit of patients despite the immediacy of folk psychological explanations of mental disorders. At the same time, practitioners need to carefully avoid the counterbalancing risk of effacing the human and interpersonal side of psychiatry and clinical psychology, which we believe, will remain centrally important to the successful clinical encounter.

Acknowledgements

SEH: I thank Pierre Loebel for making possible the opportunity to give these lectures, for his engaging discussions, and for his graciousness during my week in Oxford. I thank Julian Savulescu for inviting me to present the Loebel Lectures and to Doug McConnell for keeping me focused and playing an unerringly constructive role despite his disagreements with some of my views. I am grateful to all of the discussants who forced me to sharpen the arguments in defence of my admittedly often counterintuitive positions. It was also a special pleasure for me to interact with Jonathan Glover, whose work I have long valued, and the contemplation of which pushed me towards asking ever more challenging questions. I am, of course, the parent of all the confusing cognitive underbrush that remains in this chapter. To do better, I can only hope for future discussions with philosophers, neuroscientists, psychologists, and psychiatrists that approach the calibre of those I had at Oxford in November 2015.

References

Cannon, T.D. (2015). How schizophrenia develops: cognitive and brain mechanisms underlying onset of psychosis. *Trends in Cognitive Sciences*, **19**(12), 744–756.

Challis, C. and Berton, O. (2015). Top-down control of serotonin systems by the prefrontal cortex: a path toward restored socioemotional function in depression. *ACS Chemical Neuroscience*, **6**(7), 1040–1054.

Cisek, P. and Kalaska, J.F. (2010). Neural mechanisms for interacting with a world full of action choices. *Annual Review of Neuroscience*, **33**(1), 269–298.

Custers, R. and Aarts, H. (2010). The unconscious will: how the pursuit of goals operates outside of conscious awareness. *Science*, **329**(5987), 47–50.

de Carvalho, M.R., Rozenthal, M., and Nardi, A. (2009). The fear circuitry in panic disorder and its modulation by cognitive-behaviour therapy interventions. *World Journal of Biological Psychiatry*, **11**(2 Pt 2), 1–11.

Dennett, D. (1991). *Consciousness Explained*. Boston, MA: Little, Brown and Company.

DeRubeis, R.J., Siegle, G.J., and Hollon, S.D. (2008). Cognitive therapy versus medication for depression: treatment outcomes and neural mechanisms. *Nature Reviews Neuroscience*, **9**(10), 788–796.

Etkin, A. and Wager, T.D. (2007). Functional neuroimaging of anxiety: a meta-analysis of emotional processing in PTSD, social anxiety disorder, and specific phobia. *American Journal of Psychiatry*, **164**(10), 1476–1488.

Finkel, R.S., Mercuri, E., Darras, B.T., Connolly, A.M., Kuntz, N.L., Kirschner, J., Chiriboga, C.A., Saito, K., Servais, L., Tizzano, E., Topaloglu, H., Tulinius, M., Montes, J., Glanzman, A.M., Bishop, K., Zhong, Z.J., Gheuens, S., Bennett, C.F., Schneider, E., Farwell, W., and De Vivo, D.C. (2017). Nusinersen versus sham control in infantile-onset spinal muscular atrophy. *New England Journal of Medicine*, **377**(18), 1723–1732.

Foa, E.B., Franklin, M.E., and Moser, J. (2002). Context in the clinic: how well do cognitive-behavioral therapies and medications work in combination? *Biological Psychiatry*, **52**(10), 987–997.

Fox, M.D., Buckner, R.L., White, M.P., Greicius, M.D., and Pascual-Leone, A. (2012). Efficacy of transcranial magnetic stimulation targets for depression is related to intrinsic functional connectivity with the subgenual cingulate. *Biological Psychiatry*, **72**(7), 595–603.

Fromm-Reichmann, F. (1948). Notes on the development of treatment of schizophrenics by psychoanalytic psychotherapy. *Psychiatry*, **11**, 263–273.

Garland, E.L., Fredrickson, B., Kring, A.M., Johnson, D.P., Meyer, P.S., and **Penn, D.L.** (2010). Upward spirals of positive emotions counter downward spirals of negativity: insights from the broaden-and-build theory and affective neuroscience on the treatment of emotion dysfunctions and deficits in psychopathology. *Clinical Psychology Review*, **30**(7), 849–864.

Glover, J. (2014). *Alien Landscapes?: Interpreting Disordered Minds*. Cambridge, MA: Harvard University Press.

Greenberg, B.D., Malone, D.A., Friehs, G.M., Rezai, A.R., Kubu, C.S., Malloy, P.F., Salloway, S.P., Okun, M.S., Goodman, W.K., and **Rasmussen, S.A.** (2006). Three-year outcomes in deep brain stimulation for highly resistant obsessive–compulsive disorder. *Neuropsychopharmacology*, **31**(11), 2384–2393.

Greene, J. and **Cohen, J.** (2004). For the law, neuroscience changes nothing and everything. *Philosophical Transactions of the Royal Society of London. Series B, Biological Sciences*, **359**(1451), 1775–1785.

Haggard, P. (2008). Human volition: towards a neuroscience of will. *Nature Reviews Neuroscience*, **9**(12), 934–946.

Haggard, P. and **Lau, H.** (2013). What is volition? *Experimental Brain Research*, **229**(3), 285–287.

Hilker, R., Helenius, D., Fagerlund, B., Skytthe, A., Christensen, K., Werge, T.M., Nordentoft, M., and **Glenthøj, B.** (2018). Heritability of schizophrenia and schizophrenia spectrum based on the Nationwide Danish Twin Register. *Biological Psychiatry*, **83**(6), 492–498.

Holtzheimer, P.E., Husain, M.M., Lisanby, S.H., Taylor, S.F., Whitworth, L.A., McClintock, S., Slavin, K.V., Berman, J., McKhann, G.M., Patil, P.G., et al. (2017). Subcallosal cingulate deep brain stimulation for treatment-resistant depression: a multisite, randomised, sham-controlled trial. *The Lancet Psychiatry*, **4**(11), 839–849.

Hyman, S.E. (2012). Revolution stalled. *Science Translational Medicine*, **4**(155), 155cm11.

Hyman, S.E. (2018). The daunting polygenicity of mental illness: making a new map. *Philosophical Transactions of the Royal Society of London. Series B, Biological Sciences*, **373**(1742), 20170031.

Insel, T.R. (2017). Digital phenotyping. *JAMA*, **318**(13), 1215–1216.

Kable, J.W. and **Glimcher, P.W.** (2009). The neurobiology of decision: consensus and controversy. *Neuron*, **63**(6), 733–745.

Kahneman, D. (2011). *Thinking, Fast and Slow*. New York: Farrar, Straus, & Giroux.

Kong, C., Dunn, M., and **Parker, M.** (2017). Psychiatric genomics and mental health treatment: setting the ethical agenda. *The American Journal of Bioethics*, **17**(4), 3–12.

Lambert, J.-C., Ibrahim-Verbaas, C.A., Harold, D., Naj, A.C., Sims, R., Bellenguez, C., DeStafano, A.L., Bis, J.C., Beecham, G.W., Grenier-Boley, B., et al. (2013). Meta-analysis of 74,046 individuals identifies 11 new susceptibility loci for Alzheimer's disease. *Nature Genetics*, **45**(12), 1452–1458.

Libet, B., Gleason, C.A., Wright, E.W., and **Pearl, D.K.** (1983). Time of conscious intention to act in relation to onset of cerebral activity (readiness-potential). *Brain*, **106**(3), 623–642.

Macosko, E.Z., Basu, A., Satija, R., Nemesh, J., Shekhar, K., Goldman, M., Tirosh, I., Bialas, A.R., Kamitaki, N., Martersteck, E.M., Trombetta, J.J., Weitz, D.A., Sanes, J.R., Shalek, A.K., Regev, A., and **McCarroll, SA.** (2015). Highly parallel genome-wide expression profiling of individual cells using nanoliter droplets. *Cell*, **161**(5), 1202–1214.

Martin, A.R., Kanai, M., Kamatani, Y., Okada, Y., Neale, B.M., and Daly, M.J. (2019). Clinical use of current polygenic risk scores may exacerbate health disparities. *Nature Genetics*, **51**(4), 584–591.

McCarroll, S.A., Feng, G., and Hyman, S.E. (2014). Genome-scale neurogenetics: methodology and meaning. *Nature Neuroscience*, **17**(6), 756–763.

Naesström, M., Blomstedt, P., and Bodlund, O. (2016). A systematic review of psychiatric indications for deep brain stimulation, with focus on major depressive and obsessive-compulsive disorder. *Nordic Journal of Psychiatry*, **70**(7), 483–491.

Peterson, C., Maier, S.F. and Seligman, M.E.P. (1995). *Learned Helplessness: A Theory for the Age of Personal Control*. New York: Oxford University Press.

Regev, A., Teichmann, S. ., Lander, E.S., Amit, I., Benoist, C., Birney, E., Bodenmiller, B., Campbell, P., Carninci, P., Clatworthy, M., et al. (2017). The human cell atlas. *eLife*, **6**, e27041.

Salter, M.W. and Stevens, B. (2017). Microglia emerge as central players in brain disease. *Nature Medicine*, **23**(9), 1018–1027.

Sanders, S.J., He, X., Willsey, A.J., Ercan-Sencicek, A.G., Samocha, K.E., Cicek, A.E., Murtha, M.T., Bal, V.H., Bishop, S.L., Dong, S., et al. (2015). Insights into autism spectrum disorder genomic architecture and biology from 71 risk loci. *Neuron*, **87**(6), 1215–1233.

Satterthwaite, T.D., Wolf, D.H., Calkins, M.E., Vandekar, S.N., Erus, G., Ruparel, K., Roalf, D.R., Linn, K.A., Elliott, M.A., Moore, T.M., Hakonarson, H., Shinohara, R.T., Davatzikos, C., Gur, R.C., and Gur, R.E. (2016). Structural brain abnormalities in youth with psychosis spectrum symptoms. *JAMA Psychiatry*, **73**(5), 515–524.

Schacter, D.L. and Addis, D.R. (2007). The cognitive neuroscience of constructive memory: remembering the past and imagining the future. *Philosophical Transactions of the Royal Society of London. Series B, Biological Sciences*, **362**(1481), 773–786.

Schizophrenia Working Group of the Psychiatric Genomics Consortium (2014). Biological insights from 108 schizophrenia-associated genetic loci. *Nature*, **511**(7510), 421–427.

Schmidt, C.W. (2007). Environmental connections: a deeper look into mental illness. *Environmental Health Perspectives*, **115**(8), A404, A406–A410.

Sekar, A., Bialas, A.R., de Rivera, H., Davis, A., Hammond, T.R., Kamitaki, N., Tooley, K., Presumey, J., Baum, M., Van Doren, V., Genovese, G., Rose, S.A., Handsaker, R.E., et al. (2016). Schizophrenia risk from complex variation of complement component 4. *Nature*, **530**(7589), 177–183.

Seligman, M.E.P. (1972). Learned helplessness. *Annual Review of Medicine*, **23**(1), 407–412.

Shadlen, M.N. and Kiani, R. (2013). Decision making as a window on cognition. *Neuron*, **80**(3), 791–806.

Sims, R., van der Lee, S.J., Naj, A.C., Bellenguez, C., Badarinarayan, N., Jakobsdottir, J., Kunkle, B.W., Boland, A., Raybould, R., Bis, J.C., et al. (2017). Rare coding variants in PLCG2, ABI3, and TREM2 implicate microglial-mediated innate immunity in Alzheimer's disease. *Nature Genetics*, **49**(9), 1373–1384.

Singh, T., Walters, J.T.R., Johnstone, M., Curtis, D., Suvisaari, J., Torniainen, M., Rees, E., Iyegbe, C., Blackwood, D., McIntosh, A.M., Kirov, G., Geschwind, D., Murray, R.M., Di Forti, M., Bramon, E., Gandal, M., Hultman, C.M., Sklar, P.; INTERVAL Study; UK10K Consortium, Palotie, A., Sullivan, P.F., O'Donovan, M.C., Owen, M.J., and Barrett, J.C. (2017). The contribution of rare variants to risk of schizophrenia in individuals with and without intellectual disability. *Nature Genetics*, **49**(8), 1167–1173.

Slade, E.P., Jahn, D.R., Regenold, W.T., and Case, B.G. (2017). Association of electroconvulsive therapy with psychiatric readmissions in US hospitals. *JAMA Psychiatry*, **74**(8), 798–804.

Soon, C.S., Brass, M., Heinze, H.-J., and Haynes, J.-D. (2008). Unconscious determinants of free decisions in the human brain. *Nature Neuroscience*, *11*(5), 543–545.

Stephan, A.H., Barres, B.A., and Stevens, B. (2012). The complement system: an unexpected role in synaptic pruning during development and disease. *Annual Review of Neuroscience*, **35**(1), 369–389.

Sullivan, P.F., Daly, M.J., and O'Donovan, M. (2012). Genetic architectures of psychiatric disorders: the emerging picture and its implications. *Nature Reviews Genetics*, **13**(8), 537–551.

Thompson, L. and McCabe, R. (2012). The effect of clinician-patient alliance and communication on treatment adherence in mental health care: a systematic review. *BMC Psychiatry*, **12**(1), 87.

Walton, E., Hibar, D.P., van Erp, T.G.M., Potkin, S.G., Roiz-Santiañez, R., Crespo-Facorro, B., Suarez-Pinilla, P., van Haren, N.E.M., de Zwarte, S.M.C., Kahn, R.S., et al. (2018). Prefrontal cortical thinning links to negative symptoms in schizophrenia via the ENIGMA consortium. *Psychological Medicine*, **48**(1), 82–94.

Wray, N.R., Ripke, S., Mattheisen, M., Trzaskowski, M., Byrne, E.M., Abdellaoui, A., Adams, M.J., Agerbo, E., Air, T.M., Andlauer, T.M.F., et al. (2018). Genome-wide association analyses identify 44 risk variants and refine the genetic architecture of major depression. *Nature Genetics*, **50**(5), 668–681.

Xie, J. and Padoa-Schioppa, C. (2016). Neuronal remapping and circuit persistence in economic decisions. *Nature Neuroscience*, **19**(6), 855–861.

Chapter 18

The proper place of subjectivity, meaning, and folk psychology in psychiatry

Doug McConnell

Introduction

In his Loebel Lectures and the chapter he has contributed to his volume (Chapter 17), Steven Hyman makes a strong case for an increasingly neurobiological approach to psychiatry and clinical psychology. He is surely right that, as we develop better understandings of the neurobiological aetiology of disorders, we will be able to design more effective diagnostic tools and treatments by targeting the relevant neurobiology. At the same time, these neurobiological discoveries may reveal that, historically, we have been putting too much stock in the testimony of patients and their peers, and unfairly apportioning responsibility for mental disorders to patients and their families.

Hyman argues that accurate diagnosis and effective treatment of mental disorders must be neurobiological. He makes a convincing case for this in regard to schizophrenia where neuroanatomical anomalies appear central to aetiology and, presumably, will have to be addressed by any treatment that hopes to transform or cure the disorder rather than merely treat symptoms. Hyman also emphasizes the importance of treating the patient as a person. Clinicians should sympathize with patients and attempt to understand patients' folk psychological interpretations of their disorders. However, on Hyman's view, these interpersonal aspects of treatment are ancillary; they are valuable because they mitigate the symptomatic distress of mental disorders and encourage the patient to comply with treatment, but they can only indirectly reveal and influence the underlying neurobiological causes of mental disorders.

I agree with Hyman that neurobiological considerations in psychiatry are crucial and we should expect neurobiology to continue to improve the diagnosis and treatment of mental disorders. I also agree that interpersonal interactions in the clinic should treat patients with respect, sympathy, and understanding as a way of managing symptomatic distress. Nevertheless, I argue that Hyman underplays the role of the patient and her conceptual mental content in the aetiology and treatment of mental disorder. Hyman makes three unwarranted assumptions. First, neurobiology describes the sole fundamental truth about brain activity. Second, a person's conceptual mental content is reducible to her brain states. Third, the referents of folk psychological concepts (e.g.

subjective interpretations of feelings, desires, values, etc.) are largely fictional, at best rough approximations for the neurobiology underpinning the things they refer to. I argue that conceptual mental content is irreducible to brain states and Hyman mistakes the vehicle of content for the content itself. Neurobiology and folk psychology each capture different sets of truths about the operations of the brain. Once we see how conceptual content, including the referents of folk psychology, shape brain activity, it becomes clear that content itself (or a lack of it) can be pathological and treatment will sometimes be effective, even curative, by addressing that content.[1] Therefore, diagnosis and treatment of mental disorders cannot just focus on neurobiology, they must also consider conceptual content and the complex interactions between content and the neurobiology instantiating it.

I begin my commentary by briefly setting out Hyman's position. I then show how a plausible description of the relationship between a linguistic community, natural language, and individuals' conceptual content entails that conceptual content is irreducible to brain states. I discuss the difference between descriptions of objective phenomena and expressions of subjective phenomena to argue that neurobiology and folk psychology are engaged in different enterprises with different success criteria. Therefore, folk psychology should not be seen as a largely fictitious approximation of neurobiology. Finally, armed with my different view of the relationship between patients, conceptual content, and neurobiology, I revisit the implications of neuroscientific advances for psychiatry and clinical psychology.

Hyman's view

Hyman claims that 'scientific investigation … eventually brings us closer to the true state of affairs … while folk psychology lacks such truth value' (p. 281, this volume). Therefore, it makes sense that we should preference neuroscientific methods to classify, diagnose, and treat mental disorders. To use folk psychology for these purposes would distort our understanding of mental disorders and result in relatively ineffective treatments. But, despite the inferiority of folk psychology in revealing the truth, Hyman believes it is a much more adaptive way to manage human interactions than neuroscience. This is because the effortless automatic thoughts and responses captured by folk psychology are highly advantaged over the effortful, scientifically-based conscious cognition in their speed and their access to the massive processing power of unconscious neural circuitry.

Hyman is clearly right that the methods of folk psychology are far more helpful for understanding our own minds and communicating and interpreting the mental lives

---

[1] I won't address the issue of whether the agent qua agent is really in control of his own actions. It is possible that, despite the fundamental distinction between conceptual content and brain processes, there is still no sense in which the agent exerts independent control. Some of the factors determining action just happen to have conceptual content; we don't spin our stories, our stories spin us (Dennett, 1991).

of others than trying to attain and interpret neuroscientific information about our brains and those of others.[2] Given the pragmatic value of folk psychology in mediating interpersonal interactions, Hyman retains an important role for folk psychology in the clinic. Clinicians need to interact with patients interpersonally, to do this in a smooth, respectful, sympathetic, understanding way, the clinician needs to make use of folk psychology. 'The feeling of being respected and understood may influence patients' acceptance of treatment recommendations and adherence to the prescribed regimen' (p. 281, this volume). Furthermore, 'the experience of empathy, caring, and being listened to can initiate new learning, best taken in by such interpersonal channels, signifying that they are not outcasts, but deserving of treatment and respect' (p. 282, this volume).

Hyman's characterizations of science and folk psychology lead him to promote a strict division of labour in the clinic—the scientific approach uses neurobiology to provide accurate aetiologies and effective treatments while the interpersonal approach uses folk psychology to build rapport and mitigate distress. He states that '[i]nteractions with the patient as subject should not be taken to illuminate disease pathogenesis' (p. 288, this volume) presumably because the inaccuracies of folk psychology will distort the true neural picture of what is going on. Likewise, it would be impossible to build a respectful, sympathetic rapport with a patient through neuroscience alone. Hyman acknowledges that this division of labour is not yet perfect because the limitations in technology and neurobiological understanding force the clinician 'to rely on the testimony and behaviour of patients and their social milieu for clues to what might be happening at the brain-level' (p. 277, this volume). But, ideally, clinicians will eventually swap those folk psychologically tainted clues for biomarkers because 'all human beings … lack direct introspective access to the functioning of their brains [so] ideas, theories, and explanations of aetiology or causation grounded in introspection and subjective report or in the attributions and inferences of family members, clinicians, and others are at best hazy proxies for actual brain mechanisms and at worst outright false.' (p. 277, this volume).

Nobody would dispute that neurobiological practice is the best method for revealing neurobiological truths and folk psychology is poor at revealing neurobiological truths. Therefore, once Hyman assumes that neurobiology represents the only fundamental truth about human minds, it follows that folk psychology is inferior to neuroscience for revealing aetiology and guiding treatment design. It also entails that the truth value of folk psychological statements depends only on how well they convey what is happening neurobiologically; folk psychological statements don't do this very well so they

---

[2] Hyman ignores the fact that sometimes we think effortfully and consciously in folk psychological terms, for example, when we try to predict the next move of a serial killer or interpret the feelings of a love-interest through his or her actions. Presumably the neurobiologist also sometimes uses familiar neurobiological concepts automatically and effortlessly when engaged in neurobiology. As I will argue later, the reason folk psychology is more helpful for interpersonal interactions than neuroscience is not because it is more suited to unreflective thought but because it is designed to communicate our subjective worlds while neuroscience is not.

can be written off as largely fictional. The only reasons folk psychology persists is that it remains a useful simplification given that human brains cannot do complex neuroscience in real time and because neuroscience still has a long way to go to give us a complete understanding of the human brain.

Normatively governed conceptual content shapes the brain

The first of Hyman's assumptions that I will challenge is that conceptual content is reducible to brain states. We are each born into a world of sociocultural norms that govern, among other things, morality, conceptions of a good life (e.g. raising family, pursuing a career), and language use. At birth, the individual is ignorant of these norms, they are not built-in to his biology but his brain is well adapted to learn them. As individuals learn these norms they tap into the historically accumulated store of cultural knowledge and gain the ability to communicate and cooperate with others.

It is through learning the norms of natural language that individuals develop the capacity to think with conceptual content. Natural language provides a set of conceptual tools for carving up the world into categories and specifying meaningful links between those categories. Knowing the concept *Dog*, for example, renders dogs salient qua dogs, as a category of things distinct from other similar looking animals in other categories (badgers, cats, foxes). Knowing a concept also entails knowing a set of meaningful connections between that concept and others, knowing the concept *Dog* entails knowing that dogs are creatures with teeth that bark, chase sticks, and so on. Therefore, when an individual who knows the concept *Dog* interacts with dogs, his experience of them is informed by that concept which allows him to link his experience with the store of cultural knowledge and meanings around dogs.[3]

Importantly, when individuals use conceptual content they are beholden to the norms governing use of that content in the linguistic community. To understand a concept is roughly to engage with it successfully in the aspects of natural language where the concept is expressed, for example, to refer to the right set of things as dogs and conceptually connect dogs with the right things. Where what is 'right' is judged by the linguistic community. When I remark on a dog running across the street, for example:

> The concept *Dog* and the rules governing it (as taught to me and current in my conversations with others) determine the contents of my mind in this situation and … the correctness of my view of it is governed by criteria not intrinsic to my own experience. … Conceptualising objects correctly is, therefore, not a matter for private (or even

---

[3] The intentionality or 'aboutness' of experience and goal-directed action needn't be conceptual. All animals display intentionality in their interactions with the world and concept users continue to experience, desire, and act in non-conceptual ways. For concept-users, conceptual and non-conceptual experience interact in complex ways. For example, the experience of pleasurable rewards creates non-conceptual 'incentive salience desires' that can drive action and influence the agent's conceptual judgement of their best interests (Dill and Holton, 2014).

subjective) determination but requires the discursive subject to fit into the praxis that is language. (Gillett, 2009, pp. 115–116).

This is a crucial point because it entails that the correct use of conceptual content doesn't depend on the thinker's neurobiology alone but on the alignment between the individual's use of the concept and the social norms governing that concept.

Of course, people need certain physiological capacities if they are to instantiate concepts in their brains. A red/green colour-blind person cannot properly group the sets of stimuli that society categorizes with the concepts *Red* and *Green*. The possibility of sharing a language depends on there being certain biological similarities between us but this shared biology underdetermines the variety of concepts that communities develop. Furthermore, concepts create feedback loops which can have exponential effects on concept users and their world (Hacking, 1996). An individual who discovers he is categorized as a schizophrenic will change in reaction to that concept, perhaps fear of stigma leads him to be less social. When others learn of his status as a schizophrenic, their reaction to him will also change, perhaps they suspect him of being paranoid. As a result, he might take on further self-conceptualizations such as being reclusive and paranoid, then those concepts in turn have feedback effects. For a detailed discussion of these dynamics see Tekin (2011).

We face a puzzle once we accept both that the rules for concept use are normatively fixed and cannot be derived from an individual's neurobiology and that the neurochemical laws governing brain processes are biologically fixed and ignorant of cultural norms. Given that concepts are instantiated in the brain, how is it that an agent can follow social norms while the causal processes instantiating the meaning are ignorant of those norms? It seems that neurons somehow encode normatively governed meanings so that patterns of neural firing have causes in the brain that are consistent with the meaning encoded. Causal processes that obey sociocultural norms of meaning, however, are fundamentally different than biological causes which only follow natural laws. However the brain actually manages to manipulate conceptual content, it is clear that it does because people structure their thought and action using concepts. Therefore, the norms governing conceptual thought must drive the activity of neurons somewhat independently of the biochemical forces in the brain. Equally clearly, much of what the brain does is non-conceptual, even when the agent is thinking conceptually. 'The inescapable conclusion seems to be that the realm of words or significations, and therefore sociocultural reality, and the environmental or physical determination of content combine to shape the processing structure of the brain' (Gillett, 2007, p. 148).

On this view, neurobiological processes influence conceptual content, but that content also exerts an independent influence on neurobiology. When agents use conceptual content, they are affected both through the biology of the neurons required to manipulate that content and through the meaning of the content. It is because I understand something of what it *means* to be diagnosed as a schizophrenic, that is, the concepts that it connects me with, that I feel a surge of anxiety upon hearing my diagnosis. Likewise, many non-conceptual brain processes don't just have biological affects, they change the conceptual content at play, for example, a cue-driven dopamine surge directs attention to the presence of a drug dealer, a stroke wipes out access to certain episodic memories, and so on.[4]

The truth of folk psychological referents

Once we acknowledge the independent influence of normatively governed conceptual content, we can no longer expect neurobiology to provide the only fundamental truths about what is happening in the brain. There is more than one aspect of mind/brain reality that language might aim at. One might refer to the physical, objective world but one might also refer to the normative world or particular instances of conceptual thought shaped by that normative world. Each of these linguistic practices target different truths; they have different success criteria. Consider, for example, the various linguistic practices made possible by the concept *Neuron*. One might simply use the concept, that is, to coordinate activities related to neurons in the world, such as neuroscience, which may include pointing out instances of neurons in the world. Success here requires using the concept according to the norms governing it. One might refer to the concept of *Neuron* itself, for example, to explain how to use the concept. Success here requires distinguishing the concept from other concepts, providing something like a dictionary definition. Finally, one might also refer to the role the concept *Neuron* is playing in one's own thought or that of others. Success here depends on whether I or others are really structuring thought and action with that concept. I can judge whether others are using the concept *Neuron* by whether they structure their speech and action according to the norms governing the concept. I can judge whether I am using the concept myself if I know the concept and I can be confident I know the concept when I have been trained to use it by other competent concept users.

When we try to work out what is happening in the minds of others or in our own mind we engage in folk psychology. One method of folk psychology is to assess whether a particular concept is in use or not. We can learn a lot about the mental lives of others by how they use (or fail to use) concepts. Someone who correctly uses the concept *Neuron*, for example, must have beliefs about neurons and other concepts connected to neurons, for example, *Brain*. Someone who doesn't know the concept *Neuron* cannot have beliefs about neurons or a range of more sophisticated beliefs that depend on knowing about neurons. However, folk psychology is not limited to making such indirect inferences. We can learn a lot more about what is happening in people's minds, including our own, by using concepts that are specifically designed to communicate our subjective worlds. Linguistic practices with concrete, objective referents we could call 'descriptive' and linguistic practices with subjective referents we could call 'expressive' (Harré, 2007). All sciences are descriptive in this sense and the folk also engage in non-scientific descriptive practice when they describe where the

---

[4] Of course, there will be a vast range of typical brain processes that never have any discernible impact on conceptual content but that are nevertheless required for a typically functioning brain.

television remote is, what a music group sounds like, and so on. In expressive prac-tice we use folk psychology to understand and express our subjective experience and understand others' expressions of their subjective experience. Our subjective worlds are private in the sense that they are unavailable for others to describe in the way we describe concrete objects.[5] The meaning of the concept *Pain* cannot be established by pointing at the object pain because the internal feelings of pain are never present in the public sphere to be pointed at, only expressions of pain are.[6] Given the private source of what we express, the subject has a degree of authority in his expression that he doesn't have in describing the objective world. Descriptions and the objective tar-gets of description are logically independent of each other but expressions and what they express are not. It doesn't make sense to say 'I know that I am in pain' because one cannot be mistaken about being in pain. One just says, 'I am in pain' (Harré, 2007). Subjective authority in expression is not absolute, however; expressive concepts are still governed by norms. Indeed, this is essential if we are to teach and correct people's use of expressive concepts. It is possible to form norms for categorizing subjective phenomena because humans tend to feel similar ways when they are in similar cir-cumstances, for example, when a person hops around yelling after a brick drops on his foot, we know he is in pain from our experience of things falling on us and our expres-sions of pain. These similarities in how we each experience the world entails that we can sometimes read others' subjective worlds better than they can themselves. When we struggle to understand and communicate our subjective worlds, others can help us by telling us how they felt in similar kinds of circumstance, for example, 'I know I felt anxious and alienated from others when I was diagnosed with schizophrenia, do you feel like that?' Inaccurate self-expressions are suspected when we see mismatches be-tween someone's claims and other, more plausible folk psychological interpretations of their behaviour. When we see the look of disgust on a child's face when he bites into a raw onion, we are sure that he doesn't like that taste even though he tells us that he likes it. Rather, than believe his testimony we suspect he is saying that to save face; he's not so silly that he would bite into an onion if he didn't like it! Similarly, someone might be deluded in thinking that he did something out of kindness when everyone can see that the more likely explanation is that he did it out of self-interest. Our lack of direct access to others' subjective worlds, however, means that when we try to correct or improve others' self-expressions we must make educated guesses based on whatever information is publicly accessible, for example, others' patterns of socioculturally situ-ated behaviour. We might become convinced that, unusually, this child really does like raw onions when we see him eating them despite having other options and nobody around to prove anything to. In contrast, there is no deference to subjective authority when we judge the truth of descriptive language, for example, if a particular animal counts as a dog or not. All the information necessary to judge the accuracy of objective

---

[5] I don't deny that we also talk about 'describing' our subjective worlds, however, I think that the practice of describing the objective world is fundamentally different from the practice of describing a subjective world.

[6] Fake expressions of pain and descriptions of people in pain, including descriptions of the neural correlates of pain, are parasitic on genuine expressions of pain.

descriptions is publicly available and so scientific assessments can overrule the claims of any individual.

The difference between descriptive and expressive concepts is, however, irrelevant to the very real influence both kinds of concepts have in concept-user's minds. Whether someone is really structuring their thought and action with a concept depends on whether they are following the norms for that concept not whether the referents are concrete or subjective.[7] Just as people structure their thought with concepts like *Neuron*, it seems undeniable that they structure their thought with expressive concepts like *Pain*, *Value*, *Belief*, *Desire*, and *Intention*. If someone says, 'I feel like making a bet, so I'm going to the bookmakers' the folk psychological concepts at play provide insight into how this agent is conceptually structuring his thought and action. He wants to make a bet, he intends to make a bet, he believes that a bet can made at the bookmakers, and so on. But must we really rely on the rather messy business of folk psychology to find out what is happening in other minds or can we get a more accurate picture by describing the neural processes underpinning their concept use?

The relationship between folk psychology and neurobiology

Hyman claims that we must settle for rough and ready folk psychology in our interpersonal interactions because the limitations of human cognition and perception mean that we cannot process the complex but more accurate neurobiological picture of those interactions. On his view, folk psychology is *only* maintained because it provides an adaptive proxy for what is really happening at the neurobiological level. This entails that we should abandon folk psychology if we happened to develop the perceptual and cognitive skills to use neurobiology to communicate our subjective worlds instead.

As argued previously, however, the neural processes underpinning conceptual thought, no matter how accurately described, cannot capture the norm-governed content of concepts. This is because norms are sociocultural entities revealed and inculcated through interpersonal practices not neurobiological entities revealed by observing biological processes. Neuroscientific work can detect and improve inaccurate brain descriptions, but it cannot detect and improve inaccurate concept-use (whether those concepts are expressive or descriptive). We can only detect correct concept-use through interpersonal interactions where we judge whether an individual is following the sociocultural norms governing the concept, and we can only correct concept-use by inculcating norms through shared practice. Therefore, although Hyman is right that folk psychological understandings of oneself and others are often inaccurate, we cannot correct our own folk psychological understandings nor those of others by looking at the brains involved. The fundamental reason that folk psychology cannot be replaced by neurobiology, then, is that each practice targets different truths. Folk psychology aims at truths in our (inter-)subjective worlds while neuroscience is

---

[7] Descriptive linguistic practices can also refer to imaginary things (e.g. unicorns) and there are normative rules for using these concepts correctly. So expressive linguistic practice is not alone in having concepts without physical referents.

one of several scientific practices that aims at true descriptions of objective reality.[8] Therefore, one should not see folk psychology as a rough proxy for neurobiology. It is possible, however, to find *associations* between subjective phenomena, such as concept use, and brain descriptions, but these associations are likely to be quite weak, so that one couldn't hope to infer either precise conceptual content from brain data or neurobiology from conceptual content. To illustrate this, imagine trying to develop a device that could read conceptual content off the brain. We would have to identify associations between patterns of neural firing and instances of each concept in use. To do this we would need to calibrate the machine so that it could distinguish the brain states associated with each concept from the background neural noise. Therefore, in developing the neurobiological markers for each concept, we would still depend on folk psychology to judge when the subject is or is not using a concept. That issue aside, we would face a further problem given that each individual has a unique, holistic network of conceptual content instantiated in a unique way in his brain. If a patient thinks, 'I'm a failure because I failed to meet my father's standards', for example, the associated conceptual network of memories, expectations, and values, and the neural firing underpinning it depend on the unique history of this father–son relationship, the standards of this father, the specific failures in this life, and so on. If our scanner has been calibrated using a population, for example, an averaged neural firing pattern for when people think 'I'm a failure because I failed to meet my father's standards', then the brain scan would only reveal the content of the target patient's thought to the extent her brain activity matched that of the population average. Furthermore, the variation between each member of the population used to calibrate the machine might entail that the average of their neural firing patterns would be too vague to specify the conceptual content operating in the patient's mind. Such a scanner would almost certainly provide less resolution on the patient's conceptual content than what we could discover through folk psychology. Alternatively, we could calibrate the scanner specifically to the target patient but, given that we rely on folk psychology to calibrate the scanner anyway, we may as well abandon the scanner and just use folk psychology.

Hyman is correct that folk psychological concepts are adaptive; most concepts are adaptive because they mark groupings of stimulus features and cognitive associations that society has found useful in the past (Gillett, 2007); words convey 'good tricks' (Dennett, 1995). But folk psychological content is not adaptive because it provides a simplified representation of what is happening in one's brain. It is adaptive because it is the *only* linguistic practice that allows the agent to understand and express his subjective world and to understand the subjective worlds of others. Neurobiological concepts, in contrast, are adaptive because they help us understand the neurobiology of brains, not because they elucidate subjective experience. Trying to use neurobiology to interpret subjective worlds or trying to use folk psychology to describe the objective world would *both* be maladaptive practices because each involves taking a sophisticated set of tools and using them for purpose for which they were not designed.

---

[8] Therefore, there is a fundamental barrier to Glover's suggestion (Chapter 19, this volume) that we might aim to somehow merge the language of folk psychology with that of neuroscience.

I also agree with Hyman that people don't have introspective access to their own brain processes, including the brain processes that underpin their manipulation of conceptual content. Hyman makes a lot of this because, on his view, this means that people cannot access the fundamental neurobiological truth about the mind. People do, however, have some introspective access to their subjective experience and conceptual content and, despite their cognitive biases and limitations, they can, much of the time, reliably say what they feel, believe, desire, value, and so on. In other words, people don't have introspective access to the neural vehicles of their conceptual content, but they typically have some introspective access to the content itself. Furthermore, as discussed earlier, people can also make fairly accurate guesses about the subjective worlds of others because others structure their lives according to public norms. If we accept that conceptual content can capture truths about subjective thought and experience, then it follows that people can introspect truths about their own subjective worlds and infer truths about the subjective worlds of others. I turn now to the implications of my objections for Hyman's vision of psychiatry and clinical psychology.

Reconciling the normativity of mental disorder with neuroscientific psychiatry

By acknowledging the reality of sociocultural norms, we can resolve a contradiction at the heart of Hyman's view of psychiatry. It is nearly universally accepted that the distinction between mental health and disorder is set by normative standards governing experience, thought, and action. We realize that something is wrong when someone reports mental distress of greater intensity or duration than normal, perceives things that nobody else does, reasons in a way that doesn't make sense, exhibits extreme swings in emotion, consistently uses drugs in a highly self-destructive way, and so on. This entails that a person's neurobiology can only be called pathological because of its connection to violations of folk psychological norms (Banner, 2013). If what we ultimately care about when it comes to mental health are such person-level phenomena rather than the brain-level phenomena, then abnormal brain types that *never* lead to normative transgressions have no place in a list of mental disorders (Nordenfelt, 2007, p. 29). We may well discover biomarkers that guarantee the future development of a mental disorder in the same way we say someone has Huntington's disease before the onset of symptoms. However, such biomarkers only count as biomarkers for mental disorder because they predict the relevant normative transgressions in the future. If the biomarker didn't predict the likelihood of the relevant normative transgressions, then it wouldn't be a biomarker of mental disorder.

The view that mental disorders are inherently normative introduces a tension to Hyman's view that neuroscience reveals the true picture of the world while the world of folk psychological norms is an adaptive fiction. If mental disorders are inherently normative, person-level problems, then they are fictional, part of our shared delusion about the importance of people, agency, responsibility, and so on. One might still see neuroscience as the best approach to psychiatry because of its power to reveal the truth, but, if mental disorders are normative, this entails that neuroscience is being applied in service of our shared delusions and brought to bear on fictional problems (albeit fictional problems that we are desperate to solve). As a rule, we shouldn't allow fictional concepts to guide our truth-seeking practices. If folk psychological norms are fictions than using them to set the agenda for neuroscience is like letting astrologers decide how to spend NASA's budget. Neuroscience will be hamstrung in its ability to reveal the truth if the targets of its investigation are set by non-scientific fictions. It would be better to let neuroscience set its own targets. How can we resolve this tension? One method would be to give up on the idea that mental disorder is inherently normative and search for a value-neutral, neurobiological definition of mental disorder thereby naturalizing psychiatry. There have been attempts to do this, but they do not seem promising. Naturalistic boundaries for mental disorders, such as those set by biostatistical averages or evolutionary fitness, just don't correlate with the boundaries we take to distinguish the healthy from the pathological (Bolton, 2008; Varga, 2015). A better way to resolve the tension, in my view, is to abandon the view that neurobiology provides the sole fundamental truth about the brain and upgrade the metaphysical status of our norms from adaptive fiction to reality. If we make that move, then our conceptions of mental disorder and mental health remain normative, but they are no less real because of that.[9]

If one accepts that mental disorders are inherently normative, it commits one to the view that the most effective treatment is whatever enables the patient to accord with the norms of mental health as swiftly and robustly as possible. However, it does *not* commit one to any specific view about the aetiologies of mental disorders or the form effective treatments will take. Neither does it commit one to the view that mental disorders should be classified and diagnosed according to the ways in which sufferers violate norms. Rather, the best classificatory and diagnostic systems for mental disorder will be whatever accurately and quickly match the patient with the most effective treatments (that may involve classifying mental disorders by aetiology rather than by presentation as Hyman claims). There are, however, reasons for thinking that the most effective form of psychiatry will not be one where all mental disorders are classified and diagnosed according to their neurobiological causes and where the most effective treatments are all neurobiological in focus.

The therapeutic importance of conceptual content

Once we recognize that conceptual content has effects in the brain independent of what is captured by descriptions of the neurobiology instantiating that content, it follows that conceptual content (or lack of it) can be an independent cause of pathology and a target for disease-altering, even curative, treatment. It is therefore a mistake

---

[9] The norms governing what counts as mental illness need to be justified, of course. Not all normative categorizations are true, consider the mistaken pathologization of homosexuality, for example. The challenge for normativist approaches is to justify the set of normative transgressions that signify mental illness suitable for psychiatric care, and distinguish them from other kinds of normative transgression, such as immoral action suitable for the judiciary and deviant behaviour that doesn't need any societal response. We need to make sure we are not pathologizing unusual behaviour, excusing immoral behaviour, or constructing mental disorders that don't exist. I'm confident this can be achieved but I cannot pursue these issues here.

to think, as Hyman does, that there should be a strict division of labour in the clinic where neurobiology provides accurate aetiologies and effective treatments while folk psychology only builds rapport and mitigates distress.

It is not difficult to imagine an example of mental disorder where pathological conceptual content features centrally in aetiology and should be addressed primarily in treatment. For example, inauthentic or unrealistic values may be at the root of some people's mental disorders. Imagine an effeminate man who desperately wants to live up to his authoritarian father's old-fashioned ideals of what a 'proper man' should be but has been unable to. His inability to either conform to his father's ideals or reject the importance of those ideals results in consistent failure, a loss of self-worth, and eventually leads to serious depression. In this case, clinicians need to elucidate the patient's beliefs and values and assess their role in his mental disorder. As discussed previously, the individual has some introspective access to his subjective world, therefore, as a starting point, clinicians should listen to the patient's introspective reports. Patients can be unsure and inaccurate in their self-expression so clinicians should use folk psychology to assess the patient's expressions by asking questions and suggesting possible alternative or novel content for the patient to consider. Treatment of this disorder should help the patient adjust his beliefs and values in ways that better support his mental health. This might involve helping him recognize and give up on inauthentic values, develop more authentic values, and forgive himself for failing to achieve inauthentic goals. A neurobiological assessment of the patient's brain, no matter how sophisticated, will be unable to reveal the norm-governed values that are central to the mental disorder nor make the normative distinction between authentic and inauthentic values. So, Hyman's diagnostic approach of favouring the neurobiology and ignoring the folk psychology would be blind to the causes of this kind of mental disorder. Similarly, neurobiological treatments can play little role in making specific adjustments to the patient's conceptual content. Neurobiological interventions can lower the barrier to changes in conceptual content, for example, pharmacotherapy making it less painful to address certain memories; however, such interventions don't recommend any specific content, it remains for the patient to decide which specific changes to content are made.

Mental disorders caused predominantly by pathological conceptual content might be relatively rare. It should be much more common, however, that pathological content is one of several independent contributors to mental disorder and so should be one of several foci in treatment (Bolton, 2007, pp. 120–122; McConnell and Snoek, 2018). Mental disorders are often likely to be caused by a combination of neurobiology and conceptual content because neurobiology and content interact extensively. For example, an initial brain pathology, say, a genetic susceptibility to alcoholism, might lead to pathological conceptual content, 'I can't control my drinking'. Subsequently, that pathological content can become an independent cause that compounds the disorder. Believing oneself to be a hopeless addict, for example, can make it harder to recover than if one is just overly responsive to drug-using cues. All else equal, an addicted person with a highly fatalistic self-concept is arguably more likely to remain addicted than someone without such a concept (Pickard, 2012; McConnell and Anke, 2018). Once pathological conceptual content has become an independent causal factor it can ensure that the disorder remains, even once the original pathological neurobiology is successfully treated.

Because neurobiology and conceptual content interact, it will often be the case that mental disorders have mixed aetiology; there won't be a single root cause of a disorder that is just neurobiological or just based in conceptual content. Diagnosis and treatment need to consider conceptual content to the extent that conceptual content or lack of it contributes to disease aetiology.[10] Hyman considers but dismisses the role of the patient's folk psychological self-understandings. He claims that the patient's lived experience and interpersonal interactions can be thought of 'as *mechanistic* contributors to pathogenesis and healing' (p. 269, this volume, italics added). We can now see, however, based on the previous arguments, that conceptually structured thought and experience have effects according to what the content *means*, and meaning is grounded in sociocultural norms, not biological mechanism.

None of this is to say that some mental disorders might be best explained and treated by neurobiology. The evidence that Hyman presents to explain the aetiology of schizophrenia indicates that it is strongly influenced by neurobiological factors. There may be very little that can be done in terms of conceptual content that will effectively treat this disorder. In those cases, it is likely that any treatment hoping to cure or significantly transform the disease (rather than address symptoms) will have to target the neurological causes. But Hyman has painted himself into a corner where he is forced to treat *all* mental disorders the way he treats schizophrenia. Addiction, depression, post-traumatic stress disorder, and anxiety disorders, for example, are more likely to be significantly influenced by the patient's conceptual content. By ignoring how the socioculturally grounded meanings of conceptual content influence the brain and failing to recognize the power of folk psychology to understand and adjust that content, Hyman cuts himself off from an essential way of diagnosing and effectively treating an important aspect of many mental disorders. Clinicians need to be aware that mental disorders may have a variety of different causes, some neurobiological, some involving conceptual content, and often both. To the extent that conceptual content can be an independent cause of mental disorders we should use discursive therapies grounded in folk psychology to treat them. Psychiatry and clinical psychology should certainly welcome advances in neurobiology and, to the extent that neurobiological truths improve treatment, we should expect neurobiology to become more prevalent in the clinic. This increased focus on neurobiology should not come at the expense of folk psychology, however, because folk psychology is our only means of communicating our subjective worlds.

---

[10] A similar point could be made about the potential for the environment to be an independent contributor to mental disorder. A case of addiction could be cured, for example, if the addicted person could be moved from a stressful environment with many drug-using cues to one where there were many non-drug-using rewards and few drug-using cues. We could, therefore, think of environmental management as a focus for treatment in addition to considerations of neurobiology and conceptual content.

References

Banner, N.F. (2013). Mental disorders are not brain disorders. *Journal of Evaluation in Clinical Practice*, **19**(3), 509–513.

Bolton, D. (2007). Meaning and causal explanations in the behavioural sciences. In: B. Fulford, K. Morris, J. Sadler, & G. Stanghellini (Eds.), *Nature and Narrative* (pp. 113–126). Oxford: Oxford University Press.

Bolton, D. (2008). *What is Mental Disorder?: An Essay in Philosophy, Science, and Values*. Oxford: Oxford University Press.

Dennett, D. (1991). *Consciousness Explained*. Boston, MA: Little, Brown and Company.

Dennett, D. (1995). *Darwin's Dangerous Idea*. London: Penguin.

Dill, B. and Holton, R. (2014). The addict in us all. *Frontiers in Psychiatry*, **5**(Oct), 1–20.

Gillett, G. (2007). Form and content: the role of discourse in mental disorder. In: B. Fulford, K. Morris, J. Sadler, and G. Stanghellini (Eds.), *Nature and Narrative* (pp. 139–154). Oxford: Oxford University Press.

Gillett, G. (2009). *The Mind and Its Discontents* (2nd ed.). Oxford: Oxford University Press.

Hacking, I. (1996). The looping effects of human kinds. In D. Sperber, D. Premack, and A.J. Premack (Eds.), *Causal Cognition: A Multidisciplinary Debate* (pp. 351–394). Oxford: Oxford University Press.

Harré, R. (2007). Subjectivity and the possibility of psychiatry. In B. Fulford, K. Morris, J. Sadler, and G. Stanghellini (Eds.), *Nature and Narrative* (pp. 127–138). Oxford: Oxford University Press.

McConnell, D. and Anke, S. (2018). The importance of self-narration in recovery from addiction. *Philosophy, Psychiatry, and Psychology*, **25**(3), 31–44.

Nordenfelt, L. (2007). The concepts of health and illness revisited. *Medicine, Health Care and Philosophy*, **10**(1), 5–10.

Pickard, H. (2012). The purpose in chronic addiction. *AJOB Neuroscience*, **3**(2), 40–49.

Tekin, S. (2011). Self-concept through the diagnostic looking glass: Narratives and mental disorder. *Philosophical Psychology*, 24(3), 357–380. doi:10.1080/09515089.2011.559622

Varga, S. (2015). *Naturalism, Interpretation, and Mental Disorder*. Oxford: Oxford University Press.

Chapter 19

Psychiatry, folk psychology, and the impact of neuroscience— a response to Steven Hyman's Loebel Lectures

Jonathan Glover

Introduction

In 2001, Steven Hyman left the US National Institute of Mental Health (NIMH) and took up the post of Provost of Harvard University. He told us that when he left the NIMH he saw little progress in fundamental scientific understanding of psychiatric conditions. It is encouraging that he has returned to psychiatric research because now he believes this has changed. His stimulating Loebel Lectures reflect this optimism and give reasons for it.

The lectures revolve round a contrast between our folk psychology and what neuroscience is starting to reveal.

Our folk psychology is our unscientific picture of what goes on in people's minds when they perceive, remember, think, feel, decide, and act. It is based on introspection and on intuitive 'reading' of other people. Following much current practice, but with some reluctance, I use this phrase 'folk psychology'. The term suggests something unscientific and primitive, crying out to be replaced. My sympathies are with Peter Strawson's comment that it is the psychology of such simple folk as Shakespeare, Tolstoy, Proust, and Henry James.

In contrast to folk psychology is the fine structure neuroscience is starting to reveal: the brain mechanisms underlying perception, memory, thought, emotion, decision, and action. Hyman says that mapping out this fine structure has the promise of changing our understanding and treatment of psychiatric disorders.

Out of this emerges Hyman's philosophical claim that neuroscience radically challenges the status of our folk psychology. The brain mechanisms conflict with our intuitive picture of our own psychology in surprising ways. The neuroscientific account is true: it describes what is really going on. So our folk psychology, being in conflict with neuroscience, is largely false.

The incompatibility is sometimes local: the brain mechanisms involved in traumatic memory, in addiction, or in schizophrenia are not what we would have predicted intuitively. It is also global. Neuroscience's big picture of the brain is mechanistic: its activity is that of a large number of interacting mechanisms. But the picture we have of our own agency, our own decisions and actions, seems incompatible with mechanism. The suggestion is that here again the progress of neuroscience is likely to prove our folk psychology false.

Hyman's conclusion is not that clinical treatment should abandon folk psychology. In psychiatry these false beliefs cannot simply be pushed aside. Treatment is unlikely to work if patients are expected to see themselves as machines. Although neuroscience has such promise for treatment, psychiatry cannot attend only to synapses, protein complexes, or circuits in the brain. Attention has to be paid to the way people's problems are bound up with their subjective experiences and personal narratives. And since the false intuitive picture cannot be integrated into the true neuroscientific picture, the clinician has to switch backwards and forwards between the two.

These comments will start by expressing some support for the optimism about neuroscience leading to better psychiatric treatments. They will then turn to discuss the philosophical claims.

First, support for the optimism. Preceded by a slight caution: it is not easy to predict the future of scientific medicine. In the early days of molecular genetics, some were optimistic about the likely impact on treatment by discovering the gene for schizophrenia. Now we know that 'the' gene for schizophrenia does not exist. Well over 250 genetic variants relevant to schizophrenia have been found, each one contributing only a part of the genetic role in the disorder. This more complicated genetic picture could be repeated in neuroscience. We may be in for a much slower process of developing clinical applications than we would like to think.

But slower progress is still progress. Short-term pessimism can fit with long-term optimism. The timescale for the optimism was not spelled out in the lectures. If quite a bit of it was long term, I share it. Our grandchildren may benefit quite a lot more than our children. But, whatever the exact timescale, it would be odd if fuller understanding of the hugely complicated machinery of the brain *didn't* help us put right ways in which it goes wrong.

This response will concentrate on the philosophical claim, first expressing some agreement (less than total, but still substantial) that neuroscience challenges our intuitive ideas in surprising ways. I will disagree (to a substantial extent but not entirely) with the philosophical claim that our intuitive picture of our own psychology is largely false. The lectures are surely right that psychiatric treatment cannot ignore the intuitive way people think of themselves. But we may not have to switch back and forth between incompatible pictures. There is a case for choosing instead the fusion found in binocular vision to model of how the intuitive and scientific pictures can fit together.

Two challenges to folk psychology from neuroscience: post-traumatic memory and addictions

One of the exhilarating aspects of the lectures was their showing how neuroscience can disturb simple expectations based on our folk psychology. One striking case (stressed in the lectures as delivered but not in the text in this book) was post-traumatic memory. The folk psychology is one track: we remember the facts of the traumatic event and this leads to emotional disturbance. But the emerging neuroscientific account is two track. The first track, involving the hypothalamus, leads us to remember the facts of what happened. The second track, involving the amygdala, is implicated in the emotional disturbance. Lesions in the hypothalamus can wipe out the factual memory, leaving the disturbance intact. And lesions in the amygdala do the reverse. Here, under the influence of neuroscience, our simple one-track folk psychology needs to become two track.

Our folk psychology has been again too simple about addictions. It has assumed that addictive behaviour, such as an alcoholic's drinking, is caused by the pleasure involved. William James (1890/1950, p. 541) noted the puzzle that alcoholics stay addicted even if they dislike the taste of alcoholic drinks. Folk psychology again has to give ground. Hyman's own work is part of the story. Some addictive drugs mimic neurotransmitters such as dopamine. As Hyman (2005) has put it, addictive drugs hijack ordinary systems of motivation and learning. (I like the vivid hijacking image.) Long after William James, dopamine release at the appropriate places was assumed to be the correlate of pleasurable experiences. But neuroscience now gives a more complex account.

When monkeys have been taught to recognize a signal that juice is coming, it is not drinking itself that matters. It is the signal whose onset triggers high levels of dopamine release. So this firing seems the embodiment, not of pleasure but of enthusiastic anticipation. Understanding this about the hijacking is plausibly relevant to treatment. And the structure of the ordinary systems of motivation and learning that addictive drugs hijack turns out to be more complex than our folk psychology supposed.

Will our folk psychology go the way of the biblical account of the rainbow?

> And I will remember my covenant, which is between me and you and every living creature of all flesh; and the waters shall no more become a flood to destroy all flesh. And the bow shall be in the cloud; and I will look upon it, that I may remember the everlasting covenant between God and every living creature of all flesh that is upon the earth. (Genesis, 9:15–16)

The Bible explains the rainbow as the sign of God's covenant with Noah that there would never again be a flood covering the whole earth. This account has poetry the scientific story lacks. But, outside the private world of fundamentalists, it is not believed. It cannot compete with the testability and explanatory scope of what physics tells us.

Our intuitive psychology can also be poetic. Will it go the same way? This debate has taken place at different stages of science's history. When scientific developments give a picture substantially diverging from previous 'common sense', responses can be conservative, reformist, or revolutionary.

The conservative response rejects the science. The Church's response to Galileo is an obvious case. The response of Creationists to Darwin is another, encapsulated in a reported (or possibly misreported) question to T.H. Huxley. Bishop Wilberforce 'begged to know, was it through his grandfather or his grandmother that he claimed descent from a monkey?'(Sidgwick, 1898, pp. 433–434, quoted in Lucas, 1979).[1]

The reformers accept most or all of the new science and argue that, if some reforms are made to beliefs, the two are compatible. Usually it is the traditional religious beliefs that have to give ground. God did create the world, but did so as part of a universe in which it revolved around the sun. Or God created the world in a way that meant life would evolve on Darwinian lines. More rarely, the science is made to adapt to the religion. One version of that came from Philip Gosse. The fossil evidence is as Darwinians claim, but the Genesis story is still true. God just planted the fossils to look Darwinian in order to test our faith.

The revolutionary response is to abandon previous beliefs that do not fit the new science. In the cases of the rainbow, Galileo and Darwin this seems much the best bet.

But not all the philosophical debates about such issues give such a clear win to the revolutionary approach. In Britain in the 1930s, there was a debate whether the physics of the time showed the common sense picture of everyday physical objects was false. Contestants were the physicist Sir Arthur Eddington and the philosopher Susan Stebbing.

Nearly 90 years before Steven Hyman's Loebel Lectures, Eddington gave his 1927 Gifford Lectures on *The Nature of the Physical World*. He brought out the gulf between common sense and physics, by a consciously comic dramatization of some of the things common sense leaves out:

> I am standing on the threshold about to enter a room. It is a complicated business ... I must make sure of landing on a plank travelling at twenty miles a second round the sun—a fraction of a second too early or too late, the plank would be miles away ... The plank has no solidity of substance. To step on it is like stepping on a swarm of flies. Shall I not slip through? No, if I make the venture one of the flies hits me and gives a boost up again; I fall again and am knocked upwards by another fly; and so on. I may hope that the net result will be that I remain about steady; but if unfortunately I should slip through the floor ... the occurrence would be, not a violation of the laws of nature, but a rare coincidence. (Eddington, 1931, p. 342)

Susan Stebbing, in her 1937 book *Philosophy and the Physicists*, is severe about this passage, seeing confusion coming from everyday language being muddled up with philosophical or scientific language. She did not worry about Eddington slipping through the floor, saying his use of language is gravely misleading.

> I cannot doubt that it reveals serious confusion in Eddington's own thinking about 'the nature of the physical world'. Stepping on a plank is not in the least like 'stepping on a swarm of flies'... The plank is solid... it will support our weight ... What can be meant by saying that 'the plank has no solidity of substance'? (Stebbing, 1937, pp. 42–45)

She goes on to make the point that 'solid' is just the word used to describe one way in which a plank, a block of marble, and a cricket ball differ from a sponge, a soap bubble, or holes in a net.

---

[1] Lucas casts some doubt on whether Huxley really asked this question.

This rebuke is heavy-handedly literal. Of course Stebbing is right: in the ordinary use of the word, the plank and the bit of marble are undeniably solid. But Eddington obviously knew this. It would be astonishing to see Eddington entering a room like an acrobat leaping and straining at a really hard high-speed manoeuvre. This writing was not intended to be taken literally. It was probably not a good strategy for communicating. But it was meant to convey the strangeness of the world physics reveals. The underlying differences between solid planks and permeable things such as sponges, or things easily burst like soap bubbles, would never have been expected by common sense. Picking up on sloppy language or poor analogies is a thing philosophers do. But it is a pity when, following the less imaginative side of G.E. Moore, there is a too comfortable satisfaction with common sense. It can minimize the wonderful intellectual disturbance science can create.

Eddington said that for each table (or chair, pen, etc.) there were two: the everyday one and the scientific one. The everyday table was substantial: solid, coloured, and relatively permanent. But the scientific table was mostly empty space, in which were scattered 'numerous electric charges rushing about with great speed'. His conclusions about the everyday table parallel Hyman's about folk psychology. Only the scientific story is true, but the false unscientific story cannot be in practice be eliminated. Eddington said:

> I need not tell you that modern physics has by delicate test and remorseless logic assured me that my second scientific table is the only one that is really there ... On the other hand I need not tell you that modern physics will never succeed in exorcising that first table— strange compound of external nature, mental imagery and inherited prejudice- which lies visible to my eyes and tangible to my grasp. (Eddington, 1931, pp. xii–xiv)

These days there are no conceptual conservatives who reject what physics says about tables and planks. There are few revolutionaries who think the solidity of these items is illusory. Most of us are conceptual reformers. We do not slip through the floor because it *is* solid. But the best account of its solidity is the one given by physics.

In the present early stages of neuroscience, we should be cautious in what we accept. From outside the field it is not always easy to distinguish dramatic overhyped claims from genuine advances. Quite likely there are neuroscientific equivalents of 'the' gene for schizophrenia. But it would be bizarrely conservative to reject scientific accounts of the role of the hypothalamus and the amygdala in traumatic memory because they do not fit our folk psychology. The serious debate about the truth (as against the indispensability) of folk psychology is between revolutionaries and reformers. Will folk psychology go the way of the Genesis accounts of the rainbow and of the origin of humans? Or will it, like the solidity of the floor, survive through adjustment and accommodation to what science will tell us?

Some parts of folk psychology adapt to neuroscience more easily than others. The folk psychology of perception includes both kinds. The most general prescientific model of seeing was probably never fully spelt out. But it may have been a bit like the model I had as a child. The eyes are two holes, like windows in the head, through which I peer out from inside. This is uselessly non-explanatory. What is this 'I'? Does 'peering out' mean that inside the skull, behind the 'holes' is a smaller skull with its own 'holes', with the whole infinite regress that follows? This folk psychology model cannot survive being explicitly stated. It is just as well that neuroscience has replaced it with complex filtering and analysing mechanisms from the retina through to the visual cortex. And what we know of the role of binocular vision in depth perception even gives us a plausible account of why we have two eyes rather than one.

The primitive folk psychology of seeing may have presupposed a model of peering through holes in the skull. But few noticed this. It does not figure in how sophisticated folk psychologists think of particular perceptual activities. Consider Marcel Proust on recognizing someone:

> Even the simple act which we describe as 'seeing someone we know' is to some extent an intellectual process. We pack the physical outline of the person we see with all the notions we have already formed about him, and in the total picture of him which we compose in our minds those notions have certainly the principal place. In the end they come to fill out so completely the curve of his cheeks, to follow so exactly the line of his nose, they blend so harmoniously in the sound of his voice as if it were no more than a transparent envelope, that each time we see the face or hear the voice it is these notions which we recognise and to which we listen. (Proust, 1981, vol. 1, p. 20)

It was before modern neuroscience that Proust complicated the 'simple act' of seeing someone we know. Neuroscience may unravel the brain mechanisms that enable seeing to be shot through with pre-existing interpretations. Some of those mechanisms may take us by surprise. Some may not. And, if they do surprise us, there is no reason to *assume* that Proust's account must be unsustainable. It is not riddled with problems like the model of peering through holes in the skull.

Our intuitive ways of thinking about our own and other people's minds are complex. Neuroscience may well undermine some parts of them and fill out others. Neither reformers nor revolutionaries should expect total victory.

Conceptual revolution versus reform

Folk psychology should be able to adjust to the revisions required so far by the neuroscience of addiction and of post-traumatic memory.

Hyman's claim that normal systems of motivation and learning are hijacked by addictive drugs extends our folk psychology. It changes the picture and perhaps the treatment. It falsifies the belief that addictive drinking is initiated by enjoying the taste, replacing that trigger by an anticipatory response. Folk psychology should accommodate it without great strain. Revising our view of addiction, like revising our view of the solidity of the plank, may improve the overall picture.

Similarly, neuroscience shows the intuitive one-track model of post-traumatic memory is too simple. Evidence suggests we need a two-track model. As with addiction, the model needs to become more complex and fine grained. It was Thomas Kuhn (1962), in his book *The Structure of Scientific Revolutions*, who most influentially applied the political metaphor to science. The needed revisions look more like Kuhn's 'normal science' than like the fundamental paradigm shifts of his scientific revolutions. In normal science, we do not say that a field's existing paradigm is false, or that explanations within it lack truth, when progress requires substantial local revisions. A paradigm is declared false when the changes needed go beyond revisions to revolution.

There is a problem, in politics or in science, about deciding whether something is a revolution. The boundary is blurred between revolution and major reform. The continuum of degrees of change gives historians of politics or of science some free play about where to draw it. So it is reasonable to question the claim I have just made that these neurological developments are only normal science. What would count as a neuroscience-inspired revolution in thinking about the human mind? Two areas with the strongest claim to a revolutionary impact of neuroscience are schizophrenia and explanations of human agency.

Schizophrenia and delusions

Hyman's stimulating challenge is particularly forceful in his discussion of the science and treatment of schizophrenia. Here especially he communicates the enthusiasm that brought him back from Harvard to fundamental psychiatric research and to the hope it will transform treatment.

He stresses the *cognitive* impairments in schizophrenia. In late adolescence and young adulthood, the normal brain becomes more efficient by a process of 'pruning' weaker synapses that make little contribution to its activities. Often the onset of schizophrenic symptoms occurs around the same time as the pruning. Perhaps the two are linked, with the pruning getting out of normal control and eliminating not just weaker synapses but also needed stronger ones. In schizophrenia, the loss of brain tissue, especially in the prefrontal and temporal regions of the cerebral cortex, results in many fewer synapses. This is likely to reduce the ability to process information in ways needed for cognitive control of emotion and action.

So far, so plausible. But Hyman also brings out what makes research now potentially more exciting than before: the implications of links with genetics. Over 250 locations in the genome have been found to influence the risk of schizophrenia. Many of them may affect synapses. The one with the largest risk factor for schizophrenia influences how far the protein C4 is expressed in the brain. C4 is involved in marking weak synapses for elimination. Obviously the future of neuroscience is hard to predict. But it is easy at least to hope that research in this area may move us towards the beginning of a causal story linking genetics, neuroscience, and at least one central feature of schizophrenia. If this hope is somewhere near right, it is obvious that most or all of the likely causal story is not open to introspection. Whatever version of the genetics and neuroscience story turns out to be correct, its total absence is a *huge* gap in folk psychology. Filling it gives hope of a revolution in the science of schizophrenia.

But it may not be a revolution that wipes out all our folk psychology in this area. Delusions, so dramatic a feature of schizophrenia and other disorders, still greatly puzzle us. Neuroscience will surely tell us much that is now unknown to our intuitive 'human' thinking about them. And anyone who has heard someone producing the 'word salad' Hyman mentions is likely to share his scepticism about humanly intuitive accounts of what is more like a computer with a mechanical breakdown spewing out random symbols on the screen. But, despite its limitations, folk psychology is more than falsehoods waiting to be replaced by science. Many delusions may be open to a degree of human interpretation or questioning not fruitfully applied to a word salad.

While waiting in a psychiatric hospital for someone I had come to visit, I fell into conversation with another patient. He used the phrase 'very atelligent' to describe the person I was waiting for. '*A*telligent?' I queried. 'Yes', he said. 'Atelligent' was the right word, but to confuse us, 'they' put it about falsely that the correct word was 'intelligent'. We cannot yet explain this combination of paranoid delusion with inventing a word of which James Joyce might not have been ashamed. It is far from word salad. Our folk psychological thinking can get enough grip on what is said to raise the question of how intellectual deficits of a major delusion can coexist with such functioning creative powers. Answers will probably come from neuroscience. But the question is raised for anyone listening attentively and intuitively.

Sometimes folk psychology can raise questions about the completeness of a neuroscientific account of a delusion, or suggest where we might look for answers. Someone with Capgras delusion thinks, bizarrely, that a person emotionally close has died and been replaced by an identical impostor. One explanation draws on neuroscience's discovery of two anatomically separate systems of recognition. One analyses the person's appearance, voice, posture, and so on. The other involves an emotional response signalling familiarity. If the emotional system fails, this may explain why someone with Capgras delusion accepts the identical appearance yet denies it is of the person they are close to (Young, 1990). This is plausible as far as it goes. But our ordinary intuitive understanding of people, independent of any neuroscience, suggests it is not the whole story. If usually I am pleased to see you, but today my response is quite cold, there are some likely explanations. Perhaps I have a hangover. Or perhaps because you, uncharacteristically, are slapping me on the back. Perhaps last time we had a bad-tempered argument I have forgotten. And so on. But one explanation I will not reach for is that you have died and been replaced by an identical impostor. Since this is so unlikely, the full explanation of the delusion needs to look also for a damaged sense of plausibility. And this clue comes, not from neuroscience, but from our folk psychological understanding of the world and of normal thinking about it.

The folk psychology and neuroscience of agency

> The neurobiological view as we will develop it and the folk psychological or interpersonal view are deeply incompatible. The folk psychological view takes as true the potent, indeed ineluctable, human intuition of a self with effective agency and ascribes truth value to illness narratives based on a person's values, motivations, decisions, and actions. Neurobiology sees such narratives as 'just so' stories and understands pathogenic mechanisms to be unavailable to introspection. (Hyman and McConnell, p. 269, Chapter 17, this volume)

The neuroscience of agency may be another field where the changes forced on our everyday thinking are closer to being revolutionary.

What model do we presuppose in our everyday intuitive thinking about decision and action? What do we think goes on when people weigh up reasons and decide to act in one way rather than another? Will our intuitive model survive progress in neuroscience, with its likely emphasis on processes that are often unconscious and perhaps always mechanistic?

This is the scene of some of the deepest clashes between the reforming and revolutionary views about the impact of neuroscience. Reformers say about voluntary action roughly what has been said here about addiction and traumatic memory. They say that we still freely take conscious decisions to do things and that these decisions do control our actions. But they accept that the neurological fine structure of this is more complex than introspection lets us know.

Opposed to this are some influential revolutionary approaches. Hyman says current research suggests that the intuitive human experience of free will and agency is not the cause, but a product of the circuits that plan and initiate volitional actions. He cites Benjamin Libet and colleagues' classic 1983 study of people just about to act. They found that an electrical change, the 'readiness potential' (located in the pre-supplementary motor area), takes place 350 milliseconds before people report first being aware of the urge to act. Their suggested interpretation was that action is initiated by this readiness potential of which we are unaware. The later conscious event we think of as the decision to act is really only a signal that we are about to act (Libet et al., 1983; Libet, 1999). (Though it may be a trigger for a possible change of mind in the last 200 milliseconds before the act.)

Libet's line of thought has been supported by Daniel Wegner in his book *The Illusion of Conscious Will*. He too suggests that what we experience as a conscious decision does not really cause our action. He says we often make mistakes about how much or little we ourselves contribute to actions. He cites alien hand syndrome, automatic writing, and 'possession by spirits'. He thinks we make these mistakes because we know little about the causal processes involved in action. He goes on to argue that we have just assumed that 'conscious will' causes actions, but the true causal story needs controlled empirical investigation. His own view is that the real causes lie in neural systems. He suggests the experience of 'deciding' may just give us a preview of what we are about to do: not part of the motor but a mere gauge on the control panel (Wegner, 2002, p. 137).

However blurred the boundary is between conceptual reform and revolution, these thoughts have a strong claim to be revolutionary. Central to how we see ourselves is our sense of our own agency. The belief that actions are brought about by our conscious decisions is deep. It goes as far back in our history as we can see. The thought that actions are not initiated by decisions we are conscious of, but by decisions taken previously at some unconscious level in the brain, goes against all this.

However, these revolutionary proposals could well be wrong. Psychologically, human voluntary action is a very complicated affair. And the networks of brain circuits on to which we hope to map it are very complex. So first attempts to map specific aspects of action on to specific brain events are like shooting from the hip. Here, as elsewhere, John Donne's advice to be circumspect but persistent applies:

> On a huge hill
> Cragged and steep, Truth stands, and he that will
> Reach her, about must and about must go … (Donne, Satire 3)

The interpretation of Libet's experiments is controversial. Perhaps it is hasty to assume the 'readiness potential' in the pre-supplementary motor area is the neurological embodiment of an unconscious decision to act. There are inputs to the pre-supplementary area from the basal ganglia. Studies since Libet's show that in the basal ganglia there are neural precursors of action that come earlier than the readiness potential (Loukas and Brown, 2003; Haggard, 2008). Is it clear that either the readiness potential or these precursors embody the decision to act? Might not either or both embody some anticipatory preparation for a decision still under consideration?

Wegner is right that causes of actions need empirical investigation and that there is much neuroscience of action still undiscovered. But it is hard to see why evolution should have produced the cumbersome process of unconscious decisions followed by the illusion of conscious ones. Why reach for this clunking story rather than accept that decisions we think we make really are effective? Even now the more plausible view may be that 'conscious will' is not an illusion.

Not Descartes but Spinoza

Hyman's view of the folk psychology of agency as 'just so' stories does not depend entirely on particular studies such as Libet's. He thinks it rests on deep theoretical mistakes. He contrasts what neuroscience and genetics may bring to research with what he sees as the 'Cartesian' alternative: *psychiatrists, psychologists, and patients, like all human beings, are intuitive Cartesians. Humans experience themselves as being a self that is intuitively different from the body.* This is *erroneous Cartesian thinking, based on the deeply ingrained human folk psychological experience of being a self with agency that relies on the brain but is intuited as separate.* He says the reason why it is mistaken is that there is *no evidence for circuits or brain structures that might serve as a locus for the subjective self; no functional circuitry that might serve as a virtual homunculus that could make decisions and exert agency.*

It is still probably right that most human beings are intuitive Cartesians, with a folk psychology that assumes the self or the mind is different from the body. But the dominant programme in current neuroscience aims to explain our thoughts, feelings, and decisions in terms of brain mechanisms, without reference to dualist interaction with any non-physical 'self'. Going back to the parallel with politics, the conservative response to this is to deny the programme can succeed. But in the light of current neuroscience, this looks disconcertingly like the conservative response to Galileo or Darwin. The live options seem to be reform or revolution.

Steven Hyman is a revolutionary. It may be helpful for psychiatrists to humour or support their patients by not saying they reject the intuition of a self with effective agency is true. But really, he believes, the story is false.

When Eddington steps on the floorboard, we do not have to choose between the conservative denial of physics and the revolutionary denial that the floorboard is solid. We choose the reformist alternative. The floorboard *is* solid and modern physics tells us why it is.

In the neuroscience of agency, the conservatism of Cartesian interactive dualism can be opposed by the revolutionary denial that actions come from conscious decisions.

But, as with the floorboard, these are not the only options. Why can we not move from Descartes to Spinoza? His view of the mind leaves no room for 'interaction' between mind and body: *The mind and body are one and the same thing, which is conceived now under the attribute of thought, now under the attribute of extension. The result is that the order, or connection, of things is one, whether nature is conceived under this attribute or that; hence the order of actions and passions of our body is, by nature, at one with the order of actions and passions of the mind.*

Spinoza thought he had solved Descartes' mind–body problem. We now see that this problem is not one but a cluster. What are the neural correlates of conscious experiences? How did consciousness evolve? What is the contrast between ourselves and apparently unconscious computers? Why is consciousness necessary at all? There are also scholarly debates about what Spinoza's sometimes obscure claims come to. And there are sceptical doubts about whether it is possible to avoid questions such as 'two different attributes of *what*?'

Although philosophical questions remain, a pragmatic Spinozism gives a helpful framework for neuroscience. The brain's functions are to be understood in terms of physics, genetics, neurochemistry, and so on. There is no mysterious interaction with 'mental' objects that have no physical reality. The brain is not a closed system but is open to environmental and other influences. Neuroplasticity is real: taxi drivers who frequently consult maps of a city in their memory but rarely construct new maps may find the 'map-consulting' part of the hippocampus grows at the expense of the 'map-making' part. And, as the science gets there, increasingly we will be able to speak of experiences, emotional states, memories, decisions, and so on as being 'embodied' in particular locations in a person's brain, without bothering about metaphysical issues about the nature of 'embodiment'. Pragmatically, this gives us a framework that lets us deny dualist interaction without denying consciousness.

Spinoza applied his framework to agency: *All these things indeed show clearly that both the decision of the mind and the appetite and determination of the body by nature exist together—or rather are one and the same thing; which we call a decision when it is considered under, and explained through, he attribute of thought, and which we call a determination when it is considered under the attribute of extension.* We pragmatic Spinozists need not deny that decisions exist, or that they are causes of actions. But (as we would now say) they are embodied in neurological mechanisms.

Causal mechanisms and human choices

The phrase 'neurological mechanisms' points to a deep theoretical question. Is seeing what we do in terms of neurochemical, genetic, or other mechanisms compatible with seeing ourselves as people, as having agency?

Certainly there is a widespread view that agency and free decisions depend on the absence of complete causal mechanisms of decision and action. And, no doubt related to this, is the widespread view that some of these causal 'gaps' do exist, leaving room for human agency to transcend causal predictability. But the assumption that agency requires causal gaps in the mechanisms of action should be challenged. It is false.

Suppose the mechanistic neuroscientific project one day were to succeed. This would show that the brain is a vastly complicated set of mechanisms, interacting with environmental and other factors. Understanding the mechanisms would enable us to explain and (in principle) to predict human decisions and actions. This would give a determinist picture of what we do.

The determinist picture need not undermine agency. The right contrast is not between causal predictability and agency. Unpredictability is not free agency. In the eighteenth century David Hume pointed out that actions that are in principle unpredictable are random. To the extent that someone's decisions and actions are like this, they are not under the control of causes. And 'causes' here includes reasons. 'Why did you vote that way? What reasons did you have?' 'To me the case for each side seemed equally balanced. So I didn't have a reason. I just found myself voting that way.' This does not seem to be freedom. Nor is it the kind of political agency that citizenship classes should encourage. If this is the alternative, determinism should seem less worrying.

There is another reason for being relaxed about determinism. It does not support passivity. People with psychiatric disorders need to escape from *fatalism*. If true, fatalism would show there is no point in deliberation and decision. Whatever will be, will be: my efforts make no difference. My deliberation is powerless to influence my decision; my decision is powerless to influence my action; my action is powerless to influence the world. None of this grim picture follows from determinism.

You see a friend at a party, obviously drinking heavily. You know he plans to drive home, so you suggest he gets a taxi instead. But he refuses. He says neuroscience shows all our decisions and actions are the product of causal mechanisms. So whatever will be, will be. There is no point in trying to decide or act differently. Then he drives away drunk, crashes his car, and kills someone. If the fool had listened, instead of talking rubbish about fatalism, his victim would still be alive. It is not his determinism that should take part of the blame for the crash, but his false belief that determinism entails fatalism.

Our agency is compatible with determinism. But there is something in our folk psychology of action that determinism *does* undermine. This is an idea that is rarely expressed. It is implausible as soon as it is made explicit. But there is still a fairly widespread assumption that we have total control over what we do and what we are like. On this view freedom of choice goes '*all the way down*'.

We are responsible for the harm we do unless some excuse shows either that we did not understand or could not control what we did. We do not escape responsibility by saying that our selfishness, laziness, hatred, or love of cruelty caused us to do the harm. We are held responsible for shaping ourselves so that these features either fade away or at least are kept under control. That they persist in uncontrolled forms reflects badly on our past decisions not to confront them. But these past decisions: how did they come to be so wrong? Perhaps they reflected bad decisions even longer ago. But, if we go back far enough, we will reach decisions largely or entirely caused by factors outside our control. These causes may be our genes, or not being loved as a child, or some horrible event that happened to our mother in pregnancy. We do not create ourselves out of nothing. Our degree of responsibility for who we are is limited by the things we have to take as given. For good or bad, how we turn out is partly, in Bernard Williams' felicitous phrase, a matter of 'moral luck'.

Eroding the often unexamined assumption that freedom of choice goes all the way down has implications. It should challenge a penal system still partly based on retribution for wrongdoing. On this, Steven Hyman's thoughts about the impact on folk psychology are right. Neuroscience, through unravelling some of the causes of decisions and actions, is undermining an influential part of our folk psychology. Although this part is mistaken, it is romantically optimistic: I am the captain of my soul *all the way down*. But, through the penal system, it also does great harm. We should hope that the impact of neuroscience *is* revolutionary here.

Psychiatry that includes agency

Our folk psychology, including our intuitive sense of our own agency, can be important for psychiatric treatment. As Hyman says, giving some people neurochemical causes of their condition may undermine their sense of agency. Clinicians' concern about this sense of being dehumanized and powerless may sometimes support not talking about neuroscience to people they treat. As one person recovering from a disorder put it:

> I do not find the neurobiological theory of mental illness as helpful to my recovery because it deprives me of any sense of self-determination and responsibility. When I think I am a group of chemical reactions, each with its own scheme and plan, I feel dehumanized and powerless. I feel that I am thinking, feeling and acting at the whim of those chemicals, not through any effort or responsibility of my own. (Fisher, 1999, p. 131)

One strategy for clinicians is to switch back and forth: folk psychology for the patient and neurochemistry for their own serious thinking about the disorder. Perhaps one danger of this is that it may reinforce a tendency to treat patients' role as purely passive.

One young woman looked back on her eating disorder: 'Anorexia is not merely about body dysmorphia. There is a far deeper-reaching perversion of the mind that occurs when you are caught in the grips of this beast. You forget yourself' (Halban, 2008, p. 25). Another wrote of her anorexia that 'I came to lose all understanding of my own centre and my own edges' (Bowman, 2006, p. xiv). In these comments there is something to explore. A considerate psychiatrist might not express his or her responses if they were: *There is no Cartesian mind, no 'self' to forget, and 'my own centre' can only refer to neural circuits you know nothing about.* But better not to have these thoughts, even unexpressed, but to ask questions: *What goes on when you forget yourself? What is your centre when you haven't lost understanding of it?* The resulting conversation might help the person become active in their own escape from anorexia.

People who have played a role, either in escaping from a disorder or at least in taking some control so that it does not ruin their lives, sometimes give accounts we can learn from.

One is Simon Champ's account of his illness and of his changing self-interpretation and self-creation (Champ, 1999). At first, fighting his schizophrenia was central to his identity. Later, while still identifying with it, he saw it as more positive. Later still, gaining more control over it, 'I was recovering my personhood and saw the illness as influencing rather than defining me'. He reacted against the passivity of 'suffering' from schizophrenia, and campaigned angrily against society's attitudes to people with it and its treatment of them. 'As I worked through the anger I felt at the treatment I had received, I felt a renewed sense of hope for my own life.' Before, his sense of identity had been linked to ideas about having a job and masculinity. Thinking, he saw that he could make contributions that do not depend on paid work. And he saw that 'real men do indeed cry'. Coming to terms with schizophrenia has called for a deep communication with himself 'that has given me a thread that has linked my evolving sense of self, a thread of self-reclamation, a thread of movement toward a whole and integrated sense of self, away from the early fragmentation and confusion I felt as I first experienced schizophrenia'. He says reclaiming himself as not just picking up the self before the illness, but meant creating a concept of himself that integrated the experience of schizophrenia. Twenty-three years after developing schizophrenia, he felt he had changed, but he had still come home: 'I'm complete again, as I used to be then' (Champ, 1999).

Simon Champ clearly has exceptional capacity for self-reflection. Of course many with psychiatric disorders, even some with something like his ability, do not reach the point of being able to do what he describes. But first-person accounts suggest that we may under-rate how many people with psychiatric disorders are capable of a degree of self-creation that can make a real contribution to dealing with their condition.[2] Switching between these folk psychological thoughts and choices and the picture given by neuroscience is one plausible option. The alternative is to see the two accounts in the way we see Eddington's floorboard. The first-person account is true to the 'big picture' psychology, and the neuroscience account gives the fine structure that makes it true.

Upshot

We need to see where developments in neuroscience support 'normal science' reforms to our folk psychology and where they require revolutionary change to some central features. It is from the neuroscience of agency that the great revolutionary challenges are likely to come. It has been suggested here that the colonization of agency by causal mechanisms may, and probably should, have some revolutionary impact. It is likely to be on folk psychology's unexpressed assumption of having control over what we are like that goes 'all the way down'. This impact is likely to be felt most in forensic psychiatry.

In other parts of psychiatry, the neuroscience of agency is perhaps more likely to lead to 'normal science' reforms. These may be beneficial. Helping people liberate themselves from psychiatric disorders does not require causal gaps in neurochemical mechanisms. It requires conveying the energizing awareness that the mechanisms can be the embodiment of the decisions we take and act on.

We need a model of agency that is compatible with mechanistic explanations. The man at the party rejected the warning about drink-driving because he thought brain

---

[2] There are many. Two classics are Jamison (1995) and Sainsbury (2000).

mechanisms over-rule our decisions and actions. What he left out was the thought that some brain mechanisms are likely to be the neurophysiological or neurochemical embodiments of deliberation. Others are likely to embody the resulting decisions. Yet others are likely to embody the translation of decisions into action. An adequate neuroscience has to show how the brain and its activities can be the physical embodiment of what we think of as the mind and its activities. No doubt neuroscience will continue to surprise us. But we need not assume in advance that it will support the impoverished model of a mind reduced to passivity and fatalism.

In this area, the complications revealed by neuroscience may enrich rather than destroy our everyday intuitive thinking about decision and action. If so, clinicians may not have to alternate between attending to neuroscientific truth and listening to the 'false' folk psychology the patient accepts. Instead, the two perspectives may combine. I like the model of binocular vision in depth perception. To help some people who have psychiatric problems, we may need, as in binocular vision, to combine both perspectives. Here too, binocularity may give a better chance of seeing depth, this time seeing to the depths of people.

References

Bowman, G. (2006). *A Shape of My Own: A Memoir of Anorexia and Recovery*. London: Penguin.

Champ, S. (1999). A most precious thread. In: P. Barker, P. Campbell, and B. Davidson (Eds.), *From the Ashes of Experience: Reflections on Madness, Survival and Growth* (pp. 113–126). London: Whurr.

Donne, J. (1590s). *Satire 3*.

Eddington, A. (1931). *The Nature of the Physical World*. Cambridge: Cambridge University Press.

Fisher, D. (1999). Humanity and voice in recovery from mental illness. In: P. Barker, P. Campbell and B. Davidson (Eds.), *From the Ashes of Experience: Reflections on Madness, Survival and Growth* (p. 127–33). London: Whurr.

Halban, E. (2008). *Perfect: Anorexia and Me*. London: Vermilion.

Haggard, P. (2008). Human volition: towards a neuroscience of will. *Nature Reviews Neuroscience*, **9**(12), 934–946.

Hyman, S.E. (2005). Addiction: a disease of learning and memory. *American Journal of Psychiatry*, **162**(8), 1414–1422.

James, W. (1890/1950). *The Principles of Psychology*, Vol. **2**. New York: Dover.

Kuhn, T.S. (1962). *The Structure of Scientific Revolutions*. Chicago, IL: Chicago University Press.

Libet, B., Gleason, C.A., Wright, E.W., and Pearl, D.K. (1983). Time of conscious intention to act in relation to onset of cerebral activity (readiness potential): the unconscious initiation of a freely voluntary act. *Brain*, **106**(Pt 3), 623–642.

Libet, B. (1999). Do we have free will? *Journal of Consciousness Studies*, **6**(8–9), 47–57.

Loukas, C. and Brown, P. (2004). Online prediction of self-paced hand-movements from subthalamic activity using neural networks in Parkinson's disease. *Journal of Neuroscience, Methods*, 193–205.

Lucas, J.R. (1979). Wilberforce and Huxley: a legendary encounter. *The Historical Journal*, **2**(2), 313–330.

Proust, M. (1981). *Remembrance of Things Past*, Vol. **1** (Translated by C.K. Scott Moncrieff and T. Kilmartin). London: Chatto and Windus.

Jamison, K.R. (1995). *An Unquiet Mind: A Memoir of Mood and Madness*. London: Picador.

Sainsbury, C. (2000). *Martian in the Playground: Understanding the Schoolchild with Asperger's Syndrome*. London: Book Factory.

Sidgwick, I. (1898). A grandmother's tales. *MacMillan's Magazine*, **78**(486), 433–434.

Stebbing, L.S. (1937). *Philosophy and the Physicists*. Harmondsworth: Penguin Books.

Wegner, D.M. (2002). *The Illusion of Conscious Will*. Cambridge MA: MIT Press.

Young, A.W. (1990). Accounting for delusional misidentifications. *The British Journal of Psychiatry*, **157**, 239–248.

Chapter 20

The biopsychosocial model, *DSM*, and neurobiology

S. Nassir Ghaemi

Introduction

The biopsychosocial model (BPS) has been the conceptual status quo of psychiatry for two generations, ever since George Engel gave the keynote address at the American Psychiatric Association in 1980 (Engel, 1980), the same year of the publication of the radical change in psychiatric diagnosis implemented in the third edition of the *Diagnostic and Statistical Manual of Mental Disorders* (*DSM-III*). The timing of the two events was more than a coincidence. The BPS model codified a relativistic eclecticism (Ghaemi, 2007) that is the guiding philosophy of *DSM-III* and its two follow-up editions, *DSM-IV* (1994) and *DSM-5* (2013). Since 1980, the *DSM* editions have been based on 'pragmatism', meaning a utilitarian judgement made by *DSM* committees and leaders about what criteria are best for social, economic, and professional purposes (Phillips et al., 2012). *DSM* revisions were not, and are not, based on scientific evidence as their primary criteria for definition and change (Decker, 2013). The BPS model can be seen as providing a rationale for this pragmatic, utilitarian approach, since the BPS model argues that multiple factors can be taken into account when understanding illnesses; scientific research is one among many factors; it is not privileged (Ghaemi, 2007).

In two chapters in this volume contributed by Kendler and Gyngell and by Hyman and McConnell, one senses the tension between a scientific sensibility and unscientific aspects of psychiatry. The BPS model is invoked at times to explain or resolve this tension. Whether it does so acceptably is a question this commentary will address.

The BPS approach is based on a conceptual eclecticism (Ghaemi, 2007). The claim is that 'mental illness' is multifactorial, and thus the result of 'multilevel' interactions, which can be explained best by a BPS approach, as opposed to reductionism. The metaphor invoked is that psychiatric 'disorders' live in a 'dappled' causal word. Each of these quotations raises questions about terms that need to be well defined so as to determine if they are meaningful, and what they mean. The phrase 'mental illness' is as meaningless as the phrase 'physical illness'. There is no single physical illness, as there is no single mental illness. There are a number of physical illnesses, which differ from each other in some ways and resemble each other in other ways; so too with a number of mental illnesses. The general term is too vague to be meaningful. So too with the word 'disorder'. It was introduced in the *DSM-III* in 1980 to be vague on purpose

(Decker, 2013); the leaders of that task force wanted to be 'atheoretical', which meant not ascribing aetiology to diagnoses. They intentionally wanted to avoid the phrase 'disease' because it implied biological aetiology, and they wanted to avoid the phrase 'reaction' since it implied psychological aetiology. The word 'disorder' was given for every diagnosis to make each equal to the next, as an eclectic relativism would imply.

The belief of the BPS model was that all medical illnesses had biological, psychological, and social aspects to their aetiologies and pathogenesis. When George Engel proposed the model systematically for the first time (Engel, 1977), he contrasted it to the 'biomedical' reductionist model. The claim was that illnesses were not purely biological, or purely psychological, or purely social. This claim is false as relates to aetiology: there are many purely biological diseases, such as Mendelian genetic states like Tay–Sachs disease or Down syndrome. There are psychological conditions such as divorce-related anxiety, or temporary paralysis with trauma. There are social aetiologies such as war-related traumatic experiences. Hence, when stated strongly in relation to aetiology, the BPS model is false. When stated in relation to pathogenesis, it could be correct or false depending on the illness. For instance, the pathophysiology of Huntington's disease is driven genetically, with little environmental alteration of its course. It's important to note that Engel, who was a gastroenterologist who had trained in psychoanalysis, meant to apply the BPS model to all medical states, not just in psychiatry. One could claim, though, that the BPS model may not apply across medicine, but that it applies well to psychiatric 'disorders'.

Genetic studies of depression and substance abuse do not identify aetiology that goes in one direction or the other, that is, purely genetics or purely environment, but rather that both aspects are involved and interact. In other words, the aetiologies of depression and substance abuse are multifactorial, hence the dappled nature of causality and the need for a broad eclectic BPS model. These conclusions are presupposed in their assumptions, though, and merely reflect the inadequacies of *DSM* clinical phenotypes. To explain:

'Depression' is not a diagnosis; it's not a disease; it's a constellation of signs and symptoms, like fever, chills, and night sweats. To simplify, it's like fever. It's not a disease itself, but it can reflect other diseases, or it can happen idiopathically without any disease-based origin. If we did extensive genetic and environmental research on 'fever' as our clinical phenotype, we would find a great deal of overlap, interaction, and lack of reductionistic aetiology. We might conclude that the causal nature of fever is dappled.

If the term 'depression' is replaced with major depressive disorder, the situation is no better. As documented by documents from the proceedings of the *DSM-III* task force (Shorter, 2008; Decker, 2013), the term 'major depression' has no scientific meaning, because the criteria were based on pragmatic opinions of task force members. Key criteria, such as duration of the episode, and use of psychomotor changes, were based on preferences, not the best scientific evidence. The 1980 criteria hardly changed 14 years later, or 33 years later. They have hardened into calcified definitions. Validity has not increased because it hasn't budged. Still, with almost four decades of worship of the same criteria, reliability actually declined for major depressive disorder in the *DSM-5* field trials, compared to the *DSM-III* and *-IV* (Regier et al., 2012). Research about onset of an episode of 'major depression' based on stressful life events interacting with childhood sexual abuse is difficult to interpret, when the concept of 'major depression' has questionable scientific legitimacy.

The same general problem arises in the discussion about 'resisting hard reductionism': 'Despite extensive attempts to find single root causes for disorders such as schizophrenia, major depression and alcoholism—none have been found' (Kendler and Gyngell, p. 39, this volume). An analogous claim in internal medicine physician would be: 'Despite extensive attempts to find single root cause for disorders such as diabetes, fever, and overeating—none have been found'. Maybe the problem isn't that the causes of 'major depression' and alcoholism are dappled, but that those are not 'diseases' or even 'disorders' or even legitimate clinical phenotypes. Schizophrenia is different; it has more legitimacy, and is almost entirely genetic, but, like diabetes, it is polygenic. Alcoholism isn't a good test of a disease, just like overeating, since there are important social and cultural components for the observed behaviour, and often it is a consequence of other diseases.

It is suggested that the opposite of the BPS approach is 'hard reductionism', including the claim that all psychiatric disorders are ultimately genetic. This need not be the case. It could be that some psychiatric illnesses are ultimately genetic, and this claim is based on meta-analysis of the twin study literature, published by Kendler with other colleagues (Bienvenu et al., 2011). The authors review the twin study literature which shows that schizophrenia and bipolar illness are over 80% genetic in heritability, which is similar to Alzheimer's dementia, and that many other *DSM* psychiatric definitions are much less genetic; then they conclude that these genetic data do not support the disease concept for any psychiatric diagnosis. It is not obvious how this conclusion can be drawn for the two that are mostly genetic, though it makes sense for the rest. The rational conclusion would seem to be that some psychiatric diagnoses—specifically two—are mainly genetic, and others are not (assuming that the *DSM* phenotypes are valid, which is not the case).

The *DSM* is cited as a 'soft medical model'. As shown previously, the *DSM* system is not a medical model at all, but rather a pragmatic social construction, created for social, economic, and cultural purposes. Scientific aspects are secondary and buried within the larger social construction. Further, the 'hard medical model', or any medical model, need not be 'linked to a single clear aetiological mechanism'. The medical model approach—applied to systemic lupus erythematosus, atherosclerosis, coronary artery disease, rheumatoid arthritis, migraine, Crohn's disease, or generalized epilepsy—has no idea about a single clear aetiological mechanism. And yet it is still a medical model, not a pragmatic social construction like the *DSM*, created on utilitarian grounds and written by administrative leaders of the American Psychiatric Association, as opposed to a consensus of the research community.

A solution of 'empirically informed pluralism' has much to commend it, but not for the reasons given. The BPS assumption—that 'no one of these influences has special causal privilege over the other'—is the whole problem. It is up to scientific research to show which features have causal privilege. The difficulty here is that the false *DSM* system has led past scientific research into a dead end, leading thoughtful observers to conclude that there are no privileged features.

The problem is not 'the seductive simplicity of reductionism and hard medical models'. The problem is the failure to recognize unscientific social constructionism in the *DSM* system. The problem is not that we are too reductionistic; it is that we have been pseudoscientific, applying *P*-values to false clinical phenotypes. Plenty of non-Mendelian complex illnesses exist in medicine, as in psychiatry, such as coronary artery disease and cancers. The dappled nature of causality, and hardness versus softness, need not be invoked. Rather, we need to give up 'pragmatic' social construction, drop false *DSM* concepts, and get honest in our clinical research. Then our results will relate to reality, not to our profession's social constructions. We may find that some psychiatric conditions are purely genetic diseases, that some are purely environmental experiences, and that some are a mix. They may not be all eclectically dappled after all.

Another way of thinking about the BPS model is based on the long divide between basic and clinical researchers, the former working with animals or with objectified aspects of human research (genetics, neuroimaging), the latter working with humans in their clinical presentations (symptoms, diagnoses, course, treatment). Recent leaders in the National Institute of Mental Health have come from the basic research world, and in 2013, dropped the *DSM-5* in favour of a purely non-clinically-based diagnostic system (Research Domain Criteria). They viewed the failures of the *DSM* as failures of clinical research; they didn't understand that the *DSM* never applied clinical research with scientific integrity, but only in the service of the American Psychiatric Association's pragmatic social constructions. The main problem with the basic neurobiology-based approach to psychiatry is that billions of dollars and decades of effort are spent on gathering interesting genetic and biological data, but there is no link to clinical practice. Mechanism has no meaning, and never will, if clinical research is devalued and ignored, as in the Research Domain Criteria system. The BPS model won't solve the problem when all the emphasis is on the 'B' and the rest is reduced to folk psychology.

What is needed is honest scientific research, dropping the Research Domain Criteria as well as the *DSM*. The results of that research may well support some of the axioms of the BPS approach, finding that some psychiatric conditions have important psychosocial causes, and in other cases it will find that reductionistic approaches are more valid. Such research finally might be able to integrate clinical diagnoses with their genetic or other biological roots. It will bring mechanisms much closer to their human meanings, beyond the common-sense assumptions of folk psychology, and deeper into a more profound understanding of the human meaning of psychopathological states.

Pierre Loebel and Julian Savulescu, in their introduction to this book, laid out an honourable purpose, seeking to make sense of psychiatric conditions holistically. They hoped the BPS model could serve this purpose. The model has done so in part, but also, after half a century of effort, it has failed to do so in the end. The goals are worthy and the seekers of those goals have integrity. But perhaps their intentions will be best served by something else, a successor to the past BPS model, built on a rejection of a false *DSM* diagnostic system as well as a purely neurobiological approach to research. In the end, what Loebel and his colleagues want to do is to preserve a place for humanism in psychiatry, and to link clinical practice to solid scientific research. These laudable principles can be achieved only by a radical departure from the *DSM*-based neurobiological conventional wisdom of the present and the past.

References

Bienvenu, O.J., Davydow, D.S., and Kendler, K.S. (2011). Psychiatric "diseases" versus behavioral disorders and degree of genetic influence. *Psychological Medicine*, **41**(1), 33–40.

Decker, H. (2013). *The Making of DSM-III: A Diagnostic Manual's Conquest of American Psychiatry*. Oxford: Oxford University Press.

Engel, G.L. (1977). The need for a new medical model: a challenge for biomedicine. *Science*, **196**(4286), 129–136.

Engel, G.L. (1980). The clinical application of the biopsychosocial model. *American Journal of Psychiatry*, **137**(5), 535–544.

Ghaemi, S.N. (2007). *The Rise and Fall of the Biopsychosocial Model*. Baltimore, MD: Johns Hopkins University Press.

Phillips, J., Frances, A., Cerullo, M.A., Chardavoyne, J., Decker, H.S., First, M.B., Ghaemi, N., Greenberg, G., Hinderliter, A.C., Kinghorn, W.A., LoBello, S.G., Martin, E.B., Mishara, A.L., Paris, J., Pierre, J.M., Pies, R.W., Pincus, H.A., Porter, D., Pouncey, C., Schwartz, M.A., Szasz, T., Wakefield, J.C., Waterman, G.S., Whooley, O., and Zachar, P. (2012). The six most essential questions in psychiatric diagnosis: a pluralogue part 2: issues of conservatism and pragmatism in psychiatric diagnosis. *Philosophy, Ethics, and Humanities in Medicine*, **7**(1), 8.

Regier, D.A., Narrow, W.E., Clarke, D.E., Kraemer, H.C., Kuramoto, S.J., Kuhl, E.A., and Kupfer, D.J. (2012). DSM-5 field trials in the United States and Canada, part II: test-retest reliability of selected categorical diagnoses. *American Journal of Psychiatry*, **170**(1), 59–70.

Shorter, E. (2008). *Before Prozac: The Troubled History of Mood Disorders*. New York: Oxford University Press.

Chapter 21

Objectification: Ethical and epistemic concerns about neurocentrism in psychiatry

Jan Christoph Bublitz

Introduction

This chapter explores the ethical concept of objectification with respect to neurobiological explanations and treatments commonly found in psychiatry. Although a key reference point in humanist thought, objectification is an underexplored concept, particularly in relation to contemporary naturalistic views of the human mind. The ethical demand to not-objectify persons, understood as respect for persons' subjectivities, seems to stand in tension with neurobiological modes to explain, access, and alter minds primarily at the neurobiological level. Psychiatry traditionally and paradigmatically operates within this tension; its contentious parts (medicalization, coercive interventions) are prime examples of it. It may thus provide interesting insights for a yet to be developed broader theory of objectification. Driven by advances of the neurosciences, neurobiological modes of treatment and corresponding explanations[1] have found increasing traction in many parts of psychiatry. Biological psychiatry seems to have returned to centre stage (Akil et al., 2010; Walter, 2013; Insel and Quirion (2005) formulated an influential programmatic take on psychiatry as 'clinically applied neuroscience').[2] Although psychological and social levels are duly acknowledged, the degree to which they are deemed relevant for treatment or explanation of disorders often remains dubitable (e.g. Frances, 2014; Davies, 2017), as they are frequently overshadowed by visions of biology-based 'high-precision psychiatry' (van Os et al., 2013). This chapter is not concerned with feasibility, failures, or promises of these approaches,

---

[1] 'Neurobiological', 'biological', or 'neural level' are used interchangeably and summarily for what comprises a range of diverse levels, from genes to cells, neuron assemblies, brain circuits, networks, to connectomes. It also includes all physiological, electrochemical processes in the brain. These levels can be treated as one for present purposes because they are at least in principle fully explainable by the natural sciences (biology and physics).

[2] The degree to which current practices in psychiatry are in fact biologically oriented is an empirical question about which this chapter remains silent. There is no single answer as different schools and traditions, institutions, and healthcare systems place varying emphasis on specific methods or kinds of explanations.

but with their ethical side. Neurobiological explanations and interventions might be ethically more problematic than others in light of the idea of objectification.

Psychiatry is the very discipline of changing minds through neurobiological interventions (henceforth, neurointerventions). These methods to alter minds are routinely viewed with suspicion and unease by critics, patients, and the public at large. Many consider neurointerventions such as pharmacology or electric or magnetic brain stimulation methods as in principle more ethically worrisome than other, less direct interventions such as "talking cures". But the reasons for this difference often remain implicit or underdeveloped. A supposed lack of good arguments buttressing such worries has led many ethicists to conclude, to the contrary, that the nature of mind interventions is ethically irrelevant. All that matters is the benefit and risk profile, the sum of positive and negative effects of particular interventions. Apart from them, interventions should be treated ethically on a par (Levy, 2007).

This chapter lays out a contrasting position by fathoming one feature that renders neurointerventions problematic in principle (apart from contingent side effects). The main suggestion is that neurointerventions *objectify* persons, and that this mode of treating others is prima facie ethically wrong. Objectification captures and illuminates an ethically problematic aspect of neurointerventions and partially explains why they differ from more indirect and less troublesome interventions such as psycho- or cognitive behavioural therapies (for a related argument, see Focquaert and Schermer (2015)). As a consequence, non-objectifying interventions should, *ceteris paribus*, take priority over neurobiological ones, especially in coercive treatments and in the way healthcare is institutionally structured and provided. In addition, exclusively neurobiological or reductionist explanations of mental phenomena objectify persons and are, for the time being, *epistemically* deficient. By themselves, they should neither guide public policies, nor individual treatment decisions. However, to be clear at the outset: in many instances, people can *consent* to being objectified, which negates or mitigates the ethical charge.

Objectification is a recurrent trope in criticisms of biological psychiatry, but it is rarely explicated in more detail. Critics seem to take its meaning and inherent wrongness for granted (Schwartz, 1999).[3] By contrast, biologically minded circles in psychiatry routinely dismiss the accusation. Interestingly, however, they often neither argue against the idea that psychiatry objectifies, nor that this is wrong. Their argument is rather grounded in what is apparently understood as a purely scientific point (although it is, in fact, a metaphysical position): the idea of a primacy of the neurophysiological or brain level in explaining and treating mental disorders, which shall be called *brain primacy* or *neurocentrism* (a term borrowed from Satel (2013)). It is related to the key premise of biological psychiatry that mental disorders *are* brain disorders. Accordingly, every effective psychiatric-psychological treatment has to operate on (or

---

[3] The critique is sometimes formulated along lines as 'biologism' (Stier et al., 2014) and reverberates in complaints that psychiatry is 'inhuman', 'impersonal', or fails to treat the person holistically. In Szasz's words: 'Whereas primitive man personifies things, modern man 'thingifies' persons. We call this mechanomorphism: modern man tries to understand man as if it "it" were a machine' (Szasz, 1991, p. 199).

through) neurobiology. But then, so the often implicit reasoning goes, nothing seems particularly worrisome about neurobiological interventions; they are not fundamentally different to, say, psychotherapies, which also demonstrably change the brain. Against this backdrop, concerns specifically about neurobiological interventions appear ill-grounded. They seem to betray unscientific views about the human mind, or even confused metaphysics, beliefs in *Cartesian* dualism or disembodied idealism, notions which psychiatry and neuroscience have fortunately and finally discredited. Or so it seems.

Such metaphysical dismissals of the ethical problem of objectification are themselves misplaced and frequently commit what one may call the *anti-Cartesian* fallacy. From the rejection of substance dualism and the acceptance that all mental phenomena are in some way related to the brain, it neither follows that they are best explained at the neurobiological level, nor that interventions are *only* causally effective there. And even if that were the case, the charge of objectification might still stand. Rather than evading it by speculative metaphysics, it has to be rebutted in the ethical arena through normative discourse.

This chapter traces this line of argument and consists of two quite distinct parts. The first (see 'On objectification') seeks to provide some contours to the idea of objectification by drawing on Marxist and feminist sources. A tentative conception, according to which a key feature of objectification is disregard of subjectivity, is then suggested (see 'Towards a conception applicable to psychiatry'). The second part rehearses several metaphysical objections against the suggested construal which draw on the idea of brain primacy. But there is no scientific or metaphysical fact to sustain it. As a societal institution, psychiatry should not confuse a *research* hypothesis with valid premises for its practices. Observing the limits of one's methods and resulting findings is itself a supreme virtue of science (see 'Reductionist objections and misleading metaphysics'). As a consequence, prioritizing one treatment modality over another is warranted neither on scientific nor metaphysical grounds. Whether a particular mode of intervention promises success is solely an empirical matter. Then, the prima facie ethical wrongness of objectification may establish a defeasible *ethical priority* of non-objectifying interventions, and further normative desiderata (see 'Normative consequences').

Surely, interventions into minds differ in terms of their risk/benefit profiles, and some mental conditions are best treated, or only treatable, by neurobiological means. These contingent empirical matters are highly relevant for individual treatment decisions, but not for the present purpose of establishing a more abstract argument based on the nature of neurobiological approaches. Moreover, the chapter is mainly interested in ethically contentious scenarios such as coercive interventions, where the charge of objectification is particularly relevant. The ethical and legal grounds of coercive treatments are still not settled, as indicated by the ambivalent report of the UN Rapporteur on torture (United Nations, 2013), a decision by the European Court of Human Rights (2013), ongoing controversies about the UN Convention on the Rights of People with Disabilities (UN Committee on the Rights of Persons with Disabilities (CRPD), 2014), and drafts by the Council of Europe (2015) of an additional protocol to the Oviedo Convention on Biomedicine. At the moment, objectification is not a relevant consideration in these debates, but it might (and should) become one in the future.

The chapter is explorative and associative rather than deductive as it seeks to unearth interrelations between yet unconnected strands of thought about objectification. It formulates an *ethical* and *external* perspective on neurobiological practices in psychiatry under the salient idea of objectification. Neurobiological interventions and explanations are presented in a concededly pointed and a somewhat coarse manner, so that the chapter neither provides all-things-considered judgements, nor does justice to the often diverse, multilevel, and pragmatic practices found in diverse psychiatric institutions throughout the world. It should thus not be misread as a direct critique of psychiatric practices, but rather as a contribution to the *ethics of psychiatry*, in the spirit of Engel's (1977) seminal article.

On objectification

How does neurobiological psychiatry *objectify* patients? Answers require a substantive ethical account of objectification. But unfortunately, there is none. In its absence, distilling common elements from diverse strands of thoughts and applying them to the present context seems the most promising strategy. In the history of ideas, various conceptions have evolved in distinct, though internally interwoven strands from Kantian over Marxist to feminist thought. Elements of these theories were taken up in psychological research of the last two decades and also resurface in legal scholarship on human dignity. Of yet, the concept has not been thoroughly applied to neurobiological interventions and biological psychiatry, which may come as a surprise given that the concept is frequently (if only latently) invoked in its criticisms (a recent exception with respect to *self*-objectification through taking antidepressants is Hoffman (2013)). The following may thus serve as a case study for a broader theory of objectification. Such a theory may have implications for other questions, such as the merging of minds and machines through brain implants and brain–computer interfaces, likely entering psychiatry in the near future (Clausen, 2009; Steinert et al., 2019). Moreover, a better understanding of the idea of the person in the digital age, the relation between virtual personae and embodied beings, seems to require novel perspectives in which objectification may play a role. Even criminological issues concerning the explanation and prevention of criminal behaviour bear some structural similarities with those in psychiatry. Some authors suggest neurobiological interventions for the 'treatment of crime' (Douglas, 2014), or moral enhancement (Persson and Savulescu, 2012).[4] A theory of objectification may prove helpful in conceptualizing and assessing such uses.

Objectification is among the more elusive concepts of Continental philosophy. It reverberates in different contexts and has clearly negative connotations, but lacks well-defined theoretical foundations. It has several facets and might well be a cluster

---

[4]   In a recent controversy around coercive treatments of offenders with neurointerventions, objectification has been invoked (Shaw, 2014; Holmen, 2018) but with a different thrust. The present construal would apply to those debates as well.

concept. It stands in close proximity to concepts such as instrumentalization, alienation, commodification, depersonalization, or dehumanization, which are themselves vague and may overlap to some degree. In a first approximation, objectification can be understood as a particular mode of treating other persons—'thinglike', as objects. Engaging with persons in this mode is normatively prima facie wrong. It fails to respect them in a distinct way, as beings who are more than objects, in their distinct quality as persons or subjects. This approximation trades on the (not unproblematic) distinction between objects and subjects, and expresses the ethical demand that persons be treated as the latter.[5] Rector (2014, p. 9) understands it 'as a *spectrum of misapprehension* ... When we objectify others, we misperceive them as being less than what they are in their totality'. Against this backdrop, let us visit some selected key theories of objectification.

Kantian roots

One of the most famous lines of thought which draws upon a dichotomy between things and persons and was influential for later conceptions originates in Kant. According to a famous, yet crude dichotomy, things have value whereas humans have dignity (Kant, 1785/2002). In a Kantian perspective, humans are of dual nature: as bodily things or objects they are bound by the laws of nature, yet at the same time, they can give laws to themselves through the faculty of reason. This ability sets them apart from mere things. It is the source of dignity and responsibility, and it grounds the moral demand to treat others (and ourselves) as beings who set ends for themselves and not merely as physical objects. Treating persons as things or objects means failing to recognize them as self-end-setting beings. The most salient instance of objectification is instrumentalization, using others as a mere means for one's ends. But the wrongness of objectification does not logically depend using someone *for the purposes of others*. Disrespecting autonomy is wrong even when it does not advance others' ends (e.g. paternalistic psychiatric interventions). Respecting persons as beings who set ends for themselves prohibits manipulative influences which call into question their authorship over mental states, decisions, or behaviours. Conversely, it implies that attempts to change the minds of others should proceed through their faculty of reason and its peculiar mode, the exchange of arguments. In modern words, respecting persons as setting ends for themselves demands engaging with them in the 'space of reasons'.

Applied to psychiatry, this view calls for reason-related interventions, mainly rational persuasion, and rejects interventions proceeding on non-rational ways. Neurointerventions that transform desires, beliefs, emotions, or behaviour directly by

---

[5] Among the problems of the subject–object distinction not further pursued here are everyday interactions in which people routinely disregard each other's subjectivities (e.g. customer to salesclerks) or the fact that objects are routinely harnessed to *extend* social interactions which Latour (1996) describes as 'interobjectivity' (a wall instead of the owner blocking entrance to a property). Slogans proclaiming the 'death of the subject' only apply to particular conceptions (autonomous, free, independent, noumenal subjects), none of which are presupposed here.

bypassing capacities to set and attain ends for oneself appear particularly dubious. If they were not sought for by affected persons themselves, they violate autonomy since newly generated mental states were not chosen by the person, but externally imposed on her. However, the Kantian picture is grounded in the (overemphasized) ideal of autonomy, which has received much attention in psychiatric ethics. The present interest lies in a standalone theory of objectification, distinct from, or over and above autonomy. It is thus left aside in the following.

Marxist origins

A further origin of objectification is Marxism, where it has undergone several transformations over the last century. It is sometimes distinguished from the stronger 'reification' (used synonymously here; cf. Bewes, 2002; Honneth et al., 2008). Here are some simplified aspects: originally, objectification denoted the peculiar way in which human abilities and powers of labour are transformed into physical objects. Through producing things, labour changes its 'state of aggregation' and thus becomes detached from the person. This may lead to alienation, first of the worker from the product of her labour, and then from herself (Marx and Engels, 2009; for a contemporary explication of alienation see Jaeggi (2014)). With some interpretation, another facet of the strange relation between persons and objects can be derived from Marx. In a famous line, he notes: 'The increasing value of the world of things proceeds in direct proportion to the devaluation of the world of men' (2009, p. 71). While one might read this as an anticipating comment on contemporary consumerist culture, his point is more complex. One aspect is that social relations between persons vanish behind relations to things. In market societies, everyone constantly establishes relations to things—buys, sells, and uses them—but tends to forget the interpersonal relations this creates or modifies, for example, to those who have produced these things, or those who cannot use them because oneself does so. Every artefact one holds in one's hands has a history of production by others, but one is rarely aware of it, it is practically erased. People interact with each other *through* objects but forget the interpersonal aspect. In this sense, the 'social relation between men [assumes] the fantastic form of a relation between things' (Marx, 1962, p. 86). Lost, in other words, are intersubjective encounters with genuine human qualities. Political campaigns highlighting miserable working conditions in the production of everyday products make these hidden social relations reappear—and often immediately change people's attitudes towards products and producers. In these cases, social interactions are impoverished because they proceed through the 'logic' of dealing with objects.

In works of neo-Marxists, the idea of a falseness of relations resurfaces. Sometimes objectification is understood as a category mistake, an error in logic, not ethics: it is simply false to treat entities as objects if they are no objects, and this may lead to false conclusions. This form of reification is familiar to psychiatry: mental disorders are sometimes perceived and described as real existing *things* or natural kinds with causal powers. *The* depression, inside the head, causes depressive symptoms, like a foreign object or a virus, and it may lift, as if it was a movable thing. Through reification, an abstract concept such as depression takes on a thinglike form of existence. As a metaphorical way of speaking, it may mislead thinking about the nature and causes of mental disorder as well as possible treatments (Hyman, 2010; cf. Ryle, 2000). But this form of reification in psychiatry is not our present concern.

Another—and now ethical—meaning can be found in critical theory which developed the Marxist critique of economic relations into a more comprehensive critique of human reason. Capitalism not only subverts social interactions, but brings with it a specific form of reasoning which colonizes more and more non-economic spheres of the lifeworld. Reason, in the strong sense of aiming at mutual understanding, is subverted to instrumental rationality in the sense of effective means–end relations (Habermas, 1984). This form of rationality increasingly structures social relations in many domains of everyday life; interpersonal encounters are underwritten by imperceptible power relations and the implicit 'logic' of market exchanges. These factors shape how people relate to one another, what they want, and expect from each other. Instrumental rationality also characterizes how we deal with spontaneous natural, social, or cultural processes. If inefficient or without added value, they are brought under technical control, are transformed or forsaken. Furthermore, people internalize instrumental rationality, which then frames how they perceive themselves. People appreciate themselves primarily in terms of their 'market' value, leading to self-doubts, self-depreciations, and undermining positive self-relations, all the more when even intimate parts of life become structured in market-like fashion (e.g. dating in the age of Tinder). Such forms of self-objectification corrupt one's self-relation and create susceptibilities to a range of pathologies (Honneth et al., 2008).

An interesting variation of self-objectification which irritates and detaches people from their emotional life springs from social demands to 'be' a certain way and to publicly exhibit certain feelings (e.g. good mood in the service sector, love and passion in interpersonal relations). To meet such emotional demands, people begin to feign feelings and deploy emotions strategically. Thereby, they begin to take an observing stance towards themselves and experience their emotions and desires as contingent and amenable, evocable, or suppressible on (external) demand. What people lose is an unmediated, non-distorted connection to their emotionality (Illouz, 2007; Hochschild, 2012). And, by extension, to themselves, as emotions are biological guides for one's values, they express one's attitudes and desires, and are a route for self-understanding. Managing emotions by external demand distorts this aspect of one's self-relation. Such processes of self-estrangement are considered to lie at the root of some contemporary pathologies, especially affective disorders such as depression (Honneth, 2008). This reasoning may connect accounts of depression that characterize it as the loss of emotional experiences that matter for the person (Ratcliffe, 2014).

In these cases, objectification is a wrong mode of treating persons that generates further problems in the minds of the objectified. It is driven by large-scale societal dynamics, not so much by individual actions. Antidotes include keeping instrumental rationality at bay by defending social domains from market-like restructuring, and by promoting richer forms of reason and understanding. Whether these neo-Marxist views fittingly describe the interrelations and contiguities of social life, and the extent to which they may assist in explaining the contemporary maladies of the mind, remains to be seen. Post Foucault, uncorrupted self-relations appear as an overly naïve idea. But although these approaches are limited and incomplete, one may wonder why sociopsychological explanations of this kind have fallen so much out of favour in the sciences analysing the pathologies of the mind. Despite shortcomings and ideological overtones, they have some prima facie plausibility and they seem to correspond to people's experiences. The empirical claims on which they ground have, for the most part, not been falsified or debunked, but were never thoroughly tested. In fact, they are hardly testable under controlled conditions. However, this does not deny that they may be illuminating and informative for understanding and tackling today's mental health problems. Stronger recognition of sociological explanations, in more refined and actualized forms, may thus be warranted. And irrespective of their explanatory successes, neo-Marxist views provide some elements for a theory of objectification applicable to neurobiological interventions.

Feminist sources

Objectification is also an important concept in feminist thought. A rich and controversial literature addresses it primarily with respect to issues of bodily appearance, sexuality, and pornography. Objectification is conceptualized and criticized as an oppressive mode of perceiving and treating persons, especially women (Papadaki, 2015, 2010). A key example is pornography, which depicts women in ways catering to the male gaze. Reduced to bodies, detached from their personalities, and largely without concern for their true subjective experiences, women are portrayed and treated as objects for male pleasure.[6]

In a critical engagement with feminist scholarship on objectification, Martha Nussbaum has identified seven instances. Apart from denial of autonomy, the one most relevant for present purposes is what she calls 'denial of subjectivity': treating someone 'as something whose experience and feelings need not be taken into account' (Nussbaum, 1995, p. 257).[7] Others have added to this list the reduction to one's body and the denial of communicative agency, that is, being treated as someone who cannot speak or has nothing meaningful to say (Langton, 2005). Objectification through reducing persons to bodies is surely not limited to pornography, it permeates everyday social relations ('lookism', Minerva, 2017). Pressures that bodies satisfy prevailing aesthetic norms are ubiquitous and constantly reinforced through social rejection or acceptance on the basis of appearance. Repeated exposure to objectifying gazes might lead to its internalization by the objectified. This, again, may distort self-relations as objectified persons learn to perceive themselves through the perspective of others, from the outside, and may derive their self-worth from such an external perspective on themselves.

---

[6] A range of proposals for the conceptualization of objectification has emerged from these debates (see Haslanger, 2012). Regarding pornography, feminist literature has also developed an interesting converse perspective on the use of things as persons (personification), see Saul (2006).

[7] One controversy that has emerged from Nussbaum's writing concerns the question of whether some forms of objectification (e.g. in pleasurable submissive sexual roles) can be morally permissible. Individual liberty come in subtle conflict here with internalized oppressive attitudes. But apart from such specific examples, objectification is widely condemned.

These theories have inspired psychological objectification theory (Fredrickson and Roberts, 1997). A range of studies has investigated psychological processes of object-ification and their findings vindicate central elements of objectification theory (for a review, see Moradi and Huang (2008)). Notably, studies could establish connections between objectifying experiences, self-objectification of women, and further adverse psychological consequences. Self-objectification generates anxieties and shame about one's bodily appearance, a reduced level of flow, distractions in thinking and impair-ments in cognitive capacities, diminished perception of one's internal sensations (hunger, fatigue), as well as emotional numbness. These are quite severe disruptions of one's self-relation and may lead to further mental pathologies from depression to sexual dysfunction (Szymanski et al., 2011).

Interestingly, studies show peculiar cognitive processing styles in objectifying per-ception. Objectification seems to be a peculiar way of looking at 'things' by attending to parts rather than the full *gestalt*. It is a misleading *pars pro toto*, a reduction to body parts ('local vs global processing'; for a review, see Gervais et al. (2013)). Even more, they show that objectifying perception impacts moral treatment: the objectifying per-sons show less moral concern for the objectified (Loughnan et al., 2010; Gray et al., 2011). Objectification thus illuminates linkages from the modes in which persons per-ceive others to deep problems with themselves.

Recent research and conceptual work is often conducted under the heading of 'dehumanization'. The failure to appreciate the subjective side, or *dementalization*, is considered as one of two forms of dehumanization (Haslam, 2006; Haslam et al., 2013). And indeed, objectification means disregarding or denying specific aspects of humanness. This is the link to the humanist tradition. But the concept of 'dehuman-ization', even though used in a specific sense, seems to carry too many connotations to be useful in grasping rather than denouncing a phenomenon, and is thus avoided in the following (as the title of his book indicates, Szasz (1991) might object). Finally, it should be mentioned that there is a more general unease with modern medicine, standardized care, lacking personal and emotional support and insufficient commu-nication between doctors and patients, which is sometimes described as the object-ification of the patient (Haslam, 2006). It is consistent with, though distinct from, the present critic which is more narrowly focused in neurobiological approaches to the mind.

Without tracing finer developments, these conceptions mark the realm of objectifi-cation in current scholarship. It appears that the concept and its normative implica-tions are not as self-evident as critics seem to presuppose. Because of their diversity and variability, these conceptions also fall short of providing a general theory of ob-jectification. However, some common themes emerge: objectification is a mode of treating entities which are no things as if they were things. It includes taking parts for the whole; or reducing persons to bodies. Conversely, objectification fails to perceive and treat persons in the right mode. It disregards subjectivities, because it engages with persons on a purely physical, bodily level, or in a mode of instrumental ration-ality. Such treatments may seriously disrupt various aspects of persons' self-relations. Objectification often occurs within relations of unequal power.

Towards a conception applicable to psychiatry

Basic account

Let us now analyse how these elements of objectification may apply to psychiatry. At the outset, it is helpful to distinguish two reference points: Objectification can refer to *perceiving* persons as objects, and this entails *explaining* their behaviour or mental life at an objective level only, that is, on the physical and biological levels observable from the third-person perspective. Alternatively, it can refer to *treating* persons as objects, that is, to engage with them in ways that fail to properly acknowledge or bypass the subjective side, especially in attempts to alter minds. Here are two simple illustrations:

1. Suppose that A is anxious because of a personal issue. He tells his friend F about his anxiety. F responds: 'Oh sure, you are anxious, your amygdala is overactivated'. If this is F's only response, how would you characterize it? Something seems irritatingly wrong with it, something is missing. It is cold, distanced, and disrespectful. Although A's anxiety might well be proximally caused by an overactivation of his amygdala (otherwise F's response was simply false), the response is of a kind that people usually neither seek, nor expect. It refers to the wrong level, to the body rather than the person. It overemphasizes bodily causes and neglects the psychological setting in which it arises. But even more, it fails to address the subjective side, the feeling of anxiety, the content and intentional objects of the anxious thoughts, the circumstances that evoke it, the underlying reasons for the anxiety, as well as strategies to mitigate it, such as reappraising anxiety-generating thoughts. By referring only to bodily states, A's subjectivity is neglected, he is objectified. The bodily explanation is at best a poor substitute for an adequate response. Note that such references to bodily causes for mental phenomena are not uncommon in daily life. Levels of hormones or glucose are some examples. If they are taken to explain mental events or behaviours of persons exclusively, the level of the person as well as her subjectivity are curtailed in an inappropriate fashion.

2. Moving from explanation to intervention, suppose again that anxious A asks F for help. He responds by offering him a tranquilizer with 'anxiolytic effects', but is unwilling to engage in deeper discussions about the reasons for the anxiety. The tranquilizer is more appropriate, he explains to A, as the 'anxiety is ultimately generated by your brain'. Again, even if the intervention works (otherwise, it was simply unsuitable), the response is irritatingly off track. It fails to properly engage with A's anxiety.

In both cases, A may comprehensibly complain about not being understood, not being properly recognized, appreciated, or valued. Regularly – though not always – people do not seek bodily explanations, but psychological understanding; they want to talk about the contents of their experiences, seek relational responses, mainly reasons and explanations, on a psychological level. On this count, F's responses are severely impoverished because they fail to engage on this level, they rather reduce A to his body, which affords and somewhat implies ignorance of his subjectivity. In both responses, the subjective side is, as Nussbaum might say, disregarded or ignored because feelings and experiences are not properly taken into account.

These two cases exemplify basic elements of objectification and demonstrate that it is prima facie inadequate and wrong. This does not preclude that people sometimes seek merely an objectifying response, for example, when asking a doctor for a prescription. Objectification is not wrong *tout court*, only if it causes the absence of or replaces something valuable. People can consent to being objectified, but this marks the exception, not the rule. As a default mode of how persons should treat each other, or of how societal systems such as mental healthcare should be structured, disregarding the subjective side is inappropriate.

This account of objectification needs further refinement. Here, is a rough sketch: it requires laying out more precisely what respecting persons as subjects means. To this end, central and normatively relevant elements of subjectivity have to be identified. One hallmark of subjects in an interesting sense is that they have a self-relation. Humans are, as Charles Taylor once put it, 'self-interpreting animals'. It is also noteworthy that the formation of subjectivity seems to require, on a fundamental level, *intersubjectivity*, interpersonal relations. Moreover, the notion of disrespect needs clarification. It can mean, for instance, to weaken or undermine capacities relevant for subjectivity, or to disregard or not adequately engage with subject-typical aspects, an idea that has to be rendered more precise with respect to particular cases. In the present context, this means that disregard of first-person data or interventions into minds that do not engage with mental characteristics are prime candidates for objectification.

Furthermore, on the normative level, the wrongness of objectification has to be elaborated upon. A meta-question is whether the wrongness of various kinds of objectification rest on the same normative grounds. Is objectification inherently wrong, as the example of the objectification of women suggests? Or is it only wrong in so far as it causes further harms, such as distorted self-relations? Can objectified persons consent to being objectified in every case, or does this neglect structural forms objectification or internalized external objectification, as neo-Marxism would urge? These questions touch upon more general topics in normative ethics. Dignity-based approaches tend to consider objectification as a wrong in itself whereas consequentialist views may focus on outcomes (Hoffman, 2013). These are open questions for a general theory of objectification that have to be left aside in the following.

Objectifying explanations and interventions

But how does biological psychiatry objectify persons more precisely? Disregard of subjectivity—*mindlessness*—is a paradigmatic worry about biological psychiatry (Eisenberg, 1986). Whereas some view it is an inherent feature of biological approaches (Szasz, 1961), others emphasize it is merely a contingent side effect (Schöne-Seifert, 1994). Many psychiatrists espouse biological explanations as they consider them epistemically and scientifically preferable to other explanations because of the supposed primacy of the brain. But that position might be premature. The following seeks to bring the contrast between objectifying and non-objectifying explanations and interventions into stronger relief. First in general terms, second more specifically in regard to psychiatry.

Explanations are objectifying when they disregard the subjective side, the first-person perspective. Examples are causal explanations of mental phenomena in the language of biology, physics, or other natural sciences. They objectify if their *explanantia* for mental disorders are only 'objective' data observable from the third-person perspective. Such explanations take, to borrow a phrase from Daniel Dennett, a 'mechanical stance' towards observed phenomena (Dennett, 1989). The traditional counterpart to explanations of this kind are forms of meaningful *understanding* from an 'intentional stance'. Inherent to psychological (and commonsensical) explanations, this stance seeks to understand persons 'from within', their subjective side or first-person perspective. Understanding comprises, in a description by Karl Jaspers (1920), explaining how novel mental elements such as thoughts or emotions emerge from previous elements or psychological conditions. It does so mainly by establishing *meaningful* connections between mental elements (which are not primarily those of physics or biology). Understanding can proceed by various ways, from carefully listening to introspective self-reports and observing behaviour to dialogical and even inquisitive methods. It may involve joint attempts in making meaning, construing narratives, or speculating about non-conscious factors and psychodynamics. Notably, people use specific capacities to understand other persons, among others, they simulate other minds (mindreading, mentalizing). These intersubjective mechanisms are not yet fully empirically studied nor theoretically grasped: what is empathy more precisely, how does mindreading work, do people construct theories of other minds, or simulate or simply interact with them?[8] But these vagaries do not undermine the more general point, the distinction between explanation and understanding. It has been one of the venerable topics of philosophy of science (Feest, 2010). For centuries, the question whether explanations of human behaviour and social interaction require methods different to those of the hard natural sciences led to great controversies (the historical affirmative answer is the *raison d'etre* for the 'humanities').

Whereas understanding persons is inherently intersubjective and requires taking a 'second-person perspective', the natural sciences have a notoriously distanced relation to subjectivity and try to free themselves from it in at least two respects: by eliminating the subjective role of the scientist or observer to establish 'objective', observer-independent scientific facts. And, when the observed entities are humans, by relying on measurable and verifiable data, which excludes subjective or phenomenological aspects. Self-reports are the most subjective form of data to be accommodated ('heterophenomenology'; Dennett, 2007). However, it is not about the subjective experience per se, but about observable reports of it ('after administration of an anxiolytic substance, patient A reports no longer feeling anxious'). This is the closest a strong positivist natural science, third-person approach can approximate the mind. It has to eschew deeper engagement with subjectivity. Accordingly, approaches only accommodating data observable form the third-person perspective are, as critics point out, to some degree inherently – and not only coincidentally – *mindblind*.

---

[8] Social neuroscience has contributed interesting ideas and data such as mirror neurons, embodied simulation, or brain coupling (Gallese, 2007; Hasson and Frith, 2016).

Second-person approaches, by contrast, are explicitly intersubjective by recognizing that all sides involve subjects, with their own perspectival perceptions and distortions. Second-person approaches inevitably draw upon individual background assumptions, experiences, expectations, and, more generally, the mental life of the observer, leading into iterative processes of understanding but also hermeneutic circles. Michael Pauen usefully captures the difference between the second- and third-person perspectives as:

> the difference between a perspective on some object, whatever the object may be, and an 'object' that is recognized as an epistemic subject herself, that is, recognized as someone who has a perspective of her own and is a possible partner of an interactive process. (Pauen, 2012, p. 11)

In the best case, data from different perspectives complement each other. Often, however, they will stand in some contrast as they derive from incompatible explanatory schemes. So far, no framework has succeeded in reconciling causal processes unfolding according to the laws of nature with intentional phenomena and psychological dynamics. The ambitious aspirations of naturalistic programmes are yet to be realized. For the time being, we have to live with *several possibly incompatible explanatory schemes*. The intentional stance, the engagement with reasons, thoughts, and emotions of a person, and the biological-mechanical one. Restricting one's view to *one* of these perspectives is epistemically defective in so far as relevant information from the other is ignored. The disctinction between explanation and understanding coarsely maps the one between objectifying and non-objectifying measures. Strict neurobiological approaches are objective in terms of science, but also objectifying when they cleave to a third-person perspective. Taking an intersubjective stand in perceiving and treating others is, by contrast, usually not objectifying as it (if only implicitly) acknowledges subjectivities.

Objectification in psychiatry

These tensions also characterize psychiatry, located at the intersections of the subjective and the bodily, and traditionally oscillating between psychological and biological approaches in both explanations and interventions. The distinction between explanation and understanding is deeply engrained in the methodology of psychiatry (Phillips, 2004; Thornton, 2010). Phenomenology, the systematic investigation of the formal structures of experiences in the first-person perspective, has a long tradition (Jaspers, 1920; Fuchs, 2010). Freud famously wavered between neurological and psychological views (Freud, 1895; Brook, 1998). Regarding *explanations*, the litmus test is whether mental disorders are conceived of as mere brain disorders, which are in theory fully explainable on the neurobiological level, or whether additional psychological or social explanations are deemed necessary. Currently, the dominant 'medical model' pushes the field towards (pure) biological aetiologies. One of the hopes associated with neuroscience is that the current symptom-based classificatory systems can be restructured according to neural (including genetic) causes or biomarkers. Although envisioned for the latest revision of the *Diagnostic and Statistical Manual of Mental Disorders*, these attempts have proven unsuccessful so far.

The growing importance of biological approaches in explanations corresponds to increasing biological *interventions*, manifested in the trend towards medication. Among the various means and methods which aim at transforming mental states or processes, cognitive or affective, conscious or non-conscious, two kinds can be distinguished: direct (biological) or indirect (perceptual) interventions. The dividing characteristic is the pathway by which they reach the mind/brain: indirect are those stimuli which are perceived through the outward senses; direct interventions are those which work primarily on the bodily level and, for example, undergo a range of metabolic processes before they have mental effects. The controversial ethical question is whether these different pathways correspond to normatively relevant differences, and whether they relate to objectification. This chapter affirms such differences (see Bublitz and Merkel, 2014; Bublitz, 2020); for an opposing view, see Levy (2007; 2020). Psychopharmaceuticals and brain stimulation are instances of the latter; they work primarily on the neurobiological level. Their pathways into minds largely bypass psychological processes of recipients; they target the mind through the brain as a bodily organ with the instruments of biophysical sciences. Their effectiveness primarily depends on physical properties such as targeting the correct brain areas, inducing the right electric currents, or adequate levels of particular neurotransmitters. In pharmacology, relevant questions are addressed by subfields such as pharmacogenetics, -dynamics, and -kinetics; none of these fields is concerned with processes or events at the psychological level. Accordingly, pathways of neurointerventions and their mode of operation are mainly biochemical (for a fuller exposition, see Bublitz (2020)). To some, pharmacology embodies a 'technical paradigm' of accessing other minds (Bracken et al., 2012). It aligns well with a biomedical conceptualization of mental disorders as biological disorders, suggesting treatments have to repair biological defects. Subjectivity plays only a peripheral role; neurointerventions do not engage with content or meaning of mental states but target their neural underpinnings. The subjective side is often even purposefully circumvented. Neurointerventions are often deployed because intersubjective engagements are unsuccessful, less efficient, or met with resistance. This biological mode of accessing minds prima facie constitutes objectification.

Many second-person interventions, in contrast, work differently and are not (or to a much lesser degree) objectifying. Effective indirect interventions regularly have to engage with subjectivities of recipients. They perceive stimuli through their senses and process them through a range of psychological mechanisms. These interventions often work by appealing to beliefs and desires, by providing reasons or eliciting emotions, and relating to how persons make sense of the world and their situation. Classic psychotherapy, for instance, respects subjectivity in so far as it aims to provide analysands with self-knowledge. Although the process involves *a*rational and uncontrollable non-conscious mechanisms (e.g. transference) and includes overcoming resistance and ego-defences, analysands retain some control over outcomes as they have to accept interpretations and narratives and remain, in some sense, the authors of their accounts about themselves. Cognitive behavioural therapy, to take another example, involves rising awareness about one's thought patterns and emotional dispositions and responses, and provides patients with consciously deployable strategies for their transformation. These methods work with, and on, subjectivities in a qualitatively different way than neurobiological interventions. In addition, they also regularly involve intersubjective elements. Psychotherapy takes a 'relational stance', it seeks to build *therapeutic relationships* between clients and therapists, transference and countertransference are essentially relational processes. Indirect interventions often require mutual sensitivity and responsiveness, and rely on subtle intersubjective processes such as attunement. Effects brought about by such processes resonate with the personality of affected persons and engage with them as subjects.

In this way, various treatment modalities of behavioural, cognitive, or psychotherapeutic programmes could be analysed and ranked on a spectrum of objectification. Some will be more objectifying than others, ranging from full-blown denials of subjectivity over its circumvention to insensitivity or indifference. Most indirect interventions will differ from neurointerventions in terms of engagement with, or respect of, subjectivity. Although this juxtaposition between biological and indirect interventions is somewhat idealized, general differences in the way they relate to the subjective side of persons are hardly deniable. Direct interventions relate primarily to the organic physical side, bypass subjective capacities, and follow a technical instrumental mode in treating persons as biological beings, whereas indirect interventions usually resonate (to some degree) with the subjectivities of affected persons.

Perhaps—and at this stage more a suggestion than a deduction—one might say, in a neo-Marxist vein, that the difference between psychological and neurobiological interventions corresponds to the shift from reasonable forms of interaction, aiming at understanding, to instrumental forms in which specific mental states or processes are eliminated or elicited through technical intervention. Neurointerventions can also be subsumed under feminist conceptions of objectification as they tend to reduce relevant features of affected persons to (disordered) physical brain processes and concomitantly tend to ignore their subjective sides. Accordingly, the mechanical stance of biological psychiatry and the mode of operation of neurointerventions fulfil key criteria of objectification whereas indirect interventions regularly recognize the subjectivity of the other.

Patient views

These theoretical considerations correspond with views of patients. Although their experiences are diverse, a majority seemingly prefer psychological over pharmaceutical treatments, contrasting the trend to medication (three out of four, according to McHugh et al. (2013)). Moreover, many inpatients lament a lack of therapeutic engagement and psychological interventions (Wood and Alsawy, 2016). Not being heard is a repeated complaint; patients report that the *contents* of their (delusional) beliefs, their *experiences* of anxiety, the meaning and sense they give to the world, are not acknowledged, let alone taken seriously. Rather than being related to, patients experience that their subjective sides are medicated away. The existential dimension of their state-of-being seems often ignored and dismissively treated as something that ought not be. Although the term 'objectification' does not come up in interviews or reports, disregard for subjectivity captures some of the voiced concerns. Future questionnaires and surveys should ask about objectification more directly and explicitly.

Mischaracterizing psychiatry?

It might be objected that the foregoing mischaracterizes psychiatry. After all, psychiatry cares for subjectivity as it aims at alleviating or eliminating subjective symptoms of mental disorders. This objection is true and off-point at the same time. The present critique of objectification refers to modes of explanations and treatments, not to outcomes. Undeniably, neurobiological treatments can be effective and beneficial for subjectivities, in that sense. But they may nonetheless be worrisome. An objectification-based critique might be expanded to outcomes. It could analyse objectifying effects of neurobiological interventions, for example, their impact on self-relations, emotions, and intersubjective functioning, as in neo-Marxist approaches. But this line is not further pursued here.

Nonetheless, as treatments ultimately aim at restoring or improving aspects of subjectivity, and as ends might justify means, the charge of objectification may lose some of its force. Whether this is the case requires a broader ethical argument. Also, the juxtaposition presented here concededly falls short of capturing real psychiatric practices which often combine indirect and direct methods (e.g. drug-supported psychotherapy), and sometimes even include social interventions. These integrated interventions require more differentiated ethical assessments, the wrongness of objectifying parts might be mitigated by non-objectifying ones. Finally, the role of therapists and physicians is neglected here but would need further discussion. There are limits to the intersubjective engagement to reasonably be expected from them, as it affects them(Halpern, 2014). Thus, the present account is insufficient to provide an all-things-considered critique of psychiatric practices. But it shows the basis upon which it may be developed in the future.

Reductionist objections and misleading metaphysics

While the foregoing has outlined how the concept of objectification may serve to illuminate relevant differences approaches to the mind, this section addresses an objection which looms in the background and threatens to undermine the tenability of objection as an ethical concept. It is epitomized by the key tenet of biological psychiatry: the mental *is* biological. Drawing distinctions between, and ascribing different ethical values to, mind and brain then appears confused. If any takes priority over the other, it is the brain, the neurobiological level. After all, everything mental is caused by the brain, not vice versa. These central ideas of biological psychiatry cast doubts on the plausibility of a norm against perceiving or treating persons (mainly) on the biological level. More generally: we *are* biological beings and physical objects. Demanding that we do not treat each other like this may appear as denial of this fact. Accordingly, any theory of objectification has to answer what one may call the naturalist challenge: can the ethical wrongness of objectification be upheld in in light of the science of the twenty-first century—or does it collapse in light of advances of neuroscience?

Because of their belief in brain primacy, proponents of biological psychiatry may assume the latter. As an illustration, consider a typical reasoning, exemplified by a remark by one of Germany's leading psychiatrist in a popular science interview. After affirming that all mental disorders are also brain disorders, he explains:

> At their core is an imbalance in the biochemistry of cells. The organic causes of diseases were already accepted in antiquity … But with Descartes, modernity has introduced the separation between body and soul, fatal for research. Fortunately, and thanks to modern technology, we can overcome this today. (Ayan, 2011, p. 37, translation by author)

Pressed whether such emphasis on brain chemistry is not one-sided, he replies:

> No, particularly not if one seeks to cure. Individual suffering is surely embedded in the particular circumstances of patients' lives. They influence how one deals with illness and which specific forms of support from families or working environments can be mustered. The real problem, however, is rooted in brain processes, that is the point to be targeted by treatment. (Ayan, 2011, p. 37, translation by author)

With respect to alternatives to medication, he notes that methods such as cognitive behavioural therapy 'cause very unspecific effects' and may play a supportive role of medication (Ayan, 2011, p. 37, translation by author).

These remarks not merely express the truism that every mental disorder is related to the brain in some sense, but suggest more strongly that the brain level is more elementary in the explanation of disorders—the 'real problems' lie there. Alternative views are supposedly tainted by Cartesianism. Consequently, neurobiological interventions appear in some sense primary since they target the problem at its roots. From this perspective, one may indeed have trouble finding faults with objectifying treatments. Rather than anti-humanist, they appear as natural consequences of the way the world is. But is this line of argument convincing? Let us look at it in some detail by considering four variations.

All interventions are biological

One might be inclined to deny any meaningful distinctions between objectifying and non-objectifying interventions as they supposedly deny the biological base of the mind: *all* interventions with mental effects are biological. Under this premise, it may appear as if the above-mentioned distinctions do not make sense, that neurobiology cannot be the problem with some, but not other interventions. However, it is indeed true that all interventions, even paradigmatic indirect ones such as psychotherapy, are biological in the sense that they alter the brain (Linden, 2006; Buchheim et al., 2012). But this does not mean that they are *only* biological. As shown, different interventions take different causal routes and rely on different mechanisms; some engage with mental states and processes of recipients, others circumvent them. These differences allow drawing ethically relevant distinctions between interventions without denying a neurobiological base of all of them. Humans have a dual nature, they are biological beings—but not exclusively. In other words: the difference is not that some interventions are neurobiological whereas others are not, but rather that some engage with psychological higher levels whereas others engage primarily with lower levels (cf. Bublitz, 2020).

Dualism and the anti-Cartesian fallacy

One might be suspicious as this reply contains residues of dualism. But even though dualism has become synonymous with unscientific thinking and bad metaphysics in some quarters of psychiatry and neuroscience, this might not be as damning as it appears. Some forms of dualism are inevitable to adequately deal with the mind–brain relation. In a sense, *everyone is a dualist*. It is hard to deny that there are prima facie differences between psychological entities such as intentional mental states, thoughts, or experiential feelings on one, and the entities described by biology and physics on the other side. They possess different properties and seem to exist in different spheres (mental states do not have a spatiotemporal location). The dynamics by which they operate, and the rules by which they transition from one to the next also seem different. Furthermore, the first- and third-person perspectives do not coincide. Whether one describes these differences as running between levels, or as dualistic properties or perspectives, and whether one conceives of them as ontological or epistemological, one cannot but concede a prima facie difference between the mental and the biological. That is why there is a problem at all.

Recognizing these dualisms places the onus on those downplaying them. Many statements from biological psychiatry nonetheless appear antithetical to even weaker forms of dualism. Apart from general theoretic preconceptions, the main piece of evidence against dualism is the effectiveness of neurointerventions. But the indisputable fact that biological interventions can effectively change minds only refutes specific variations of dualism, those denying causal effects of matter on mind. But there are other forms such as property dualism (Chalmers, 1995), perspectival dualism (Habermas, 2007), or interactionist forms resembling Cartesian dualism (Popper and Eccles, 2012). They may find prima facie support in top-down influences of mental states on effects of neurointerventions (from the placebo effect to the 'set and setting' influences on psychedelics, cf. Beauregard (2007)). In any case, it was misleading to draw sweeping reductionist conclusions from the wrongness of substance dualism. One may call this the *anti-Cartesian fallacy*: from the falseness of Cartesian dualism, the falseness of other dualisms does not follow, let alone the truth of neuroreductionism.

Neuroreductionism and neurocentrism

Nonetheless, one may still believe in some primacy of the brain, as expressed in claims such as 'everything is caused by the brain'. There are two problems with it: while mental effects of drugs and other bodily interventions prove *bottom-up* causality from brain to mind, they cannot prove more general statements that *everything* mental is caused by the brain. Some changes in the mind may have different causes, for example, other mental events ('A's negative feelings are caused by his thought that other people dislike him'). Furthermore, the kind of causality is unclear. In a weak form, 'caused by the brain' means that the brain is a necessary condition of the mind. This is almost certainly true. Every mental state needs a physical realizer, every psychological process a neurological implementation. But this does not establish a primacy of the brain of a kind that causes deep problems for a theory of objectification. In stronger forms, 'caused by the brain' denotes a form of neuroreductionism. Its truth may threaten the plausibility of a claim against objectification, as the metaphysical and evaluative meanings of 'reducing persons' seem to hang together. Reductionism comes in many forms and strengths, and can refer to different objects. It has led to complex debates in philosophy of science and mind which have produced a great variety of plausible positions that cannot be rehearsed here (Hohwy and Kallestrup, 2008; Kendler, 2008; Roache, 2019). Here is a brief and rough look at two forms potentially undermining the idea of objectification:

1. Explanatory reductionism: mental, higher-level phenomena can be reduced to the lower, neurobiological level, in the sense that all properties of mental elements are *fully explainable* by properties of the elements at the neurobiological level. For example, the content of paranoid thoughts or the emotional numbness of depression are fully explainable by neurobiological facts (e.g. about brain chemistry or brain activation patterns). Furthermore, if reductionism extends to transitions between mental states, then psychological laws or dynamics would be fully reducible to the laws of the reductive base, the laws of physics or neurobiology. For example, the behaviour of persons and their psychological causes which attachment theory describes would then be describable in terms of physical laws, without losing any relevant information. If this generalizes, it would deny the independence of psychology from neuroscience and physics.

2. Causal reductionism: according to stronger ontological forms, the properties of the higher level are *nothing over and above* the properties of the reductive base. Especially relevant here is the claim that causality runs at the neurobiological level alone. Thus, the transition from one mental state, M1, to the next, M2, is causally affected only by their neural correlates, N1 and N2. Accordingly, N1 causes N2, but no further causal relations obtain between M1 and M2. Causal reductionism rules out mental, top-down, or other non-strictly physical forms of causation.

The truth of these (interrelated) claims might let a norm against objectification appear unreasonable. If the neurobiological level fully explains or exclusively causes all occurrences on the mental level, it seems to suggest itself to only (or primarily) engage with the former level. Understanding through finding meaningful connections between mental events would then, at best, be an intermediate step since the causally effective connections run elsewhere and follow the laws of physics or neurobiology. Why bother with phenomenology or higher-level processes, why pursue hermeneutic understanding and idiographic inquiries, and why examine objects of anxieties and their meaning for the person if one can directly engage with neurobiology? Identifying and repairing 'defects' and 'failures' at more elementary levels, in cells, neurotransmitters, pathways, circuits, or networks, seems to be the straightforward route for explaining and curing disorders. After all, even interventions such as psychotherapy are in the reductionist picture effective only because they induce the right neurobiological changes (not in virtue of the insights they provide). So, if mental disorders were nothing but disorders of the brain, it seems advisable to target them there directly. Mental information and symptoms would only be of epistemic value as they point to the *real* neurobiological problems (e.g. depressive symptoms indicate chemical imbalances; anxiety indicates amygdala overactivation). If this view was correct, objectification does not appear wrong; effective treatments may even require it. Notably, according to studies, this reasoning seems to be held by mental health clinicians who more strongly favour medication over psychotherapy if they are given a biological rather than a psychosocial explanation (for the same symptoms), and vice versa (Ahn et al., 2009; Lebowitz and Ahn, 2014).

However, whether these or related variants of reductionism are true is an unsolved question at the heart of the mind–body problem. It should be emphasized that neither biological psychiatry, nor neuroscience, has come close to answering it. Their reductive commitments stem from methodological and theoretical assumptions rather than from conclusive empirical findings. Unless one shares these assumptions, the prospects of full *explanatory* reducibility of the mental do not seem terribly high, for at least two reasons: the properties of conscious experience, the 'what it is likeness', for example, experiencing a psychosis, are not explainable at the brain level at the moment (Nagel, 1974). And without solving the 'hard problem of consciousness', it is unlikely that they ever will. Furthermore, current neurobiology is inept to account for the content of mental states, for their intentionality. These are two notorious hurdles to reductionism (Levine, 1983; Chalmers, 1995). Relevant disciplines such as biology have not seriously started to modify their theories to accommodate intentionality and experience in their terms. Nor are psychophysical bridge laws on the horizon. They are a far cry from the more or less strong correlations between neurobiological and mental processes which neuroscience has demonstrated in the last years. Thus, nothing forces us to adopt a reductionist view at present. Even more, I wish to suggest that a fully reductive and objectifying view even constitutes an *epistemic failure*, as irreducible relevant data would be ignored.

With respect to transitions from one mental event to the next, it is likewise unsettled whether they follow the laws of physics because causality runs at the physical level only. This would entail that 'meaningful relations' between mental states are, ultimately, manifestations of physical causal relata. For instance, a train of thought which may be associative to the thinker, say, consecutive thoughts about sun, summer, vacation, and beach, or job loss, family problems, and anxiety, would be exhaustively explainable by properties of the neural level (e.g. by the strength of connections between neurons encoding these concepts). But the *content* of thoughts and their meaningful relation would not add anything novel to the neuronal explanation and hence, not even be a necessary part of it. Other psychological laws or dynamics would be equally irrelevant. That is already a far-reaching claim, and the degree to which strict psychological laws exist is not even clear (cf. 'mental anomalism'). Where good psychological explanations exist, it is hard to see how they translate into laws of physics or biology. How might the latter account for, say, the interpersonal and intrapsychic dynamics which attachment theory describes? If attachment theory is correct, interpersonal dynamics, say, fear of abandonment and longing for object-stability, have to be effective in some sense (otherwise the theory is false). To explain the effectiveness, some form of higher-level causation from the mind to the biological level is a prime candidate. Surely not the only one, but one that is far too god to simply be dismissed for abstract considerations. Again, scepticism about full reducibility does not deny biological substrates of the mental. There is surely a biological side to attachment, it may shape or limit higher-level processes (Carter, 2014; Music, 2014). But reductive claims which may lead the ethical idea of objectification ad absurdum have to be stronger, asserting that the lower level is all there is, in a relevant sense (Hohwy and Kallestrup, 2008).

The view that higher-level dynamics do not possess any causal powers is also not particularly attractive for other reasons. For instance, it cannot evade the question why higher levels exist at all if they are causally inert. A plausible alternative view holds that they may possess structural (or part-whole) causal powers. Moreover, causal reductionism rules out mental causation, that is, top-down causation of physical effects by mental properties. But mental causation is a central part of successful everyday explanatory practices and is presupposed in ideas such as that persons *act for reasons* in a stricter sense, or that the will causes behaviour. Much has been written about mental causation in recent years (Pockett et al., 2006), especially with respect to free will. It seems that not much speaks in favour of the causal inertness of mental properties, apart, that is, from a naturalistic scientific view of the world that presupposes it. The main problem with mental causation is that it seems to contravene the causal closure of the world. Then, however, the strongest argument for reductionism does not derive from empirical findings, but from general considerations about science. Reductionism is, to some degree, inscribed in its logic (see Oppenheim and Putnam, 1958 but also Horst, 2007), and has of course been a successful strategy in the past. However, such broad theories as the nature of causation or the idea of laws of nature, or the causal closure of the world, are always provisional, and inferences are abductive. And thus, we should, at least for the time being, never be too convinced that they are right. And if, for instance, downward causation exists in other domains such as biology or sociology (Ellis, 2016; Paolini Paoletti, 2017), the plausibility of its rejection in the mind–brain relation would be seriously weakened. In sum: the forces that effect the transition from one mental event to another, and the logic or rules or dynamic that they follow, are not well understood. Positing the primacy of one level over another is thus not warranted by current evidence.

After all, minds might still be *emergent* phenomena of complex systems that operate by laws and dynamics distinct from those of neurobiology (for the notion of emergence see Kim (1999)). This and other non-reductive theories (e.g. supervenience; Davidson, 1995) enjoy some support in philosophy of mind. There are thus no compelling reasons for psychiatry to accept the truth of reductionism. At present, it is merely a metaphysical speculation and a research hypothesis. One should be aware of its fragility and avoid conflating a research hypothesis with established scientific facts. Consequently, the belief in neuroreductionism is impotent to cast severe doubts on the plausibility of the wrongness of objectification.

Nonetheless, parts of psychiatry flirt with, and sometimes presuppose, the truth of reductionism, or stronger positions ('the mind *is* the brain'). Other parts, such as neuropsychoanalysis, seek to combine higher- and lower-level explanations without ascribing priority to one, placing mind and brain on an equal footing (Panksepp and Solms, 2012; Solms, 2015; cf. also Kandel's (1998) 'rapprochement' programme). Many statements in psychiatry are not terribly precise about the relation between mind and brain that they presuppose and sometimes appear quite unclear from the view of philosophy of mind (Kendler, 2008; Schramme, 2013; Roache, 2019; a related but different point is made by Bennett and Hacker (2003)). Even seminal articles seem oblique to the details of the problem (Gold, 2009).[9] Pragmatic reasons may speak in favour of such a loose approach. However, especially when far-ranging consequences are attached to (denial of) specific positions (as in the opening quote of this section), more attention is warranted. This shortcoming also irritates since the critique of psychiatry drew on related metaphysical arguments (Szasz, 1974). One might have expected that appropriate engagement with that criticism would motivate a clearer view on the mind–brain problem.

Practically speaking, reductive approaches in explanation, nosology, and aetiology have not been terribly successful in the last two decades which were characterized by heavy emphasis on the neuro. For instance, biomarkers for disorders could not be identified (Kapur et al., 2012). Nor are there individual reductive success stories that let its broader truth appear very likely. Many theorists thus believe in multilevel explanations (Mitchell, 2008; Schaffner, 2008; Kendler, 2012). Of course, a reductive neuro-future of psychiatry might be around the corner, with genetic markers and big-data regrouping disorders and affording personalized 'high-precision' treatment. One may make such predictions, harbour such hopes, and push for research in that direction. But they remain hypotheticals and expectations. The unshackled optimism in the realization of reductive programmes and the belief in brain priority is neither evidence based, nor warranted by philosophy of mind, and often seems untroubled by the grave objections it faces.

Still, one might more modestly concede irreducible properties and unbridgeable gaps between mind and brain but downplay their relevance for psychiatry. It might be possible to explain the pathogenesis of disorders and treat them without accounting for every causal process, or even solving the 'hard problem of consciousness'. As long as it works, we metaphysics can be left metaphysics. However, even biological psychiatry needs to resort to supposedly reducible, subjective aspects for purposes such as diagnosing and classifying disorders.[10] And more importantly, this would not

---

[9] To exemplify this with one of the most influential recent contributions, consider Kandel's (1998) call for a 'rapprochement' of neurobiology and Freudian psychoanalysis. His first principle reads: 'All mental processes, even the most complex psychological processes, derive from operations of the brain. The central tenet of this view is that what we commonly call mind is a range of functions carried out by the brain. The actions of the brain underlie ... all of the complex cognitive actions ... As a corollary, behavioral disorders that characterize psychiatric illness are disturbances of brain function, even in those cases where the causes of the disturbances are clearly environmental in origin.' This is one principle that apparently describes one coherent approach to the mind–brain relation. However, it contains several distinct, possibly mutually exclusive positions: A *derives from* B; A is a *function* of B; actions of B *underlie* A; disorders of A *are* disorders of B. The last sentence which asserts that mental disorders are brain disorders even though causes are *clearly of environmental origin* is also anything but self-evident. Perhaps, Kandel merely wants to express a biological side to the mental. That seems almost trivially true. (Cf. Kandel (1999) where he attempts to clarify his position.)

[10] Third-person perspectives alone seem to miss important aspects (Gold, 2009; Kirmayer and Gold, 2012). Even in schizophrenia, the paradigmatic neurobiological mental disorder, a first-person perspective seems to add interesting and otherwise unobservable aspects (Sass

undermine the norm against objectification, which posits that one *should* explain and intervene at higher levels. As long as such interventions are possible, its plausibility as an ethical demand is not undermined.

What if reductionism were true?

However, even though prospects for full reductionism may not be too bright, it might be possible to reduce partial aspects such as specific mechanisms (Bechtel and Abrahamsen, 2005; Bechtel, 2007). And, given the strong appeal of reductionism on contemporary thought, its implications for the concept of objectification merit discussion. Prima vista, it may appear that the truth of reductionism implies that psychological theories as well as meaningful, higher-level connections between mental events are false and that intersubjective means to uncover and understand them are therefore futile. But this reasoning gets the argument the wrong way around. By itself, reductionism does not disprove higher-level mental processes, non-reductive connections between them, or anything that can be called a psychological theory. The reverse is true: one of the conditions of success of explanatory or causal reductionism is that it reconstructs existing higher-level connections (more precisely) at lower levels, or that causal relations only obtain there. If explanatory reductionism is true, resort to first-person data or psychological theories might become unnecessary. It does not imply, however, that first-person data or psychological theories are *false*, nor that they do not exist. Reductionism does not make psychological phenomena, dynamics, or processes disappear (in so far as it is not *eliminativism*). Rather, it aims to explain them. If connections exist, for instance, between biographical events, life problems, thought patterns, emotional dispositions, and mental disorders, then reductionism does not, and cannot, disprove them. Likewise, whether attachment theory is correct does not depend on its reducibility to neurobiology, but on independent reasons, the general conditions of the truth of scientific theories (such as describing relevant processes accurately, with better predictive and explanatory powers than alternatives). If people form the kind of emotional bonds which attachment theory describes, reductionism either accounts for them, or is false—but not vice versa.

Furthermore, even the truth of *explanatory reductionism* would not imply that engaging with others on higher-levels through non-objectifying means is epistemically wrong. Such engagements can still yield true and interesting insights. Comprehensively explaining disorders may still require taking an intentional stance, as data might not be obtained on other ways. Accordingly, the truth of explanatory reductionism neither renders non-objectifying practices futile, nor a norm against objectification implausible.

However, its truth would still have ramifications for plausible accounts of objectification. It might be that psychological explanations drawing on meaningful connections are *wrong* and turn out as pseudo-explanations masking the correct neurobiological ones. If this is true, objectifying explanations are epistemically superior to

---

and Parnas, 2007). Likewise, accounting for the mental changes in depression, a first-person account seems indispensable (Ratcliffe, 2014).

non-objectifying ones. And this directly affects norms favouring the latter. It is suggested here that no ethical theory can demand ignoring relevant data or espousing pseudo-explanations. In so far as best explanations contravene higher-level and support lower-level explanations, the demand to not objectify must yield. The truth of reductionism would thus limit the scope of the norm against objectifying explanations in those instances in which it would demand ignoring better explanations. In other words: epistemic truth must prevail over the claim against objectification. Again, non-objectifying explanations are not necessarily false, even if reductionism were true. But they might often be so. And this points to a weak spot in positions strictly opposing biological approaches in psychiatry.

With respect to *interventions into minds*, the truth of causal reductionism would not imply a priority of neurobiological ones. One may falsely believe the opposite because of the casual reductionist claim outlined previously: if causality only runs at the neurobiological level, all interventions have to be causally effective there. However, no scientific or metaphysical fact, including the truth of causal reductionism, necessitates a categorical primacy of neurointerventions. *If* the real, core, or root cause (whatever that precisely means) of a mental disorder is a brain disorder, neurobiological treatments will surely often be effective. But even then the relation between the levels of cause and intervention is contingent, not necessary. One may call this the *aetiology-treatment fallacy*: the fact that the genesis of a state of affairs can be primarily located at one particular level does not necessitate that remedies primarily intervene at that level, too. There is no necessary relation between causes of an event and subsequent interventions to transform it. Such a relation may obtain only if one understands treatments literally as antidotes counteracting or negating the 'real', original causes of an illness. But medical treatments frequently work at different levels, as the reverse *cum hoc ergo propter hoc fallacy* shows: aspirin may cure headaches, even though they were not caused by a deficit of acetylsalicylic acid. Accordingly, even if chemical imbalances cause depression, it does not follow that alleviating interventions necessarily have to be chemical. Other interventions at different levels might be equally effective, even more, or with less side effects. Transforming minds may then still require harnessing intersubjective processes or talk therapy because they induce desired changes better than direct interventions. Aetiological facts might be epistemically helpful in finding effective treatments, but they do not prejudice whether specific interventions are effective. This remains *an empirical matter*. Allusions to metaphysics, brain primacy, or reductionism, as in the quote opening this section, unfortunately suggest otherwise. They should be avoided, along with suggestive talk about 'real' causes, and be replaced with evidence-based evaluations of interventions of every kind.

Brain primacy, intersubjectivity, and social environment

Hereto, only the relations between higher- and lower-levels have been addressed. To complete the picture, here is a brief look at the external dimension. Neurocentrism tends to lead to insensitivity to environmental influences and interpersonal (social, cultural) determinants of health, as well as to effective interventions at those levels. Biological psychiatry provides an illustrative example again (although psychotherapeutic practices also tend to downplay social factors; Flick, 2016). Consider the opening sentences of a leading textbook, *Biological Psychiatry*:

> It has become fashionable periodically to ascribe much psychopathology to the evils of modern society, and the resurgence of this notion from time to time reflects the popularity of the simple. Often imbued with political overtones, and rarely aspiring to scientific insights, such a view of the pathogenesis of psychiatric illness ignores the long tradition of both the recognition of patterns of psychopathology and successful treatment by somatic therapies. Further, it does not take into account the obvious fact that humanity's biological heritage extends back many millions of years. (Trimble and George, 2010, p. 1)

Breathing the belief in brain primacy, this passage dismisses the search for causes of mental disorders in social conditions as ideological and non-scientific, refuted by the successes of neurobiological interventions and ignorant of evolution and genetics. But such a denial of social—and supposedly, environmental—causes of mental health and illness is a non-sequitur. Neither the truth of evolution nor successes of neurointerventions cast doubt on the causal powers which societal or environment factors may exert on human minds.[11] This rejection of social causes is apparently motivated by the following reasoning: evolved biological bodies cause mental disorders, evidenced by the fact that somatic interventions work. This cause apparently excludes the possibility of further societal causes. The problem with this view is a narrow understanding of causation and a false dichotomy between several causal factors. Biological and societal causes are not mutually exclusive; the presence of one does not indicate or preclude the absence of the other. Environmental events precede the brain events which cause mental disorders. Environmental or societal factors have to work through the brain, which is the more immediate, direct or *proximate* cause. But proximate causation do not negate the causality of preceding, more distal ones. Moreover, the behaviour of an individual organism is regularly not explainable without considering the environment with which it interacts. This is just as true for humans as for other animals. The perennial question that neuroscience is unable to answer by itself is *why* the brain proximately causes specific mental phenomena and behavioural responses. Answers may often refer to the environment. Strong dependency on, and adaption to, the (naturally and socially constituted) environment are, by the way, key features of evolutionary explanations.

External factors are frequently inevitable parts of comprehensive explanations as well as suitable, though neglected, targets of interventions (Levy, 2012). Sociological models about the contemporary human condition provide a range of large-scale effects that influence the mental fabric of society and individuals, and thereby affect the likelihood and onset of mental disorders. Typical candidates are the loss of meaning, issues of self-identity, changing social roles, precarious working conditions, and reduced

---

[11] This blunt rejection of social causes is not representative of psychiatry. But the role of the environment in psychiatric thought is not settled. Gestures towards the relevance of social influences abound, practice and research often proceed without further regard for it (be that for theoretical or practical reasons). Davies (2017) grasps the paradoxical situation in his comment that the biopsychosocial model is 'everywhere and yet nowhere'.

security and control over one's future (Whitley, 2008; Sik, 2018). More concretely, for instance, interrelations between increasing rates of depression, the waning quality of supportive social relationships, and overburdening societal demands appear likely ('weariness of the self'; Ehrenberg, 2010). The same is true for negative effects of the expanding commodification of social life. Moreover, and even tough scepticism about self-assessments in psychological matters is warranted, these explanations correspond to what persons themselves consider to be the causes of their depression (working conditions, current and past life stressors are the most cited factors; Hansson et al., 2010). An example of a multi-perspectival research project is provided by King and colleagues (2018). They analysed the interplay of the acceleration of everyday societal processes, resulting drives to self-optimization as well as biographical reports and psychodynamic effects in patients. Not surprisingly, these societal dynamics contribute to anxieties, low self-reliance, and doubts about one's self-efficacy, which in turn create vulnerabilities for mental disorders. Supposedly, such explanations are true. Although they are incomplete, they identify risk factors, which complement further psychological and biological facts. But even though these explanations are likely true, they do not play a significant role in psychiatric aetiologies.

Even neuroscience has come to acknowledge peculiar biological effects of social interactions such as 'brain coupling', allegedly not understandable by views restricted to one brain alone (Hasson et al., 2012). Other studies show that social rejection activates the same pain networks as physical harm (Eisenberger, 2015). Thus, even neuro-explanations of the causes of brain disorders cannot ignore the environment. Accordingly, Thomas Fuchs conceptualizes the brain as an 'essentially historical and social organ' (Fuchs, 2017). It has long been recognized that mental health and illness have social determinants, as risk factors but also as resources for recovery or resilience (World Health Organization, 2014). A recent guidance article by the European Psychiatric Association analysed several hundred publications linking mental health with economic conditions. It states:

> [T]here is a broad consensus about the deleterious consequences of economic crises on mental health, particularly on psychological well-being, depression, anxiety disorders, insomnia, alcohol abuse, and suicidal behaviour. Unemployment, indebtedness, precarious working conditions, inequalities, lack of social connectedness, and housing instability emerge as main risk factors. (Martin-Carrasco et al., 2016, p. 89)

In the same vein, Kenneth Kendler concludes a review of the risk factors for three paradigmatic disorders—schizophrenia, depression, alcoholism: 'for the three archetypal disorders examined, difference-makers are distributed across the biological, psychological and social–cultural domains, and these levels are actively inter-twined with each other in etiologic pathways' (Kendler, 2012, p. 383). Finally, even in schizophrenia, recent genome-wide studies have shown that genes contribute to disease susceptibility (Ripke et al., 2014), but no one seems to hold that genetic causes alone fully explain it. Gene–environment interaction is crucial (Caspi and Moffitt, 2006; van Os et al., 2010). Accordingly, there is no primacy of the brain over environmental factors. Mental disorders are best understood as resulting from the complex interplay of genetic, biological, psychological, and environmental factors. Even though one aspect may be more dominant in some diseases than others, one-sided explanations are 'fervent monisms' (Kendler, 2014). Recognizing interlevel connectedness leads to—following the arrow of causation—a *sociobiopsycho* model, and the 're-socialization of psychiatry' (Kirmayer and Gold, 2012). Neglecting social or environmental determinants of mental health is then as *epistemically wrong* as a premature assumption of reductionism is. Not unlikely, recent increases in the rates of depression are better explainable by changing social and economic conditions than by changes in brain chemistry.

Normative consequences

After all, no scientific or metaphysical facts demand priority of neurobiological over other interventions, or ground a principled explanatory primacy of neurobiological over psychological or social levels. Therefore, nothing forces psychiatry to dismiss non-reductive psychological or societal explanations, or second-person approaches. In light of present knowledge, this would even constitute an *epistemic mistake* as relevant data is ignored. Until the reductive project makes groundbreaking progress, a plurality of explanations on multiple levels is the most viable option (Kendler, 2008). Drawing out the implications of espousing potentially contradictory positions, rather than betting on the dissolution of this tension, seems to be the challenge of the day. As a consequence, adopting reductionism as a default position in treatment decisions, matters of public policy, or research priorities is not warranted for *epistemic and ethical reasons*. And therefore, the concept of objectification and its wrongness is not undermined.

However, while mindlessness is no option, brainlessness is surely neither. Many times, objectifying neurobiological *explanations* might be more illuminating than non-objectifying ones. Ignoring them is epistemically defective. And some mental disorders are indeed, as Jaspers put it, unintelligible through meaningful understanding. Then, lower-level and neurobiological explanations are indispensable. Ethical claims against non-objectification begin to weaken in such cases. As a consequence, non-objectifying explanations should take priority over objectifying ones, but this priority is limited by epistemic considerations. Non-objectification should not lead to accepting pseudo-explanations. Objectification might be *justified* in these cases. While this does not call into question its prima facie wrongness, it poses problems for in-principled rejections of objectifying explanations.

A more nuanced picture emerges with respect to *interventions*: their effectiveness is exclusively an empirical matter. No metaphysical fact speaks in favour of privileging one level of intervention over another. But their ethical differences favour non-objectifying ones. This means, more concretely, that among several interventions with relevantly similar cost/benefit ratios, the non-objectifying ones should be chosen. However, neurobiological interventions might sometimes be preferable for reasons of effectiveness or costs. This again raises questions about the limits of the norm against objectification. At some point, costs may become too high to uphold it. Finally, in some cases, neurointerventions will be the only available option. For instance, persuading an acutely psychotic person about the falsity of her delusions is (by definition) a futile endeavour. Then, objectifying treatment has to be balanced against the harms of non-intervention. Yet again, the lack of alternatives does not call into question the prima facie wrongness of objectifying interventions, it may provide a justification in exceptional cases.

One may accuse this position of absurdity. Some mental disorders are clearly side effects of bodily disorders (e.g. hallucinations due to malnutrition or fever). Is trying to understand feverish thoughts and working through their meaning really preferable to administering, say, antipyretics? Well, lowering body temperature and fighting causes of fever is certainly advisable with respect to bodily health. With respect to the hallucinations, a non-objectifying position indeed implies that they be engaged with if the person so wishes. Non-objectification demands that mental phenomena are taken seriously, at least before the limits of incomprehensibility are reached. Even feverish thoughts might reveal true and unexpected insights. This a bullet which critics of objectification have to bite to some extent.

Conclusion

Further from the discussion? *Firstly*, objectification can be reconstructed as disregard, ignorance of, or insensitivity to subjectivity or intersubjectivity with respect to explanations of mental or behavioural phenomena as well as interventions to transform them. Neurobiological interventions objectify affected persons because they bypass, by design, their subjectivities. Other interventions, by contrast, especially intersubjective ones, acknowledge subjectivities and engage with them in several ways. *Secondly*, objectification is a prima facie wrong mode of dealing with persons (without their consent). It therefore requires justification and should be avoided by default. Non-objectifying interventions have *ethical priority* over objectifying ones, for example, an intentional stance is ethically preferable to a mechanical stance, approaches that accommodate first- or second-person perspectives are preferable to third-person approaches. Further work grounding and explicating the concept of objectification, especially with respect to its latent tensions with neurobiology, is required and encouraged. Adequately capturing mixed or integrated psychiatric practices requires a conception that allows for graduations, minor cases, and aggravated cases. *Thirdly*, the wrongness of objectification is not as self-evident as critics suggest. Especially epistemic advantages of objectifying explanations may override ethical concerns against their adoption. The same might be true for psychiatric interventions alleviating symptoms of mental disorders for which no non-objectifying alternatives exist. Per se, objectification might not be as damning as critics assume. *Fourthly*, objectification may serve as a key element in reconstructing the popular distinction between direct and indirect interventions, and in its vindication against rejections in psychiatry and neuroethics. It opens a novel perspective by marking a central difference between second- and third-person approaches to the person, which other concepts regularly fail to grasp. Methods of changing minds can be distinguished and ranked in its light.

Fifthly, no present scientific or metaphysical finding casts serious doubts over the suggested construal or ethical relevance of objectification. Even if neuroreductionism was true, non-objectifying methods such as understanding would not necessarily be false or futile. Metaphysical claims of a primacy of the neurobiological level should regularly be met with scepticism. They might well be based on one of the fallacies presented here: the anti-Cartesian fallacy that falsely rejects anything dualistic, or the aetiology–intervention fallacy that assumes that effective interventions to transform an event have to be placed at the same level that caused it. *Sixthly*, the role of reductive premises and objectifying practices in psychiatry has to be further differentiated in light of the different roles of psychiatry. As a field of *medical research*, it can pursue and push reductive hypotheses, whereas it cannot do so *as a medical science* because of the epistemic deficits. Furthermore, psychiatry is also a *social institution* that exerts coercive powers and structures the provision of healthcare as well as individual treatment decisions. In fields of public policy, assuming neurocentrism is wrong. It should be resisted if it is invoked to downplay competing considerations or alternative programmes. If psychiatry aspires to be the discipline decisively informing political or individual treatment decisions, it has to embrace a multilevel sociobiopsycho model. No level should be privileged over others except for evidence-based reasons. If it wishes to turn into applied neuroscience, a different meta-discipline for such decision is needed. *Seventhly*, psychiatry has to take the charge of objectification seriously and should openly engage with it. More clarity in its thinking about the mind–brain relation and implications for therapy and research would be helpful.

Eighthly, patients can expect that some healthcare institution provides them with an exhaustive all-things-considered assessment of available treatment options. If psychiatry assumes this role, it has to present all options without prejudice. This may practically require overcoming the often fragmented and parallel services for psychological support. Informed decisions require patients to understand the range of options. Failures to adequately present them, including non-evidence-based priorities of some modalities over others, may call consent into question and might even ground malpractice claims. *Ninthly*, many healthcare systems favour some methods over others for financial reasons (pharmacology over psychotherapy). This is problematic in light of objectification. Healthcare systems should, *ceteris paribus*, strive to offer non-objectifying interventions, even if more costly (of course, other considerations apply).

Tenthly, objectifying *involuntary* treatments are particularly problematic and should be avoided. Cases devoid of alternatives raise the question whether objectifying interventions might be *justified*. Answers require a broader argument about coercive interventions and the importance of the claim against non-objectification. The degrees to which they are complemented by non-objectifying measures, and whether they restore possibilities of communication and understanding, are relevant considerations.

There are two overlapping yet partly incompatible perspectives on humans: the detached scientific view and the experiential, subjective side. At present, they are irreducible and sometimes incompatible. This calls for 'binocularity' (Parens, 2015) or multi-perspectival approaches. The neurocentrist temper of the times raises the worry of a shift towards one-dimensional and objectifying approaches. But there are alternatives: postmodern theory (Lewis, 2000), postpsychiatry (Kinderman, 2014), return to hermeneutics or phenomenology (Fuchs, 2017), or a resocialization of psychiatry. They may appear unattractive as they seem to entail a partial abandonment of premises and methods of the natural sciences. The belief in them is one of the reasons sustaining biological psychiatry. Psychiatry's quest to meet strict standards of natural science is comprehensible, in light of its history of abusive treatments, pseudo-explanations, ideologically laden skirmishes, as well as political and economic pressures. However, good science openly acknowledges its limits rather than implicitly oversteps them. It distinguishes between research hypotheses, theoretical assumptions, empirically validated models, and phenomena outside of its purview. The natural sciences may fail to appreciate the lived existence of humans in all its dimensions, and things visible in one perspective might be invisible from another. At some point, the belief in neuroscience turns into neuroscientism, and the idealization of a scientific method into ideology. Ironically, it was the antipsychiatric movement that pressured psychiatry into justifying its practices by the standards of the hard natural sciences, which now motivate the objectifying practices one may lament about. But there is room for psychiatry to engage with the ethical problem of objectification without becoming fully susceptible to antipsychiatric objections.

Acknowledgements

Research funding by the German Ministry for Education and Research (BMBF) through the project INTERFACES (01GP1622B) as well as the Volkswagen Foundation is gratefully acknowledged.

References

Ahn, W., Proctor, C.C., and Flanagan, E.H. (2009). Mental health clinicians' beliefs about the biological, psychological, and environmental bases of mental disorders. *Cognitive Science*, **33**(2), 147–182.

Akil, H., Brenner, S., Kandel, E., Kendler, K.S., King, M.C., Scolnick, E., Watson, J.D., and Zoghbi, H.Y. (2010). The future of psychiatric research: genomes and neural circuits. *Science*, **327**(5973), 1580–1581.

Ayan, S. (2011). Psychische Störungen sind Hirnerkrankungen. *Gehirn & Geist*, 36–38.

Beauregard, M. (2007). Mind does really matter: evidence from neuroimaging studies of emotional self-regulation, psychotherapy, and placebo effect. *Progress in Neurobiology*, **81**(4), 218–236.

Bechtel, W. (2007). Reducing psychology while maintaining its autonomy via mechanistic explanation. In: M.K.D. Schouten and H. Looren de Jong (Eds.), *The Matter of the Mind: Philosophical Essays on Psychology, Neuroscience, and Reduction* (pp. 172–198). Malden, MA: Blackwell.

Bechtel, W. and Abrahamsen, A. (2005). Explanation: a mechanist alternative. *Studies in History and Philosophy of Science Part C: Studies in History and Philosophy of Biological and Biomedical Sciences*, **36**, 421–441.

Bennett, M.R. and Hacker, P.M.S. (2003). *Philosophical Foundations of Neuroscience*. Oxford: Blackwell.

Bewes, T. (2002). *Reification, or, The Anxiety of Late Capitalism*. London: Verso.

Bracken, P., Thomas, P., Timimi, S., Asen, E., Behr, G., Beuster, C., Bhunnoo, S., Browne, I., China, N., Double, D., et al. (2012). Psychiatry beyond the current paradigm. *The British Journal of Psychiatry*, **201**, 430–434.

Brook, A. (1998). Neuroscience versus psychology in Freud. *Annals of the New York Academy of Sciences*, **843**, 66–79.

Bublitz, C., 2020. Means matter: on the legal relevance of the distinction between direct and indirect mind-interventions. In: N. Vincent (Ed.), *Neuro-Interventions and the Law: Regulating Human Mental Capacity*. New York: Oxford University Press.

Bublitz, J.C. and **Merkel, R.** (2014). Crimes against minds: on mental manipulations, harms and a human right to mental self-determination. *Criminal Law and Philosophy*, **8**, 51–77.

Buchheim, A., Viviani, R., Kessler, H., Kächele, H., Cierpka, M., Roth, G., George, C., Kernberg, O.F., Bruns, G., and Taubner, S. (2012). Changes in prefrontal-limbic function in major depression after 15 months of long-term psychotherapy. *PLoS One*, **7**(3), e33745.

Carter, C.S. (2014). Oxytocin pathways and the evolution of human behavior. *Annual Review of Psychology*, **65**, 17–39.

Caspi, A. and Moffitt, T.E. (2006). Gene–environment interactions in psychiatry: joining forces with neuroscience. *Nature Reviews Neuroscience*, **7**(7), 583–590.

Chalmers, D.J. (1995). Facing up to the problem of consciousness. *Journal of Consciousness Studies*, **2**(3), 200–219.

Clausen, J. (2009). Man, machine and in between. *Nature*, **457**, 1080–1081.

Council of Europe (2015). *Committee on Bioethics: Working Document Concerning the Protection of Human Rights and Dignity of Persons with Mental Disorder with Regard to Involuntary Placement and Involuntary Treatment*. DH-BIO/INF (2015) 7. Strasbourg: Council of Europe.

Davies, W. (2017). Social explanations in psychiatry. (Unpublished.)

Davidson, D. (1995). Mental events. In: P.K. Moser and J.D. Trout (Eds.), *Contemporary Materialism: A Reader* (pp. 127–137). London: Routledge.

Dennett, D.C. (2007). Heterophenomenology reconsidered. *Phenomenology and the Cognitive Sciences*, **6**, 247–270.

Dennett, D.C. (1989). *The Intentional Stance*. Cambridge, MA: MIT Press.

Douglas, T. (2014). Criminal rehabilitation through medical intervention: moral liability and the right to bodily integrity. *The Journal of Ethics*, **18**, 101–122.

Ehrenberg, A. (2010). *The Weariness of the Self: Diagnosing the History of Depression in the Contemporary Age*. Montreal, QC: McGill-Queen's University Press.

Eisenberg, L. (1986). Mindlessness and brainlessness in psychiatry. *The British Journal of Psychiatry*, **148**, 497–508.

Eisenberger, N.I. (2015). Social pain and the brain: controversies, questions, and where to go from here. *Annual Review of Psychology*, **66**, 601–629.

Ellis, G. (2016). *How Can Physics Underlie the Mind?* New York: Springer.

Engel, G.L. (1977. The need for a new medical model: a challenge for biomedicine. *Science*, **196**(4286), 129–136.

European Court of Human Rights (2013). Final Judgment in the Case of Pleso v. Hungary (App. No 41242/08). Strasbourg.

Feest, U. (Ed.) (2010). *Historical Perspectives on Erklären and Verstehen, Archimedes*. Dordrecht: Springer.

Flick, S. (2016). Treating social suffering? Work-related suffering and its psychotherapeutic re/interpretation. *Distinktion: Journal of Social Theory*, **17**(2), 149–173.

Focquaert, F. and Schermer, M. (2015). Moral enhancement: do means matter morally? *Neuroethics*, **8**, 139–151.

Frances, A. (2014). Resuscitating the biopsychosocial model. *The Lancet Psychiatry*, **1**(7), 496–497.

Fredrickson, B.L., Roberts, T.-A. (1997). Objectification theory: toward understanding women's lived experiences and mental health risks. *Psychology of Women Quarterly*, **21**(2), 173–206.

Fuchs, T. (2017). *Ecology of the Brain: An Organ in Relations*. New York: Oxford University Press.

Fuchs, T. (2010). Phenomenology and psychopathology. In: D. Schmicking and S. Gallagher (Eds.), *Handbook of Phenomenology and Cognitive Science* (pp. 546–573). Dordrecht: Springer.

Gallese, V. (2007). Before and below 'theory of mind': embodied simulation and the neural correlates of social cognition. *Philosophical Transactions of the Royal Society B: Biological Sciences*, **362**(1480), 659–669.

Gervais, S., Bernard, P., Klein, O., and Allen, J. (2013). Toward a unified theory of objectification and dehumanization. In: S.J. Gervais (Ed.), *Objectification and (de) Humanization: 60th Nebraska Symposium on Motivation* (pp. 1–23). New York: Springer.

Gold, I. (2009). Reduction in psychiatry. *The Canadian Journal of Psychiatry*, **54**(8), 506–512.

Gray, K., Knobe, J., Sheskin, M., Bloom, P., and Barrett, L.F. (2011). More than a body: mind perception and the nature of objectification. *Journal of Personality and Social Psychology*, **101**(6), 1207–1220.

Habermas, J. (2007). The language game of responsible agency and the problem of free will: how can epistemic dualism be reconciled with ontological monism? *Philosophical Explorations*, **10**(1), 13–50.

Habermas, J. (1984). *The Theory of Communicative Action, Vol. 1: Reason and the Rationalization of Society*. Boston, MA: Beacon Press.

Halpern, J. (2014). From idealized clinical empathy to empathic communication in medical care. *Medicine, Health Care and Philosophy*, **17**(2), 301–311.

Hansson, M., Chotai, J., and Bodlund, O. (2010). Patients' beliefs about the cause of their depression. *Journal of Affective Disorders*, **124**(1–2), 54–59.

Haslam, N. (2006). Dehumanization: an integrative review. *Personality and Social Psychology Review*, **10**(3), 252–264.

Haslam, N., Loughnan, S., Holland, E. (2013). The psychology of humanness. S.J. Gervais (Ed.), *Objectification and (de)Humanization: 60th Nebraska Symposium on Motivation, Nebraska Symposium on Motivation* (pp. 25–52). New York: Springer.

Haslanger, S. (2012). On being objective and being objectified. In: *Resisting Reality: Social Construction and Social Critique* (pp. 35–82). Oxford: Oxford University Press.

Hasson, U. and Frith, C.D. (2016). Mirroring and beyond: coupled dynamics as a generalized framework for modelling social interactions. *Philosophical Transactions of the Royal Society B: Biological Sciences*, **371**(1693), 20150366.

Hasson, U., Ghazanfar, A.A., Galantucci, B., Garrod, S., Keysers, C. (2012). Brain-to-brain coupling: a mechanism for creating and sharing a social world. *Trends in Cognitive Sciences*, **16**(2), 114–121.

Hochschild, A.R. (2012). *The Managed Heart: Commercialization of Human Feeling* (updated with a new preface). Berkeley, CA: University of California Press.

Hoffman, G.A. (2013). Treating yourself as an object: self-objectification and the ethical dimensions of antidepressant use. *Neuroethics*, **6**, 165–178.

Hohwy, J. and Kallestrup, J. (Eds.) (2008). *Being Reduced: New Essays on Reduction, Explanation, and Causation*. Oxford: Oxford University Press.

Holmen, S. (2018). Direct brain interventions, changing values and the argument from objectification–a reply to Elizabeth Shaw. *Neuroethics*, **11**, 217–227.

Honneth, A., Butler, J., Geuss, R., Lear, J., and Jay, M. (2008). *Reification: A New Look at an Old Idea, The Berkeley Tanner Lectures*. Oxford: Oxford University Press.

Horst, S. (2007). *Beyond Reduction: Philosophy of Mind and Post-Reductionist Philosophy of Science*. Oxford: Oxford University Press.

Hyman, S.E. (2010). The diagnosis of mental disorders: the problem of reification. *Annual Review of Clinical Psychology*, **6**, 155–179.

Illouz, E. (2007). *Cold Intimacies: The Making of Emotional Capitalism*. Malden, MA: Polity Press.

Insel, T.R. and Quirion, R. (2005). Psychiatry as a clinical neuroscience discipline. *JAMA*, **294**(17), 2221–2224.

Jaeggi, R. (2014). *Alienation*. New York: Columbia University Press.

Jaspers, K. (1920). *Allgemeine Psychopathologie für Studierende, Ärzte und Psychologen*. Berlin: Springer.

Kandel, E.R. (1998). A new intellectual framework for psychiatry. *American Journal of Psychiatry*, **155**(4), 457–469.

Kandel, E.R. (1999). Biology and the future of psychoanalysis: a new intellectual framework for psychiatry revisited. *American journal of Psychiatry*, **156**(4), 505–524.

Kant, I. (1785/2002). *Groundwork for the Metaphysics of Morals* (Edited and translated by Allen W. Wood). Cambridge: Cambridge University Press.

Kapur, S., Phillips, A.G., and Insel, T.R. (2012). Why has it taken so long for biological psychiatry to develop clinical tests and what to do about it? *Molecular Psychiatry*, **17**(12), 1174–1179.

Kendler, K.S. (2008). Explanatory models for psychiatric illness. *American Journal of Psychiatry*, **165**, 695–702.

Kendler, K.S. (2012). The dappled nature of causes of psychiatric illness: replacing the organic–functional/hardware–software dichotomy with empirically based pluralism. *Molecular Psychiatry*, **17**(4), 377–388.

Kendler, K.S. (2014). The structure of psychiatric science. *American Journal of Psychiatry*, **171**(9), 931–938.

Kim, J. (1999). Making sense of emergence. *Philosophical Studies*, **95**(1), 3–36.

Kinderman, P. (2014). *A Prescription for Psychiatry: Why We Need a Whole New Approach to Mental Health and Wellbeing*. New York: Palgrave Macmillan.

King, V., Gerisch, B., and Rosa, H. (2018). *Lost in Perfection: Impacts of Optimisation on Culture and Psyche*. London: Routledge.

Kirmayer, L.J. and Gold, I. (2012). Re-socializing psychiatry: critical neuroscience and the limits of reductionism. In: S. Choudhury and J. Slaby (Eds.), *Critical Neuroscience: A Handbook of the Social and Cultural Contexts of Neuroscience*, 307–330). Oxford: Blackwell.

Langton, R. (2005). Autonomy-denial in objectification. Reprinted in Langton, R., *Sexual Solipsism: Philosophical Essays on Pornography and Objectification* (pp. 223–40). Oxford: Oxford University Press.

Latour, B. (1996). On interobjectivity. *Mind, Culture, and Activity*, **3**(4), 228–245.

Lebowitz, M.S. and Ahn, W. (2014). Effects of biological explanations for mental disorders on clinicians' empathy. *Proceedings of the National Academy of Sciences*, **111**(50), 17786–17790.

Levine, J. (1983). Materialism and qualia: the explanatory gap. *Pacific Philosophical Quarterly*, **64**(4), 354–361.

Levy, N. (2007). *Neuroethics: Challenges for the 21st century*. Cambridge: Cambridge University Press.

Levy, N. (2012). Ecological engineering: reshaping our environments to achieve our goals. *Philosophy & Technology*, **25**(4), 589–604.

Levy, N., 2020. Cognitive enhancement: defending the parity principle. In: Vincent, N. (Ed.), *Neuro-Interventions and the Law: Regulating Human Mental Capacity*. New York: Oxford University Press.

Lewis, B. (2000). Psychiatry and postmodern theory. *Journal of Medical Humanities*, **21**(2), 71–84.

Linden, D.E.J. (2006). How psychotherapy changes the brain–the contribution of functional neuroimaging. *Molecular Psychiatry*, **11**(6), 528–538.

Loughnan, S., Haslam, N., Murnane, T., Vaes, J., Reynolds, C., and Suitner, C., 2010. Objectification leads to depersonalization: the denial of mind and moral concern to objectified others. *European Journal of Social Psychology*, **40**(5), 709–717.

Martin-Carrasco, M., Evans-Lacko, S., Dom, G., Christodoulou, N.G., Samochowiec, J., González-Fraile, E., Bienkowski, P., Gómez-Beneyto, M., Dos Santos, M.J.H., and Wasserman, D. (2016). EPA guidance on mental health and economic crises in Europe. *European Archives of Psychiatry and Clinical Neuroscience*, **266**(2), 89–124.

Marx, K. (1962). Das Kapital. Band I. In: *Marx und Engels Werke* (p. 958). Berlin: Dietz Verlag.

Marx, K. and Engels, F. (2009). *The Economic and Philosophic Manuscripts of 1844 and the Communist Manifesto*. Buffalo, NY: Prometheus Books.

McHugh, R.K., Whitton, S.W., Peckham, A.D., Welge, J.A., and Otto, M.W. (2013). Patient preference for psychological vs pharmacologic treatment of psychiatric disorders: a meta-analytic review. *The Journal of Clinical Psychiatry*, **74**(6), 595–602.

Minerva, F. (2017). The invisible discrimination before our eyes: a bioethical analysis: the invisible discrimination before our eyes. *Bioethics*, **31**(3), 180–189.

Mitchell, S. (2008). Explaining complex behavior. In: K.S. Kendler and J. Parnas (Eds.), *Philosophical Issues in Psychiatry* (pp. 19–47). Baltimore, MD: Johns Hopkins University Press.

Moradi, B. and Huang, Y.-P. (2008). Objectification theory and psychology of women: a decade of advances and future directions. *Psychology of Women Quarterly*, **32**, 377–398.

Music, G. (2014). Attachment, brains, nervous systems, and hormones. In: P. Holmes and S. Farnfield (Eds.), *The Routledge Handbook of Attachment Theory* (pp. 127–147). New York: Routledge.

Nagel, T. (1974). What is it like to be a bat? *The Philosophical Review*, **83**(4), 435–450.

Nussbaum, M.C. (1995). Objectification. *Philosophy & Public Affairs*, **24**(4), 249–291.

Oppenheim, P. and Putnam, H. (1958). Unity of science as a working hypothesis. *Minnesota Studies in the Philosophy of Science*, **2**, 3–36.

Panksepp, J. and Solms, M. (2012). What is neuropsychoanalysis? Clinically relevant studies of the minded brain. *Trends in Cognitive Sciences*, **16**(1), 6–8.

Paolini Paoletti, M. (2017). *Philosophical and Scientific Perspectives on Downward Causation* (Routledge Studies in Contemporary Philosophy, 91). New York: Routledge.

Papadaki, E.L. (2015). Feminist perspectives on objectification. In: E.N. Zalta (Ed.), *The Stanford Encyclopedia of Philosophy*. https://plato.stanford.edu/entries/feminism-objectification/

Papadaki, L. (2010). What is objectification? *Journal of Moral Philosophy*, 7, 16–36.

Parens, E. (2015). *Shaping Our Selves: On Technology, Flourishing, and a Habit of Thinking.* New York: Oxford University Press.

Pauen, M. (2012). The second-person perspective. *Inquiry*, 55, 33–49.

Persson, I. and Savulescu, J. (2012). *Unfit for the Future: The Need for Moral Enhancement.* Oxford: Oxford University Press.

Phillips, J. (2004). Understanding/explanation. In: J. Radden (Ed.), *The Philosophy of Psychiatry: A Companion* (pp. 180–190). Oxford: Oxford University Press.

Pockett, S., Banks, W.P., and Gallagher, S. (Eds.) (2006). *Does Consciousness Cause Behavior?* Cambridge, MA: MIT Press.

Popper, K. and Eccles, J. (2012). *The Self and Its Brain*. Berlin: Springer-Verlag.

Ratcliffe, M. (2014). The phenomenology of depression and the nature of empathy. *Medicine, Health Care and Philosophy*, **17**(2), 269–280.

Rector, J.M. (2014). *The Objectification Spectrum: Understanding and Transcending Our Diminishment and Dehumanization of Others*. New York: Oxford University Press.

Ripke, S., Neale, B.M., Corvin, A., Walters, J.T., Farh, K.-H., Holmans, P.A., Lee, P., Bulik-Sullivan, B., Collier, D.A., Huang, H., et al. (2014). Biological insights from 108 schizophrenia-associated genetic loci. *Nature*, **511**(7510), 421–427.

Roache, R. (2019). Psychiatry's problem with reductionism. *Philosophy, Psychiatry & Psychology*, **26**(3), 219–229.

Ryle, G. (2000). *The Concept of Mind* (Reprinted with a new introduction). London: Penguin Books.

Sass, L.A. and Parnas, J. (2007). Explaining schizophrenia: the relevance of phenomenology. In: M.C. Chung, K.W.M. (B.) Fulford, and G. Graham (Eds.), *Reconceiving Schizophrenia* (pp. 63–95). Oxford: Oxford University Press.

Satel, S. (2013). Distinguishing brain from mind. *The Atlantic*. https://www.theatlantic.com/health/archive/2013/05/distinguishing-brain-from-mind/276380/

Saul, J.M. (2006). On treating things as people: objectification, pornography, and the history of the vibrator. *Hypatia*, **21**, 45–61.

Schaffner, K. (2008). Etiological models in psychiatry. In: K.S. Kendler and J. Parnas (Eds.), *Philosophical Issues in Psychiatry* (pp. 48–89). Baltimore, MD: John Hopkins University Press.

Schöne-Seifert, B. (1994). Biologismusvorwürfe gegenüber Neurowissenschaften und Psychiatrie. In: O. Güntürkün and J. Hacker (Eds.), *Geist – Gehirn – Genom Gesellschaft* (pp. 123–142). Halle: Wissenschaftliche Verlagsgesellschaft.

Schramme, T. (2013). On the autonomy of the concept of disease in psychiatry. *Frontiers in Psychology*, **4**, 457.

Schwartz, M.A. (1999). The crisis of present-day psychiatry: regaining the personal. *Psychiatric Times*, **16**, 10.

Shaw, E. (2014). Direct brain interventions and responsibility enhancement. *Criminal Law and Philosophy*, **8**, 1–20.

Sik, D. (2018). From mental disorders to social suffering: making sense of depression for critical theories. *European Journal of Social Theory*, **22**(4), 477–496.

Solms, M. (2015). *The Feeling Brain: Selected Papers on Neuropsychoanalysis.* London: Karnac Books.

Steinert, S., Bublitz, C., Jox, R., and Friedrich, O. (2019). Doing things with thoughts: brain-computer interfaces and disembodied agency. *Philosophy & Technology*, **32**(3), 457–482.

Stier, M., Schoene-Seifert, B., Ruether, M., and Muders, S. (Eds.) (2014). The philosophy of psychiatry and biologism. *Frontiers in Psychology*, **5**, 1032.

Szasz, T. (1991). *Ideology and Insanity: Essays on the Psychiatric Dehumanization of Man.* Syracuse, NY: Syracuse University Press.

Szasz, T. (1974). *The Myth of Mental Illness.* New York: Harper & Row.

Szymanski, D.M., Moffitt, L.B., and Carr, E.R. (2011). Sexual objectification of women: advances to theory and research. *The Counseling Psychologist*, **39**(1), 6–38.

Thornton, T. (2010). Psychiatric explanation and understanding. *European Journal of Analytic Philosophy*, **6**, 95–111.

Trimble, M.R. and George, M.S. (2010). *Biological Psychiatry* (3rd ed.). Hoboken, NJ: Wiley-Blackwell.

UN Committee on the Rights of Persons with Disabilities (2014). Convention on the Rights of Persons with Disabilities (CRPD). https://www.un.org/development/desa/disabilities/convention-on-the-rights-of-persons-with-disabilities.html

United Nations (2013). Report of the Special Rapporteur on torture and other cruel, inhuman or degrading treatment or punishment, Juan E. Mendez. Human Rights Council, A/HRC/22/53. https://undocs.org/A/HRC/22/53

van Os, J., Delespaul, P., Wigman, J., Myin-Germeys, I., and Wichers, M. (2013). Beyond DSM and ICD: introducing 'precision diagnosis' for psychiatry using momentary assessment technology. *World Psychiatry*, **12**(2), 113–117.

van Os, J., Kenis, G., and Rutten, B.P. (2010). The environment and schizophrenia. *Nature*, **468**(7321), 203–212.

Walter, H. (2013). The third wave of biological psychiatry. *Frontiers in Psychology*, **4**, 582.

Whitley, R. (2008). Postmodernity and mental health. *Harvard Review of Psychiatry*, **16**(6), 352–364.

Wood, L. and Alsawy, S. (2016). Patient experiences of psychiatric inpatient care: a systematic review of qualitative evidence. *Journal of Psychiatric Intensive Care*, **12**(1), 35–43.

World Health Organization (2014). *Social Determinants of Mental Health.* Geneva: World Health Organization.

Part 5

The Future

Chapter 22

How to adopt
the biopsychosocial model

Rebecca Roache

Introduction

Psychiatry and the disciplines related to it continue to be targeted for investment and research, and new discoveries about the brain are being made all the time. Yet advances in understanding the brain have not so far resulted in advances in tackling psychiatric illness. We have had the 'psychopharmacology revolution' of the 1950s, the 'decade of the brain' in the 1990s, and contemporary neuroscientific research initiatives like the Human Brain Project. The last half-century has seen impressive gains in life expectancy and reductions in mortality for most infectious and cardiovascular diseases and some cancers. Yet suicide rates—associated with depression—have steadily increased, and longevity for those with serious mental illness falls more than two decades short of the general population (World Health Organization, 2002; Colton and Manderscheid, 2006; Hosseinpoor et al., 2012; Insel, 2013).

It is widely recognized that, in order to make progress in understanding and treating mental illness, we must take account of the range of factors that contribute to it, from genetic and neurological considerations, through the psychological state of the patient, to her social, cultural, and political context. While many psychiatrists attend to the full range of these factors in their efforts to make progress, there remains confusion about how the biological, psychological, and social factors relate to each other systematically. Exploring how the biopsychosocial psychiatrist can most appropriately take account of the fact that mental illness has biological, psychological, and social aspects is my focus in this chapter.

History

The biopsychosocial model was described and popularized by George Engel. Engel (1977) drew upon general systems theory—according to which the various 'levels' of conceptualizing illness (biological, psychological, social) form a hierarchy with some laws and principles applying only within a level and others applying to the system as a whole—to envisage a holistic way of understanding and scientifically studying the mind.[1]

----

[1] The wider historical motivations of Engel's view will not be explored here. For more, see Shorter (2005) and Ghaemi (2010).

Those sympathetic to Engel's approach can point to various empirical studies that support the view that the biological, the psychological, and the social are bound up together. Consider, for example, the famous work of Avshalom Caspi and colleagues (2002) showing that childhood maltreatment combined with a certain genotype (that is, a psychosocial phenomenon combined with a biological feature) predisposes males to antisocial behaviour in adulthood; the work of Julian Leff and colleagues showing that the social environment of schizophrenics has a direct effect on relapse (Leff et al., 1982, 1985); Kenneth Kendler and colleagues' (2003) study showing that an individual's risk of suffering from depressive episodes is strongly linked to suffering certain sorts of humiliation; Gerard Hogarty and colleagues' conclusion that schizophrenics who live alone have a higher relapse rate when treated with both medication and psychotherapy than when treated with medication alone (Hogarty et al., 1997a, 1997b); Charles Nemeroff and Wylie Vale's (2005) work showing that traumatic experiences increase the risk of depression in those with a certain genotype; Nancy Andreasen's (1997) efforts to combine biological and psychological explanations in understanding various mental illnesses; Glen Gabbard's (2000) elucidation of the effects of psychotherapy by considering how environmental and genetic influences combine to affect the brain; Haggard's (2008) identification of certain biological changes that underpin psychological experiences characteristic of acting voluntarily; and Apter-Levy and colleagues' (2013) consideration of the role of oxytocin in post-birth maternal depression and its subsequent negative effects on children's mental health.

In what sense, exactly, could such studies support the biopsychosocial model? What do they tell us about how we should conceive psychiatric illnesses? What sort of thing could count as evidence in favour of (or against) the biopsychosocial model? The answers to these questions depend largely on exactly what the biopsychosocial model is. Let us turn now to this issue.

The biopsychosocial model as a Kuhnian paradigm

Engel reflects at various points on what sort of thing the biopsychosocial model is. Some of his remarks conceive it as akin to a Kuhnian paradigm (Kuhn, 1962), while at other times he presents it more as a way of life that applies not only to understanding and illness, but also to explaining the social interactions and relations between and among medical staff and patients.

The Kuhnian framework is helpful for making sense of the biopsychosocial model and its place in psychiatry. According to Kuhn, a mark of a mature science is conformity to a paradigm: a set of theories, values, and assumptions widely accepted by the science's practitioners. On this view, psychiatry is not a mature science, since it does not conform to a single paradigm: that some psychiatrists emphasize a biomedical approach to mental illness, while some emphasize a psychological conception, and others emphasize an eclectic biopsychosocial view, demonstrates that psychiatry is divided by fundamental disagreements about paradigmatic matters.[2] Engel argued that, while many psychiatrists favour adopting the biomedical model as the defining

---

[2] This point is also made by Kendler (2005) and Cooper (2007).

paradigm, psychiatry (and, indeed, medicine in general) would do better to adopt the biopsychosocial model. As such, he proposed to transform psychiatry from its immature, pre-paradigmatic state into a mature science.[3]

To be clear, it is not obvious that the Kuhnian framework is the best way to conceive of the biopsychosocial model, and I will not provide an argument for doing so here. But conceiving it in this way will be a useful exercise in helping us understand what the model is and what it is for. Let us, then, take seriously the idea that the biopsychosocial model is a Kuhnian paradigm, and consider what would be involved in psychiatrists embracing it. Embracing it would involve—in Engel's words—subscribing to 'a shared set of assumptions and rules of conduct based on the scientific method'. What would this entail?

The causal view

One possibility is that this would entail psychiatrists endorsing the claim that mental illness is caused by a mixture of biological, psychological, and social factors. Something like this causal view of the biopsychosocial approach is adopted, for example, by the contributors to *Biopsychosocial Medicine*, an interdisciplinary collection of essays edited by the psychiatrist Peter White (2005). But, what exactly does this claim mean? Does it involve the view that the aetiology of *all* mental illness involves biological, psychological, and social factors? If so, and if this is an empirical claim about mental illness, then it would not be appropriate for psychiatrists to endorse it, since there is insufficient evidence to support it. The aetiology of almost all mental illnesses is poorly understood, after all.

On the other hand, we could view the claim as conceptual rather than empirical. That is, we could take the claim that, necessarily, mental illness is caused by a mixture of biological, psychological, and social factors to say something about what it is for a condition to be a mental illness, rather than (say) a somatic illness or a moral or epistemological failing. On this view, though, the claim is implausible. Take depression, for example. Being depressed involves being in a certain mood, the aetiology of which makes no difference to whether or not one is depressed. This is so both intuitively— that is, our ordinary, 'folk' idea of depression is not sensitive to how this condition is caused—and according to the diagnostic criteria of the *Diagnostic and Statistical*

---

[3] He also argues that the biopsychosocial model should be adopted by medicine more generally, but for somatic medicine (i.e. medicine excluding psychiatry) to adopt this model would not involve moving from a prescientific state to a scientific one, since—at least according to Engel's conception of somatic medicine—somatic medicine already adheres to a paradigm. In arguing that this paradigm, which 'has a firm base in the biological sciences' (Engel 1977, p. 129), should be replaced by the biopsychosocial model, Engel proposes a Kuhnian scientific revolution. Such a revolution occurs when the existing paradigm ceases to be useful in explaining new discoveries, and is replaced by a new one. That Engel proposes a scientific revolution in somatic medicine is clear from his remark, in advance of his argument that somatic medicine should adopt the biopsychosocial model, that somatic medicine is 'in crisis' as a result of its 'adherence to a model of disease no longer adequate for [its] scientific tasks and social responsibilities' (Engel, 1977, p. 129).

Manual of Mental Disorders, fifth edition (*DSM-5*). Similar observations apply to other mental illnesses, or symptoms of mental illness.[4]

Even so, one might think that it does sometimes matter for psychiatry how a mental illness is caused. Sometimes, discovery of a certain aetiology can result in a condition being reclassified so that it is no longer considered primarily a psychiatric disorder. Consider, for example, general paresis of the insane (GPI). It involves classic psychiatric symptoms including psychosis, personality changes, mood disturbances, and cognitive decline. It was considered a psychiatric disorder until the discovery in the early twentieth century that it was caused by late-stage syphilis, and that it can be treated—like the somatic earlier stage of syphilis—with penicillin. GPI is now considered a somatic disorder with psychiatric symptoms, and it falls within the remit of somatic medicine. A more recent example is the discovery by Josep Dalmau and colleagues that anti-*N*-methyl-D-aspartate (NMDA) receptor encephalitis can cause psychosis and other psychiatric symptoms (Dalmau et al., 2007). The journalist Susannah Cahalan vividly recounts her experience with the disease in *Brain on Fire* (Cahalan, 2013), and it is striking that her diagnosis resulted in her shifting from the care of psychiatrists into that of somatic physicians.

Cases in which an apparently psychiatric disorder is reclassified as somatic are rare, and it would be a mistake to read too much into what they tell us about the *concept* of mental disorder. Such reclassifications plausibly have little to do with the conceptual relevance of the aetiology of the disease in question, and everything to do with the practical issue of how it is most effectively treated. The discoveries that GPI is most effectively treated with penicillin, and that anti-NMDA receptor encephalitis is most effectively treated with immunotherapy and (in some cases) surgery, meant that the psychiatrist's specialist skills were not required. That, in cases such as these, it is possible to *alleviate* psychiatric symptoms without *understanding* them does not entail that they are conceptually distinct from the symptoms of mental disorders that cannot be treated by somatic medicine, nor that our remarks about these other mental disorders do not also apply to reclassified disorders like GPI and anti-NMDA receptor encephalitis. It only entails that understanding the psychiatric symptoms of reclassified disorders is less urgent than understanding other mental disorders, since in general understanding psychiatric symptoms is an important step towards alleviating them.

It is, then, implausible to claim that all psychiatric illness must *by definition* have a particular aetiology, and if endorsing the biopsychosocial model involves endorsing the claim that all mental illness is caused by a mixture of biological, psychological, and social causes, this model is unappealing. This is so whether we take the claim to be an empirical hypothesis or an assertion about the concept of mental disorder.

Thankfully, one may make assertions about the aetiology of mental disorders without committing to such a strong claim. We might, instead, take the biopsychosocial model

---

[4] Exceptions to this are those conditions where, by stipulation, a certain aetiology features in the diagnostic criteria. Such conditions in the *DSM-5* include trauma- and stressor-related disorders—'in which exposure to a traumatic or stressful event is listed explicitly as a diagnostic criterion' (American Psychiatric Association, 2013, p. 265)—and medication-induced disorders.

to involve commitment to the claim that it is important to remain open-minded to the possibility that the causes of mental illness could be a mixture of biological, psychological, and social factors. This is the view of Kenneth Kendler. Referring to the discovery that GPI is a form of syphilis, he cautions us that 'we can expect no more "spirochete-like" discoveries that will explain [psychiatric disorders'] origins in simple terms' (2005, p. 433). He argues that the causes of psychiatric disorders are *dappled*— that is, 'distributed widely across multiple categories' (Kendler, 2012, p. 383).

As a candidate for the central claim of the biopsychosocial model conceived as a Kuhnian paradigm, this claim is uninterestingly weak, however. Remaining open-minded about the possible aetiology of mental illnesses seems more like good scientific practice or common sense than like a substantive claim about what sort of things mental illnesses are. Given this, what is the most appropriate way to make sense of the claim that mental illness can be caused by a mixture of biological, psychological, and social factors?

Let us answer this question by first considering, as a clarificatory exercise, an unappealing account of what we might take this claim to mean. Imagine a metaphysically extravagant theorist who believes not only (with Cartesian mind–brain substance dualists) that biological and psychological occurrences involve different sorts of stuff (one physical and one mental), but also that there is a social stuff. For such a person, the claim that psychiatric disorders are caused by a mixture of biological, psychological, and social factors can be taken to mean that that these disorders arise from three separate types of substance, each of which acts on the patient.

This 'three-substance' view is not plausible, however. It would sidetrack us to consider why it is not plausible—so, let it suffice to note that, as far as I know, nobody has seriously defended it.[5] Most metaphysicians of the mind are monists. More specifically, they are *physicalists*: they believe that physical stuff is the only type of stuff in the world, and that the mind is realized or expressed in physical stuff.[6] On this view, biological, psychological, and social events *are* physical events, in the sense that the occurrence of certain physical events is sufficient for the occurrence of biological, psychological, and social events. Another way of putting this claim is that 'the world is the way it is, because the physical world is the way it is' (Kallestrup, 2006, p. 459). Yet another way of putting this claim is that the biological, the psychological, and the social are all *ontologically reducible* to the physical: if there were nothing physical, then there would *ipso facto* be nothing biological, psychological, or social, either.[7]

In the philosophy of mind literature, different sorts of physicalist account for the relationship between the mental and the physical in different ways, but one of the most popular and least controversial views involves the idea of *supervenience*.[8] The claim

---

[5] A 'three-substance' view would face all the problems faced by mind–brain substance dualists, along with a slew of other problems arising from the addition of a third substance.

[6] There are, however, difficulties in spelling out exactly what physicalism is beyond this superficial characterization. See, for example, Hempel (1970) and Crane and Mellor (1990).

[7] For more on reductionism in psychiatry, see Roache (2019).

[8] Less popular and more controversial forms of physicalism involve stronger forms of reductionism, such as *explanatory reductionism*, which holds that the language of (say) psychology

that mental properties supervene on physical properties entails that no two things that are identical with respect to their physical properties can differ with respect to their mental properties. Supervenience allows for *multiple realizability*: physically different things can nevertheless be alike mentally. This makes it possible for physically different people (or animals, robots, angels, Martians, etc.) to experience the same type of mental state; say, fear. It is not only mental properties that supervene on physical ones, and the idea of supervenience is perhaps easier to grasp in relation to other sorts of properties. For example, we might claim that aesthetic properties supervene on physical properties. This entails that, if two paintings are physically identical, it is not possible for one but not the other to be beautiful. It also allows that beautiful things can be physically diverse. These ideas about beauty and its relationship to what is physical fit with our intuitions. A physicalist takes biological, psychological, and social properties to supervene on physical properties, too.[9]

For the biopsychosocial theorist who claims that mental illness can be caused by a mixture of biological, psychological, and social factors, adopting a physicalist view risks double- (or triple-) counting causes. To see this, let us adapt a famous example from Donald Davidson, and suppose that I arrive home one night and flip the light switch. Unbeknown to me, there is a prowler inside my house, who is alerted to my presence when the lights come on. My single physical action of flipping the light switch can be described in various ways, including as the biological event of making a certain series of bodily movements, the psychological (because intentional) event of turning on the light, and the social event of alerting the prowler to my presence. Suppose that, startled by my action, the prowler falls down the stairs and injures herself. What is the cause of this event? The cause is my action, which is biopsychosocial in that it can be described as a biological, a psychological, or a social event. But it would be incorrect to claim that the event has *three separate* causes: one biological, one psychological, and one social. To do so would be to mistake three separate descriptions of a single physical event for three separate events.[10] Similarly, in citing biopsychosocial causes of mental illness, we should take care not to triple-count causes. Triple-counting causes would be correct in the three-substance world described previously, but it is not correct in a physicalist world.

The staunch physicalist might, further, question the sense of claiming that there are biological, psychological, and social causes. Since these categories supervene on the

---

can be replaced by the language of biology without sacrificing understanding (so, for example, talk of beliefs can be replaced by talk of particular brain states). Explanatory reductionism is arguably involved in Ullin Place's identity theory (Place 1956) and in Paul Churchland's eliminative materialism (Churchland 1981).

[9] For a detailed treatment of supervenience, see Kim (1993).

[10] In keeping with the Davidsonian theme, I am adopting a Davidsonian metaphysics of causation, according to which causes are events. This is not the only conception of causation— D.H. Mellor, for example, takes causes to be facts rather than events (Mellor 1995)—but the cautionary point about double-counting causes goes through on any plausible account of causation.

physical, why bother mentioning them at all? Why not keep things simple and mention causes only as characterized in physical terms? Is there anything to be gained by invoking the language of the biological, the psychological, and the social?

There is something to be gained by doing this; we consider exactly what in the following section.

The explanatory view

Taking endorsement of the biopsychosocial model (*qua* Kuhnian paradigm) to centre on the claim that mental illness is caused by a mixture of biological, psychological, and social events is, as we have just seen, unsatisfactory. As an empirical claim there is insufficient evidence for it; as a conceptual claim it is implausible; and in any case citing biological, psychological, and social causes risks double- (or triple-) counting causes unless we subscribe to the unpalatable idea that biological, psychological, and social events involve distinct substances.

Even so, for any event that we wish to explain, we can choose among multiple accurate explanations, and invariably some of these explanations—often those that refer to supervenient but not to subvenient (i.e. physical) properties—are *better* than others. This is as true when explaining psychiatric disorders as it is when explaining many other phenomena. Consider, for example, Kendler's observation that the cultural acceptability of public drunkenness is among the factors that affects one's risk of becoming alcohol dependent (Kendler, 2008). Cultural acceptability of public drunkenness is a property that supervenes on physical properties, and so the physicalist keen on theoretical elegance might claim that we can fully account for its effects on alcohol dependency by mentioning only physical properties. That is, instead of claiming that 'Cultural acceptability of public drunkenness increases one's risk of alcohol dependency', we could instead claim that 'Physical state A and/or B and/or C and/or ... n increases one's risk of alcohol dependency', where $A-n$ is a (certainly infinite) series of descriptions of all the physical states of affairs that could possibly subvene the social property of cultural acceptability of public drunkenness.

There is a sense in which an explanation of the risk of alcohol dependency that refers to cultural acceptability of drunkenness is *better* than an explanation that refers to the subvenient physical properties. But, in what sense is it better? Being able to answer this question will be an important step for the advocate of the biopsychosocial model. There are several factors to consider.

First, as noted previously, that supervenience allows for multiple realizability means that there are infinitely many physical states of the world that could subvene under cultural acceptability of public drunkenness. That we cannot know every such state is an obstacle to substituting cultural descriptions for physical ones in explanations for alcohol dependency. In this sense, reference to cultural considerations is a useful shorthand way of referring to any number of potentially subvenient physical states. However, reference to the supervenient cultural property is more than mere shorthand, since it may not be possible to eliminate the *concept* of cultural acceptability of public drunkenness from our explanations. In the example given earlier, how does the physicalist know what physical states of affairs to include in the series $A-n$ and which to omit? The only way to make such decisions, surely, would be to test whether or not candidate sets of physical properties give rise to the supervenient, cultural property in question. Given this, the physicalist would need to refer to cultural properties in order to formulate the physicalist explanation; that is, she would need to refer to exactly those supervenient properties that she meant to eliminate. Even if supervenient concepts and descriptions could be eliminated from the eventual physicalist explanation, then, they are required in order to generate it.

It is not always the case, however, that a 'higher-level' explanation (that is, one that makes reference to supervenient properties) will be preferable to a lower-level one. Imagine that Jack and Jill both suffer from depression. Jack has recently lost a loved one and is grieving. By contrast, Jill has not recently experienced anything upsetting, but she has pancreatic cancer, a disease that often presents with depression. In the absence of other considerations relevant to explaining their depression, an explanation that focuses on psychological factors (i.e. grief) is preferable to one that focuses on biological factors in Jack's case, and an explanation that focuses on biological factors (i.e. pancreatic cancer) is preferable to one that focuses on psychological factors in Jill's case.

What factors determine what sort of explanation is better than another in cases like this? The answer, in part, has to do with the fact that different explanations can furnish us with different sorts of understanding. Karl Jaspers distinguished between empathic, narrative understanding—the sort of understanding of people that we gain by relating to them *as people*, rather than as (say) organisms or lumps of physical matter—which typically makes reference to first-person, subjective, qualitative experience; and the sort of objective, third-person understanding that the sciences typically aim to provide.[11] Ghaemi, following Dilthey, refers to these types of understanding as *Verstehen* and *Erklären*, respectively. By explaining Jack's depression in terms of his grief, we use the *Verstehen* approach. As fellow humans, our understanding of Jack's grief-induced depression is immediate: having understood that he is grieving, and knowing what sort of experience grief is, we require no further information in order to see how his depression has followed from his grief. On the other hand, a *Verstehen* approach to explaining Jill's depression will be less successful, since there are no events in Jill's recent personal narrative—that is, her life described in terms of the sort of experiences and events that enable us, as fellow persons, to empathize with her—that explain her depression in the way that Jack's grief explains his. In Jill's case, we revert instead to *Erklären*: an explanation of Jill's depression in terms of her pancreatic cancer, alongside information about the correlation between pancreatic cancer and depression, better helps us to understand her depression. A higher-level explanation is preferable to a lower-level one in Jack's case, and the reverse in Jill's case, because a *Verstehen* approach (but not an *Erklären* approach) gives insight into Jack's depression and an *Erklären* approach (but not a *Verstehen* approach) gives insight into Jill's depression. We will return in a moment to consider the question of why this might be the case.

---

[11] Jaspers was influenced by other thinkers in making this distinction. For an admirably lucid attempt to place Jaspers' approach in its historical context, see Ghaemi (2010, chapters 14–16). For an illuminating attempt to cast Jaspers' empathic understanding in terms of the simulation debate in contemporary philosophy of mind, see Cooper (2007, chapter 5).

Another distinction between types of explanation is made by Cooper. She argues that, when assessing whether or not an individual's behaviour should be deemed symptomatic of a medical disorder, the behaviour is symptomatic if the best explanation of it is a *sub-personal* explanation rather than a *person-level* explanation. Person-level explanations, she tells us, 'make reference to an individual's reasons, motives and so on. When a person-level explanation is most appropriate, the behaviour comes to be understood as a purposeful action' (Cooper, 2007, p. 18). By contrast, sub-personal explanations:

> characteristically make reference to biological or sub-personal psychological mechanisms. So, someone might have a fit because something has gone wrong with a part of their brain, or they might fail to recognize faces because something has gone wrong with their face-recognition system. (Cooper, 2007, p. 18)

This reflects the distinction between *Verstehen* and *Erklären*. Cooper concludes that an individual's behaviour is symptomatic in cases where 'a sub-personal explanation looks like a *better* explanation than does a person-level explanation' (Cooper, 2007, p. 18). Under what circumstances might this be the case? Cooper goes on:

> For example, a pattern of behaviour may be more commonly seen in a particular biological kind of person (five-year-old boys, say, or menopausal women); behaviours may co-occur in ways that do not make sense from a purposeful point of view (so feelings of depression often co-occur with sleep problems); a pattern of behaviour may fail to 'fit' with the rest of a person's life history (as in dissociative conditions, where there are memory lapses between semi-independent pockets of behaviour). All such features tend to make a sub-personal explanation more plausible than a personal explanation. (Cooper, 2007, p. 18)

Thomas Szasz, who argued that there is no such thing as mental disorders except in cases where such disorders can be shown to have a physical basis, appears to be motivated partly by the view, expressed here by Cooper, that where an individual's behaviour can best be explained at the person level, this behaviour is not symptomatic of disease. Writing in the early 1960s, he argued that some conditions that were considered symptomatic of mental disease could be given what Cooper would call a person-level explanation: they could, for example, be understood as attempts by the individual to communicate her desires, or as struggles with ethical, social, or legal norms (Szasz, 1960, 1961). Szasz took the availability of such explanations to support his view that the conditions in question should not be regarded as disorders.

However, even granting that behaviours are symptomatic when a sub-personal explanation for them is better than a personal explanation, or when the best explanation cannot be found within traditional folk theories, we lack an account of what factors determine when a certain type of explanation is *better* than another type. Returning to our example of Jack and Jill, why is it the case that a *Verstehen* approach is more successful in Jack's case, while an *Erklären* approach is preferable in Jill's?

This has to do, I think, with the sorts of generalization we can make about each case. Explaining Jack's depression in terms of his psychological state—that is, his grief—is better than explaining his depression in terms of his biological state because it is widely acknowledged that *grief causes depression*. On the other hand, we may have available no generalization linking Jack's underlying biological state to his depression: there may be no truth of the form *biological state B causes depression*, where *B* is a type of state instantiated by Jack.[12] Mentioning grief, then, gives us more explanatory power than we have by mentioning Jack's biological state, because we come to see Jack's condition as an instance of the familiar generalization. The reverse is true, however, in Jill's case. While the causal mechanism by which pancreatic cancer comes to be associated with depression is not fully understood, it is nevertheless recognized that *pancreatic cancer is correlated with depression*. On the other hand, nothing about Jill's psychological state enables us to assert a similarly general truth: there may be no truth of the form *psychological state P causes depression*, where *P* is a state of Jill. Biological factors therefore give us greater explanatory power than psychological factors in Jill's case; the reverse is true for Jack's case.[13]

Before going on, I want to say something more about the sort of generalizations that underpin the explanations in the examples previously given. These generalizations need not be exceptionless laws. After all, not all cases of grief result in depression, and not everyone with pancreatic cancer is depressed. Rather, the generalizations in question may be what Alice Drewery has called *nomic regularities*, or generics. Nomic regularities admit of exceptions: '[o]rdinary usage does not insist that an exception falsifies a generic' (Drewery, 2000, p. 2). For example, 'Birds fly' is true despite the fact that some birds, such as penguins, cannot fly. Drewery explains:

> Statements of nomic regularities typically:
>
> 1. have empirical content,
>
> 2. are generalisations from particular facts or events about individuals,
>
> 3. are learnt inductively,
>
> 4. presuppose a systematic approach to the world (maybe not a science, but some way of making generalisations about the world),
>
> 5. are useful for explanation and prediction,
>
> 6. (possibly defeasibly) support counterfactuals. (Drewery, 2000, pp. 2–3)

In explaining under what circumstances a sub-personal explanation may be better than a person-level one, Cooper hints at the supporting role played by generalizations. Even so, she writes of the various types of explanation for a given behaviour as if these different types are competing; as if we can rank the person-level and sub-personal explanations in order of merit, and conclude that the behaviour is

---

[12] This might change as we learn more about the biology of grief. But, even when we achieve this, a biological explanation of the depression of someone like Jack would be less satisfactory than a psychological explanation, for reasons we will go on to explore.

[13] We may, of course, wish to explore why these generalizations are true; that is, we may want to discover why it is that grief causes depression or that pancreatic cancer is correlated with depression. Answers to these questions would doubtless enhance our understanding of why Jack and Jill are depressed, but even in the absence of such answers, that the generalizations in question are recognized as true explains why reference to grief is helpful in explaining Jack's depression and why reference to pancreatic cancer is helpful in explaining Jill's.

symptomatic if there is a sub-personal explanation that ranks more highly than any person-level explanation. However, often things are not this simple. It can happen that explanations at different levels complement each other, so that we can better understand a given behaviour by combining both person-level and sub-personal explanations than by considering either alone. For example, if you are very rude to me, recalling that I have recently inconvenienced you will go some way towards helping me understand why, since it is widely recognized that *being inconvenienced by friends causes irritability*. But if you are normally very polite even under stressful circumstances, I may feel that your having been inconvenienced does not fully explain your rudeness. However, if I also learn that you did not sleep very well last night, and therefore that you are currently having to endure being inconvenienced while unusually tired, I have a more satisfying explanation of your behaviour. After all, *tiredness causes irritability*. The explanation in terms of my having inconvenienced you is person-level, while the explanation in terms of your tiredness is sub-personal; yet these explanations complement each other rather than compete. The combination of these two explanations helps me understand your behaviour better than if I attended to either one alone.

The distinction between person-level and sub-personal explanations, while not mapping neatly onto the distinction between biological, psychological, and social explanations, is useful for understanding why a combination of these explanations is important. Biological explanations of human behaviour are invariably sub-personal, psychological explanations can be sub-personal (as in Cooper's example where someone's inability to recognize faces is attributed to a fault with their face-recognition system) or person-level (as when we refer to a person's beliefs, desires, etc.), and social explanation are—if they focus on persons at all—person-level rather than sub-personal.[14] We might take adherents of the biopsychosocial model to be committed to the claim that understanding mental illness requires attending to biological, psychological, and social *explanations*. More specifically, we might take them to be committed to the claim that if we want to maximize our understanding of mental illness, we must consider explanations from all three perspectives.

As it stands, however, this characterization of the biopsychosocial view amounts to little more than an observation that, in seeking explanations to understand a phenomenon, more is often better. This might be true, but it is uninteresting: of course more explanation is better than less, especially in cases which we struggle to understand. In addition, as it stands, this claim amounts to the sort of unstructured, anarchic eclecticism that has been attacked by Ghaemi, who compares the biopsychosocial model to a list of ingredients rather than a recipe. If it is important to consider biological, psychological, and social perspectives in trying to understand mental illness, we need some account of *why* this is important, and of *how* these perspectives combine. I offer such an account in the following section.

....

[14] An example of a social explanation that does not focus on persons might be one that explains an increase in depression in a population in terms of political or economic factors.

The biopsychosocial paradigm as a commitment to pluralistic explanation

Not everybody thinks that we need a pluralistic, multilevel approach to understand mental illness. In a famous editorial, Thomas Insel and Rémi Quirion argue that 'mental disorders [should] be understood … as brain disorders' (Insel and Quirion, 2005, p. 2221). Insel and Quirion call their position *clinical neuroscience*. How might the defender of the biopsychosocial model persuade the clinical neuroscientist that psychosocial explanations are as important as biological ones in understanding mental illness?

One strategy involves arguing that psychosocial factors simply cannot be eliminated. Matthew Broome and Lisa Bortolotti have argued that mental disorders differ from somatic disorders in that, in addition to any biological features they have, they have 'distinctive features' which 'can be adequately characterized only by using the vocabulary of the mental' (Broome and Bortolotti, 2009, p. 31). They explain that 'mental illness is mental precisely because in order to establish whether a certain behaviour is disturbed we need to apply psychological concepts. This is of course orthogonal to the question about how these disturbances are caused' (Broome and Bortolotti, 2009, p. 31). For example, in order to account for why delusions are pathological, we must make reference to normative considerations that govern our beliefs, which are violated by delusions. Delusions, unlike most other beliefs, are held for no (or for bad) reasons, and are held with a certainty that is resistant to evidence that they are false. That they violate the sorts of epistemic norms that usually govern our beliefs explains why they are pathological; they are not pathological in virtue of whatever neurobiological states underlie them.

George Graham and Owen Flanagan make a similar point in arguing that, without reference to psychosocial phenomena, the existence of some mental disorders cannot even be recognized. For example, addiction to gambling arises when a generally valuable reinforcement schedule operates in certain environments. Gambling addiction is not, then, a brain disorder: the brain of a gambling addict 'is behaving as it should from a biological point of view' (Graham and Flanagan, 2013). To conceive it as a disorder, one must consider psychosocial factors, such as the effects of persistent gambling on the gambler's relationships and financial security.

The views expressed by Broome and Bortolloti, and by Graham and Flanagan, do not embody a controversial, fringe conception of mental disorders. On the contrary, these views are reflected in the official line on mental disorders set out in the *DSM-5*, which states that '[m]ental disorders are defined in relation to cultural, social, and familial norms and values' (American Psychiatric Association, 2013, p. 14).

In addition, as I have remarked elsewhere (Roache, 2019), the presence of certain characteristic subjective, psychological experiences and/or behaviours plays a role in mental illness that is absent in somatic illness. A diagnosis of a somatic illness such as cancer, chickenpox, or multiple sclerosis is not contingent on the patient's having certain sorts of subjective experiences, or on behaving in certain characteristic ways. This is not to deny that many somatic disorders are associated with certain such experiences and behaviours (we considered earlier the example of pancreatic cancer presenting with depression); rather, the point is that the diagnosis of somatic disorders does not stand or fall with the presence or absence of certain experiences and behaviours. They stand or fall, instead, with the presence or absence of certain biological factors. This is not the case for psychiatric disorders. People who are not unhappy *ipso facto* do not suffer from depression; people who do not experience recurrent, intrusive thoughts or behaviours *ipso facto* do not suffer from obsessive–compulsive disorder; people who do not have unusual difficulties with performing intellectual tasks *ipso facto* do not have an intellectual disability; and so on. Psychological and behavioural considerations play a far more central role in determining whether or not someone has a mental disorder than they play in deciding whether or not someone has a somatic disorder.

The central role of psychological and behavioural considerations in determining whether or not someone has a mental illness means that we should be cautious in hoping for biological characterizations of mental illness. There are some who believe that such biological characterizations are possible—Insel and Quirion, for example, want to view 'mental disorders as complex genetic disorders' (Insel and Quirion, 2005, p. 2221). Yet any biological account of a given mental disorder is correct only in so far as it picks out those people who suffer the relevant psychological and behavioural symptoms characteristic of that disorder. We might—at least, some people would—be sympathetic to a purely biological account of schizophrenia that happened to deem all and only those people who suffer the characteristic psychological and behavioural symptoms of schizophrenia to be suffering from that disorder. However, if such an account could, *at least in principle*, enable people to be diagnosed with schizophrenia even if they lacked any of the psychological or behavioural symptoms characteristic of schizophrenia, then the disorder described by such account is not exactly the same disorder to which psychiatrists currently refer using the term 'schizophrenia'.[15] Diagnosis of schizophrenia, like diagnosis of other mental disorders, stands or falls with the presence or absence of certain characteristic psychological and/or behavioural symptoms; in this sense, reference to psychological and behavioural considerations is ineliminable in characterizing mental disorders.

Let us pause to consider what has been said so far about the importance of psychosocial factors in understanding mental disorder. We have noted that, often, even non-pathological human behaviour can be better understood when we attend to both person-level and sub-personal explanations than when we attend to either in isolation. Person-level explanations can be psychological and/or social, while sub-personal explanations are psychological or biological. It should not, then, be surprising that our

---

[15] This need not necessarily be a bad thing, and a move towards classifying mental illnesses in terms of biological factors would raise the possibility of being able to diagnose asymptomatic or unusually symptomatic mental illnesses, just as people are sometimes diagnosed as having asymptomatic somatic illnesses. Shea and Bayne (2010) develop a way of diagnosing consciousness in vegetative state patients; an analogous strategy could be employed to develop a way of diagnosing mental illness in patients without symptoms. (I owe these observations to Neil Levy.) While such a move is not inconceivable, however, it would mark a departure from the way we *currently* conceive of mental illnesses.

understanding of *pathological* human behaviour may also enhanced by considering a combination of person-level and sub-personal explanations. This makes sense given that those who exhibit pathological human behaviour are persons—to whom we relate as such—whose behaviour and experience are influenced by the workings of their sub-personal systems. Further, we noted that psychosocial factors are ineliminable in identifying and characterizing mental illness: we must make reference to such factors in order to explain what is pathological about mental disorders, and the question of whether or not somebody has a mental disorder cannot be settled independently of psychosocial considerations.

So much for the relevance of psychological and social factors. What about the relevance of biological factors? Biological factors are relevant, I suggest, partly because biological explanations are among the sub-personal explanations that are often useful in understanding human behaviour (pathological or otherwise), which makes investigating the biological factors underlying mental disorders important in increasing understanding those disorders; and partly because biological factors are more amenable to scientific study than are psychosocial factors. Biological factors are replicable; they are the same regardless of who is observing them (unlike psychological factors: we each, as philosophers say, have 'privileged access' to our own psychological states (Alston, 1971)); and they can be observed relatively easily using brain scans, blood tests, and so on. Understanding mental illness would be easier if we could ignore psychosocial factors and concentrate solely on the biological—and this approach, of course, would also make mental illness more closely resemble somatic illness. Unfortunately for advocates of the biomedical approach, however, it is unrealistic to hope that a purely biological account of mental disorder is possible.

Understanding mental illness and treating mental illness

The goal of psychiatry is to cure, manage, alleviate, or otherwise treat the symptoms of mental disorder. Generally, the most promising route to being able to treat mental illness involves trying to understand it better. In trying to characterize the biopsychosocial model, I have focused on its role in helping us understand mental illness. Beyond this, I have not focused on how it might help us better treat mental illness.

Why not? Because while the question of how we should understand mental disorder is largely conceptual, the question of what treatments are most effective for mental illness must be answered empirically. Failing to separate these two questions risks confusing matters.[16] The answer to the question, 'Is a biopsychosocial approach to this mental disorder the best one?' might be 'Yes' if we are concerned with *understanding*

---

[16] Engel does not explicitly separate them. He believed that taking a biopsychosocial approach is more effective than taking a biomedical approach at improving patient outcomes—but this is a contentious claim which he does not support in anything like the way he would be expected to support it were he arguing for this claim today. His argument in Engel (1978) relies on a speculative discussion of a hypothetical patient.

the disorder in question but 'No' if we are concerned with *treating* it. This could happen if we discover a successful method of treating a mental disorder that obviates the need to understand it. Imagine, for example, the discovery of a new plant whose fruit completely (and, perhaps, mysteriously) cures schizophrenic patients of their symptoms. In such a case, while understanding and explaining schizophrenia might require a biopsychosocial approach, treating it would not. In such a scenario, schizophrenia could—like GPI and anti-NMDA receptor encephalitis—be treated without the need for the skills of the psychiatrist. Were we able to treat schizophrenia as easily and effectively as this, the task of understanding the condition would be a matter of purely academic interest. Understanding mental disorder is an urgent task of practical significance only in cases where we anticipate that increased understanding will enable more effective treatment.

A good example of a case in which failure to separate the question of how we should best understand mental disorder from the question of how we should best treat it can be found in the work of Szasz, who dismisses the idea of mental illness and claims instead that so-called mental illnesses are 'problems of living'. He writes,

> In actual contemporary social usage, the finding of a mental illness is made by establishing a deviance in behavior from certain psychosocial, ethical, or legal norms. The judgment may be made, as in medicine, by the patient, the physician (psychiatrist), or others. Remedial action, finally, tends to be sought in a therapeutic—or covertly medical—framework, thus creating a situation in which *psychosocial, ethical*, and/or *legal deviations* are claimed to be correctible by (so-called) *medical action*. Since medical action is designed to correct only medical deviations, it seems logically absurd to expect that it will help solve problems whose very existence had been defined and established on nonmedical grounds. I think that these considerations may be fruitfully applied to the present use of tranquilizers and, more generally, to what might be expected of drugs of whatever type in regard to the amelioration or solution of problems in human living. (Szasz, 1960, p. 115)

Szasz's view that 'the finding of a mental illness is made by establishing a deviance in behavior from certain psychosocial, ethical, or legal norms' closely resembles the way in which I have characterized mental disorder here. However, his view that it is 'logically absurd to expect that [medical treatment] will help solve problems whose very existence had been defined and established on nonmedical grounds' is confused. Whether or not a given medical intervention is an effective treatment for mental disorder is not an issue to be settled by logic, but an empirical one. Szasz's confused analysis results from his running together the *conceptual* issue of how mental disorder is best understood with the *empirical* issue of how it is most effectively treated.

Conclusion

I have attempted here to elucidate the biopsychosocial model by conceiving of it as a Kuhnian paradigm, which involves commitment to a set of assumptions and rules of conduct. These should include the recognition that mental illness need not have a specific type of aetiology; that is, commitment to the biopsychosocial model should not involve an a priori acceptance of the view that mental illness always has biological, psychological, and social causes. Adopting the biopsychosocial model should also involve recognizing that our understanding of any given mental illness may best be advanced by considering explanations at each of the biological, psychological, and social levels. Often (depending on the illness in question), explanation at one of these levels may be more elucidating than explanations at the other levels, but considering all of them combined is likely to maximize our understanding. Psychological and social explanations are not eliminable in favour of (that is, reducible to) biological ones, largely because of the way that mental illnesses are conceived and diagnosed. Commitment to a biopsychosocial approach should not involve commitment to the view that treatment of mental illness should always involve interventions at every level. Which treatment is most effective in any given case—that is, whether a biological, a psychological, or a social approach—can best be decided empirically.

The sketch I have provided here is incomplete. There are important issues that I have not addressed, and assumptions that I have not challenged. I have, for example, not explored the precise meanings of the terms 'biological', 'psychological', or 'social', and have instead relied upon readers' intuitive grasp of them. Exactly what these terms mean is an underexplored issue in the literature on biopsychosocial psychiatry. I have observed elsewhere that more attention to this issue is likely to help psychiatrists and philosophers sharpen the tools that they use for conceptualizing and understanding mental illness (Roache, 2019). Another important issue that I have not explored here is the question of what is so special about the biological, the psychological, and the social in understanding and addressing mental health problems. If, as I have argued, and as Engel and others have recognized, our understanding of mental illness is likely to be maximized by attending to explanations at all of these three levels rather than to a subset of them, then why not also take into account explanations at other levels, too—such as the atomic? These considerations are worth exploring for anyone wishing to understand what the biopsychosocial model is and how it can be put to work in understanding and treating patients and their symptoms.

Acknowledgement

I am grateful to Neil Levy for helpful feedback on this chapter.

References

Alston, W. (1971). Varieties of privileged access. *American Philosophical Quarterly*, **8**(3), 223–241.

American Psychiatric Association (2013). *Diagnostic and Statistical Manual of Mental Disorders*, fifth edition. Washington, DC: American Psychiatric Association.

Andreasen, N. (1997). Linking mind and brain in the study of mental illness: a project for a scientific psychopathology. *Science*, **275**(5306), 1586–1593.

Apter-Levy, Y., Feldman, M., Vakart, A., Ebstein, R.P., and Feldman, R. (2013). Impact of maternal depression across the first 6 years of life on the child's mental health, social engagement, and empathy: the moderating role of oxytocin. *American Journal of Psychiatry*, **170**(10), 1161–1168.

Broome, M.R. and Bortolotti, L. (2009). Mental illness as mental: in defence of psychological realism. *Humana Mente*, **11**, 25–43.

Cahalan, S. (2013). *Brain on Fire: My Month of Madness*. London: Penguin.

Caspi, A., McClay, J., Moffitt, T.E., Mill, J., Martin, J., Craig, I.W., Taylor, A., and Poulton, R. (2002). Role of genotype in the cycle of violence in maltreated children. *Science*, **297**(5582), 851–854.

Churchland, P. (1981). Eliminative materialism and the propositional attitudes. *Journal of Philosophy*, **78**, 67–90.

Colton, C.W. and Manderscheid, R.W. (2006). Congruencies in increased mortality rates, years of potential life lost, and causes of death among public mental health clients in eight states. *Preventing Chronic Disease*, **3**(2), A42.

Cooper, R. (2007). *Psychiatry and Philosophy of Science*. King's Lynn: Acumen.

Crane, T. and Mellor, D.H. (1990). There is no question of physicalism. *Mind*, **99**(394), 185–206.

Dalmau, J., Tüzün, E., Wu, H., Masjuan, J., Rossi, J., Voloschin, A., Baehring, J.M., Shimazaki, H., Koide, R., King, D., Mason, W., Sansing, L.H., Dichter, M.A., Rosenfeld, M.R., and Lynch, D.R. (2007). Paraneoplastic anti-N-methyl-D-aspartate receptor encephalitis associated with ovarian teratoma. *Annals of Neurology*, **61**(1), 25–36.

Engel, G. (1977). The need for a new medical model: a challenge for biomedicine. *Science*, **196**(4286), 129–136.

Engel, G. (1978). The biopsychosocial model and the education of health professionals. *Annals of the New York Academy of Sciences*, **310**, 169–181; reprinted in *General Hospital Psychiatry* (1979), **1**(2), 156–165.

Gabbard, G.O. (2000). A neurobiologically informed perspective on psychotherapy. *British Journal of Psychiatry*, **177**, 117–122.

Ghaemi, S.N. (2010). *The Rise and Fall of the Biopsychosocial Model: Reconciling Art and Science in Psychiatry*. Baltimore, MD: Johns Hopkins University Press.

Graham, G. and Flanagan, O. (2013). Psychiatry and the brain. https://blog.oup.com/2013/08/psychiatry-brain-dsm-5-rdoc/

Haggard, P. (2008). Human volition: towards a neuroscience of free will. *Nature Reviews Neuroscience*, **9**, 934–946.

Hempel, C. (1970). Reduction: ontological and linguistic facets. In: S. Morgenbesser, P. Suppes, and M. White (Eds.), *Essays in Honor of Ernest Nagel* (pp. 179–199). New York: St Martin's Press.

Hogarty, G.E., Greenwald, D., Ulrich, R.F., Kornblith, S.J., DiBarry, A.L., Cooley, S., Carter, M., and Flesher, S. (1997a). Three-year trials of personal therapy among schizophrenic patients living with or independent of family, II: effects on adjustment of patients. *American Journal of Psychiatry*, **154**(11), 1514–1524.

Hogarty, G.E., Kornblith, S.J., Greenwald, D., DiBarry, A.L., Cooley, S., Ulrich, R.F., Carter, M., and Flesher, S. (1997b). Three-year trials of personal therapy among schizophrenic patients living with or independent of family, I: description of study and effects on relapse rates. *American Journal of Psychiatry*, **154**(11), 1504–1513.

Hosseinpoor, A.R., Harper, S., Lee, J.H., Lynch, J., Mathers, C., and Abou-Zahr, C. (2012). International shortfall inequality in life expectancy in women and in men, 1950–2010. *Bulletin of the World Health Organization*, **90**(8), 588–594.

Insel, T. (2013). The beginning of history illusion. NIMH Director's Blog, 9 January. https://www.nimh.nih.gov/about/directors/thomas-insel/blog/2013/the-beginning-of-history-illusion.shtml

Insel, T. and **Quirion, R.** (2005). Psychiatry as a clinical neuroscience discipline. *JAMA* **294**(17), 2221–2224.

Kallestrup, J. (2006). The causal exclusion argument. *Philosophical Studies*, **131**(2), 459–485.

Kendler, K.S. (2005). Toward a philosophical structure for psychiatry. *American Journal of Psychiatry*, **162**(3), 433–440.

Kendler, K.S. (2008). Explanatory models for psychiatric illness. *American Journal of Psychiatry*, **165**(6), 695–702.

Kendler, K.S. (2012). The dappled nature of causes of psychiatric illness: replacing the organic-functional/hardware/software dichotomy with empirically based pluralism. *Molecular Psychiatry*, **17**, 377–388.

Kendler, K.S., Hettema, J.M., Butera, F., Gardner, C.O., and **Prescott, C.A.** (2003). Life event dimensions of loss, humiliation, entrapment, and danger in the prediction of onsets of major depression and generalized anxiety. *Archives of General Psychiatry*, **60**(8), 789–796.

Kim, J. (1993). *Supervenience and Mind*. Cambridge: Cambridge University Press.

Kuhn, T. (1962). *The Structure of Scientific Revolutions*. Chicago, IL: University of Chicago Press.

Leff, J., Kuipers, L., Berkowitz, R., Eberlein-Vries, R., and **Sturgeon, D.** (1982). A controlled trial of social intervention in the families of schizophrenic patients. *British Journal of Psychiatry*, **141**, 121–134.

Leff, J., Kuipers, L., Berkowitz, R., and **Sturgeon, D.** (1985). A controlled trial of social intervention in the families of schizophrenic patients: two year follow-up. *British Journal of Psychiatry*, **146**, 594–600.

Mellor, D.H. (1995). *The Facts of Causation*. London: Routledge.

Nemeroff, C.B. and **Vale, W.W.** (2005). The neurobiology of depression: inroads to treatment and new drug discovery. *Journal of Clinical Psychiatry*, **66**(Suppl 7), 5–13.

Place, U. (1956). Is consciousness a brain process? *British Journal of Psychology*, **47**, 44–50.

Roache, R. (2019). Psychiatry's problem with reductionism. *Philosophy, Psychiatry & Psychology*, **26**(3), 219–229.

Shea, N. and **Bayne, T.** (2010). The vegetative state and the science of consciousness. *British Journal for the Philosophy of Science*, **61**(3), 459–484.

Shorter, E. (2005). The history of the biopsychosocial approach in medicine: before and after Engel. In: P. White (Ed.), *Biopsychosocial Medicine* (pp. 1–20). Oxford: Oxford University Press.

Szasz, T. (1960). The myth of mental illness. *American Psychologist*, **15**, 113–118.

Szasz, T. (1961). *The Myth of Mental Illness*. London: Paladin.

White, P. (Ed.) (2005). *Biopsychosocial Medicine*. Oxford: Oxford University Press.

World Health Organization (2002). Evolution 1950–2000 of global suicide rates (per 100,000). https://www.who.int/mental_health/prevention/suicide/evolution/en/

Chapter 23

Specifying the best conception of the biopsychosocial model

Doug McConnell

Introduction

There has been significant debate and confusion over which principles the biopsychosocial (BPS) model is committed to and the exact form of psychiatric practice it advises. The contributions to this anthology have done much to clarify and advance these debates and, in this final chapter, I build on three themes that have run through those contributions.

First, I investigate what the BPS model is committed to regarding the aetiology and treatment of mental disorder. At the very minimum, the BPS model is making two weak disjunctive claims: mental disorders are caused by biological, or psychological, or social factors, or some combination of them; and mental disorders will be most effectively treated by biological, or psychological, or social treatments, or some combination of them. However, the BPS model might also make stronger conjunctive claims: mental disorders are always caused by a combination of biological, psychological, and social factors; and mental disorders will always be most effectively treated by a combination of biological, psychological, and social treatments (Sinnott-Armstrong and Summers, Chapter 6, this volume). Roache (Chapter 2, this volume) has argued that the BPS model must restrict itself to the weaker claims because psychiatry would have no reason to develop complex multilevel aetiologies or to insist on multimodal treatments if a perfectly effective single-level treatment were discovered (e.g. a new drug). Roache's argument, however, only shows that the conjunctive claims are not true a priori. I draw on empirical evidence showing the complex interplay between biological, psychological, and social factors (e.g. Kendler and Gyngell, Chapter 2; Viding Chapter 10; Cecil, Chapter 12; Holton, Chapter 13, this volume) to argue that we should expect the conjunctive aetiological claim to hold true of psychiatry for the foreseeable future. The conjunctive treatment claim faces more serious objections. I argue that it must be weakened to state that ideal treatment of mental disorders will typically, but not necessarily, be a conjunction of biological, psychological, and social interventions.

A second theme centres on how the BPS model relates to the constitution and classification of mental disorders. I agree with Sinnott-Armstrong and Summers (Chapter 6, this volume) that the BPS model would be wrong to claim that mental disorders are constituted by combinations of biological, psychological, *and* social characteristics. In my view, the BPS model doesn't offer any guidance in regard to mental disorder constitution but it would be best complemented with a view that takes mental disorders to be constituted either by psychological aspects alone or a combination of psychological and social aspects. When it comes to classification, we could classify mental disorders according to their psychological or psychosocial constitutions (i.e. their symptomatology) or we might aim to classify them by aetiology (where biological factors remain relevant). I argue that the BPS model provides no guidance on whether to classify mental disorders according to symptomatology, aetiology, or some compromise between the two. What it does say, however, is that, to the extent we use aetiology to classify mental disorders, we should not restrict ourselves to a bioreductive aetiology but must consider biological, psychological, and social causal factors.

The final theme I address is whether the BPS model is a purely scientific endeavour or a way of conjoining a humanist approach to psychiatry with a scientific one. I argue that limiting ourselves to a scientific BPS model would be a mistake. Subjective experience, meaning, value, and social norms have wide-ranging influences on mental health so psychiatry cannot be optimally effective if it ignores them (Fulford, Chapter 8; McConnell, Chapter 18, this volume). In any case, a purely scientific BPS model is not really possible because scientific investigation of much of the psychosocial world must wait on the intersubjective processes by which meaning, values, and norms develop (Thornton, Chapter 15, this volume). Therefore, we should conceive of the BPS model as an attempt to integrate biological, psychological, and social sciences on the one hand with a concern for subjective experience, meaning, and values-based care on the other hand. This thoroughgoing pluralism does not just resist bioreductive approaches to psychiatry but scientific reductionism more broadly.

Aetiology

The weakest aetiological claim the BPS model could make is the disjunctive claim that mental disorders are caused by biological, or psychological, or social factors, or any combination of them (Sinnott-Armstrong and Summers, Chapter 6, this volume). In other words, any of these things alone or in combination could contribute to the development of a mental disorder so the psychiatrist should consider them all when developing aetiology. This claim is relatively uncontroversial since only those who think that psychological or social factors were fictional or epiphenomenal would deny it.

A stronger, more interesting claim is the conjunctive claim that mental disorders are always caused by a combination of factors at each of the psychological, biological, *and* social levels (Sinnott-Armstrong and Summers, Chapter 6, this volume). Therefore, to fully understand a mental disorder, we must understand the causes at all three levels. If we only look at one or two of these causal levels, for example, just psychology, or just psychology and biology, we will always miss out on something in the remaining level(s) and so we will lack a *full* understanding of the disorder.

This claim might seem implausibly strong because surely *some* mental disorders will be caused by factors at just one level, for example, just biological factors. A case of schizophrenia, for example, might be primarily caused by genetic abnormalities

that result in excessive synaptic pruning; perhaps the subsequent psychological phenomenon of paranoia and social phenomenon of stigma are effects of those physiological causes and do not causally contribute to the disorder themselves (Hyman and
McConnell, Chapter 17, this volume). Or, to take another example, a case of depression could be caused by the psychological realization that one has wasted much of
one's life pursuing inauthentic values; the subsequent changes in brain chemistry and
social isolation are effects of this psychological event.

In response to this we should first note that it is uncontroversial to accept the conjunctive claim that all mental disorders have *effects* at the biological, psychological,
and social levels. This follows from several commonly held assumptions. First, mental
disorders necessarily manifest at the psychological level and involve behaviour that
breaches social norms governing mentally healthy behaviour (Broome and Bortolotti,
2009; Banner, 2013). Second, all psychological events (healthy or disordered) have
psychological effects, even if many of those effects are relatively insignificant. The psychological effects of breaching social norms are, however, usually significant because
a breach of norms demands justification and risks social opprobrium. Third, when a
person breaches social norms it has social effects because it is an essential part of there
being a norm that people recognize when it has been breached.[1] Fourth, people, psych-
ologies, and societies are biologically instantiated so it is impossible to have a mental
disorder (or any lived experience) without that having biological effects.

Not all the effects of a mental disorder are relevant to psychiatry, however. For example, the patient might start eating lunch slightly earlier on Thursdays in order to fit
it around appointments with his psychiatrist. When the effects of a mental disorder
have no impact on the patient's mental health they are irrelevant to a full *psychiatric*
understanding of the disorder. Given that the BPS model is intended as a framework
for psychiatry, it should narrow its focus to effects of mental disorders that are relevant to mental health. Effects that are relevant to mental health include symptoms that
may not causally contribute to the course of the disorder (e.g. an instance of hallucination or a panic attack) and effects that themselves contribute to the chronicity and/
or acuity of the disorder (e.g. a growing sensitivity to cues for drug-use). So the BPS
model might narrow the claim to—all mental disorders have effects relevant to the
patient's mental health at biological, psychological, and social levels. Before assessing
the truth of this claim it is also worth considering a related aetiological claim which
limits itself to consideration of the original causes of a mental disorder plus the subset
of effects that causally contribute to the course of the disorder. Presumably it would be
uncommon for the original causes of a mental disorder to arise simultaneously in several different causal levels. Proponents of the BPS model would probably be happy to
concede this point. However, they might still hold that all mental disorders are caused
by a conjunction of biological, psychological, and social factors because some of the
effects of the original cause of a disorder come to causally contribute to the disorder.
So are either of these conjunctive claims true? Do all mental disorders have effects
relevant to mental health at each of the biological, psychological, and social levels? Are

---

[1] It is true that the actions of individuals who are totally isolated from society will have no social
effects but I set these cases aside.

all mental disorders caused by a conjunction of biological, psychological, and social factors?

One problem for both these claims is that a mental disorder could, in theory, be detected and successfully treated prior to the full set of causes and symptoms developing. In such a case, the mental disorder may have only, say, biological causes and may not yet have had any significant effects relevant to mental health. Roache (Chapter 2, this volume) provides a similar objection to the conjunctive aetiological claim based on the goals of psychiatry. Psychiatry is not like physics, for example, where pursuit of knowledge is the overriding goal. The central goal of psychiatry is to prevent, cure, and manage mental disorders. Aetiology and knowledge of the effects of mental disorders are only relevant to psychiatry as long as it helps achieve that goal. To illustrate this point, she suggests the following thought experiment:

> If we were to discover an obscure plant that, when eaten, could cure every type of mental disorder without any adverse side effects, then there would no longer be any need for psychiatrists to try to understand how and why mental disorders arise. (Roache, Chapter 2, p. 11, this volume)

If we have 'magic bullet' treatments like this, then we don't need to know exactly how those treatments disrupt the usual causes and effects of mental disorders. So, even if a full psychiatric understanding of the progression of an untreated mental disorder presently requires consideration of biological, psychological, and social causes and symptoms, future psychiatry does not necessarily need that full understanding. Whether psychiatry needs that full understanding or not depends on contingent factors such as the efficacy of the treatments that happen to be available. Therefore, the proponent of the BPS model should concede the a priori claims that mental disorders are *necessarily* caused by conjunctions of biological, psychological, and social factors and *necessarily* have biological, psychological, and social effects relevant to mental health.

There is, however, a weaker a posteriori version of the conjunctive aetiological claim that might be maintained. Given our present limitations in detecting and treating mental disorders, those disorders develop so that they are caused by factors at all three causal levels and have effects relevant to mental health at all three casual levels. These limitations will remain for the foreseeable future so we will continue to have a set of disorders caused by a conjunction of biological, psychological, and social factors that should be treated by psychiatry.[2] What is the empirical evidence supporting this a posteriori version of the conjunctive claim?

---

[2] One might think that once we develop completely effective treatments for a disorder (such as the obscure plant example) the disorder will no longer count as a mental disorder and so will no longer be within the purview of psychiatry. This appears to have already happened in the case of syphilis, for example. Now that syphilis is effectively treated by antibiotics we consider it an infection that should be treated by a physician not a mental disorder requiring a psychiatrist. When we know enough about a mental disorder to treat it as a somatic condition we may no longer need to know the biological, psychological, and social causes and symptoms of that condition. If it is a necessary condition of something being a *mental* disorder that we don't have a ready cure for it, then psychiatry will, by definition, be striving to improve the treatment of suboptimally understood disorders and so necessarily needs to know the biological,

The empirical evidence strongly suggests that highly effective, rapid, cheap treatments with no side effects are not likely to be discovered any time soon. Despite massive investments of time and money:

> We are still a long way from effectively treating mental health problems in childhood or adulthood. Even the best treatments are relatively limited (helping at most 50% of the sufferers) and significant proportion of individuals who suffer from mental health problems either do not improve or relapse following treatment. (Viding, Chapter 10, p. 155, this volume)

Clearly, each instance of mental disorder could be prevented or cured more effectively and rapidly than it is at present. Rational design of better treatments must proceed via aetiological understanding because we cannot effectively intervene in the causes of disorders until we know what those causes are; therefore, we need to know more about mental disorder aetiologies.

The aetiological data we have to date strongly indicates that mental disorders are caused by a combination of biological, psychological, and social factors. Many studies have shown that not only do mental disorders have both biological and (social) environmental risk factors, those factors interact to amplify or dampen the risk of a mental disorder (Kendler and Gyngell, Chapter 3; Viding, Chapter 10; Cecil, Chapter 12, this volume). These multilevel causal influences have been shown in depression (Kendler et al., 1995, 2006; Nemeroff and Vale, 2005), addiction (Kendler et al., 2011, 2012, 2014), and schizophrenia (Tienari et al., 2004), among others. The variety of environmental factors that contribute to the development of mental disorders are diverse but include characteristics of peer groups and parents, cultural factors like sex-specific norms about smoking, and stressful life events (Kendler and Gyngell, Chapter 3, this volume). Furthermore, studies of gene–environment interactions in psychiatric syndromes typically indicate that 'individuals with particular genotypes are relatively insensitive to risks in their environment, whereas others are much more susceptible' (Kendler and Gyngell, Chapter 3, p. 11, this volume). The picture is further complicated by the fact that people's genes influence their social environment. A systematic review of the heritability of 35 different environmental factors showed that differences in genes explain between 15% and 35% of the observed variation in environmental factors such as divorce, maternal warmth, and peer-group deviance (Kendler and Baker, 2007; see also Kendler et al., 2006). In other words, genetic differences explain, in part, why some people develop social environments that are more likely to lead to mental disorder. A genetic predisposition to poor impulse-control, for example, might make one vulnerable to temptations that put one's job, marriage, and friendships at risk. Importantly, the social and psychological effects of genetic causes are not always merely effects, often they causally contribute to the disorder, entrenching it and adjusting its character through feedback mechanisms. For example, a paranoid attitude initially driven by biology can drive social stigma but then the paranoid

---

psychological, *and* social causes of mental disorder. However, this just pushes the question back from which aetiologies psychiatry should be interested in to which conditions count as mental disorder and are thus suitable for psychiatric treatment.

individual might correctly pick up on that stigma which tends to reinforce the utility of being suspicious of others which in turn entrenches pathological neural firing patterns in the brain.

There is also highly suggestive evidence that patients' understanding of their own illnesses contributes to symptomatology. Richard Holton (Chapter 13, this volume) summarizes a range of the evidence in support of this including a threefold increase in the incidence of bulimia nervosa correlating with the cultural changes at the end of the twentieth century (Currin et al., 2005; Hudson et al., 2007), and culturally specific presentations of anorexia nervosa, post-traumatic stress disorder, schizophrenia, and depression (Watters, 2010; Kitanaka, 2012). This is related to the more general phenomenon of how a patient's beliefs about themselves protect or make them vulnerable to mental disorders. When people believe themselves to be powerless or worthless, those beliefs can contribute to mental disorder (Pickard, 2014; McConnell, 2016; Kennett et al., 2018; McConnell and Snoek, 2018). Certain self-beliefs can also be protective. Consider the example provided by Kendler and Gyngell (Chapter 3, this volume) of a child of an alcoholic father whose personal experience of his father's effect on his family led him, as a child, to make a life-long pledge to not drink alcohol. That pledge drew its strength from his personal context. He believed that to drink would be to risk becoming like his father. Importantly, these beliefs are not formed in isolation but depend on proximal and distal social factors. Proximally, the content of those beliefs depends on what friends and family inculcate. Distally, the content depends on the archetypes society makes available for the agent and their proximal social milieu to use in developing self-concepts (MacIntyre, 1984; Schechtman, 2007).

Even if we work out the typical aetiology (or range of aetiologies) for a kind of mental disorder, each disorder is likely to be caused slightly differently in each patient's case. For example, addiction might typically be caused by an environment high in addictive substances and low in non-drug-using opportunities, combined with genetic predispositions to addiction, poor impulse control, low self-esteem, a self-concept as a hopeless drug user, exposure to social stigma, and so on. Any particular individual suffering from addiction, however, will be affected by a different combination of these factors; some suffer stronger cravings, some live in more tempting environments, some have fewer non-drug-using options, some identify more strongly with being an addict, some face more stigma, and so on. Furthermore, the relative influence of these factors changes developmentally—as the individual gets older, different factors become more causally efficacious and other factors less so (Kendler and Gyngell, Chapter 3, this volume). Unless we discover a treatment that cures a disorder (without adverse effects) no matter the personal variations in biological, psychological, and social aetiological factors, psychiatry will have to concern itself with the details of that personal aetiology to select the most appropriate treatment. Furthermore, unless these treatments cost very little (which seems unlikely given the costs of synthesizing chemicals, conducting psychotherapy, or adjusting social environments) we will need to know personalized aetiologies to avoid wasting resources where they won't be effective.

In summary, the proponent of the BPS model should stop short of saying mental disorders are necessarily caused by a conjunction of biological, psychological, and social factors and that they necessarily have biological, psychological, and social effects relevant to mental health. Nevertheless, given the current aetiological evidence and the poor prospect of 'magic bullet' treatments, we should expect such conjunctions of aetiological factors and effects to be relevant to the understanding of mental disorders for the foreseeable future.

Treatment

The claims the BPS model might make in regard to treatment are analogous to the claims about understanding a mental disorder. The weak disjunctive claim is that mental illnesses will be effectively treated by biological, or psychological, or social interventions, or any combination of them. That is, the psychiatrist should remain open to any form of treatment and shouldn't necessarily commit to providing combinations of treatments (e.g. pharmacology and psychotherapy).

Sinnott-Armstrong and Summers (Chapter 6, this volume), however, believe that the BPS model can make the stronger conjunctive claim about treatment: in order to *fully* treat a mental illness, we will need to treat each of its biological, psychological, and social causes and effects. This view of treatment might, initially seem to follow from accepting the conjunctive claim about aetiology. If mental disorders are caused by factors at all three levels, then a complete form of treatment must combine treatment at all three levels—biological causes will be most effectively treated biologically, psychological causes will be most effectively treated psychologically, and social causes will be most effectively treated socially. However, as Roache (Chapter 2, this volume) points out, this doesn't necessarily follow. It is possible that 'magic bullet' treatments which intervene at a biological level could be effective independent of the causal levels involved in aetiology. Furthermore, we don't need to imagine 'magic bullet' treatments to see that treatments that initially operate at one causal level can exert influence across other causal levels. For example, when antidepressants work (without concomitant psychological or social intervention) presumably they generate the brain conditions conducive to the patient making the further psychological and social moves required to establish better mental health. Similarly, psychotherapy and cognitive behavioural therapy don't just counteract the psychological causes of disorder but also influence the biological and social factors contributing to the disorder. In other words, the interplay between the biological, psychological, and social that enables the original cause of a mental disorder to generate more causes at other levels can be exploited in treatment. 'The best treatment approach is the one that produces the best results, regardless of the extent to which it is fully biopsychosocial' (Roache, Chapter 2, p. 14, this volume). Therefore, the BPS model should restrict itself to the weaker, disjunctive treatment claim.[3]

In response to this objection, the proponent of the conjunctive treatment claim can use an analogous defence to that provided for the conjunctive aetiological claim. This involves conceding that the conjunctive treatment claim is not true a priori, perfectly

---

[3]   Similarly, Ghaemi claims that the BPS model flounders when a one-to-one correlation between type of cause and type of treatment fails to hold (2010, p. 113). This criticism assumes that the BPS model is committed to the conjunctive view about treatment.

effective treatment or prevention *could* operate through a single modality, but reiterate that we are in a world where all the treatments available for mental disorders are suboptimal. Given this reality, it makes sense that we combine the partially effective treatments we have to get the best results that we can. That entails using a conjunction of biological, psychological, and social interventions:

> [T]here is strong evidence that treatments work better when they target all three levels together. There is less relapse to opioid use when a patient is not only on naltrexone but also moves to a neighbourhood with fewer drug cues, engages in regular talk therapy sessions, and has job training plus help in finding and keeping a job (cf. Ahmed, et al., 2013). (Sinnott-Armstrong and Summers, Chapter 6, p. 85, this volume)

Similarly, a review of attention deficit hyperactivity disorder treatment shows that a combination of behavioural interventions and medication has better outcomes than either treatment alone (Murray et al., 2008). Given the strain that having a child with attention deficit hyperactivity disorder places on parents, we would also expect even better results if there were also social interventions to support the parents. Evidence also suggests that combinations of pharmacology and psychotherapy tend to be more effective for major depressive disorder (Craighead and Dunlop, 2014). It certainly seems plausible that patients would be able to make the healing psychological moves more efficiently if pharmacotherapy was complemented with appropriate psychotherapy and support was provided for the patients' social networks.

Sinnott-Armstrong and Summers (Chapter 6, this volume) point out that a complete BPS treatment often doesn't happen, not because healthcare professionals disagree with the conjunctive claim as an ideal form of treatment, but because they lack the resources to provide such treatment to everyone. In cases where a single mode of treatment is likely to be effective but a multimodal treatment will marginally increase the chance and speed of healing, it often makes sense to conserve resources and just use the single treatment. The conjunctive claim about ideal psychiatric treatment must be tempered with a concern for distributive justice.

One might object that there are obvious counterexamples to the conjunctive treatment claim. There already are single modality treatments that can cure addiction, for example. If we move an addicted person to an environment where they will never have access to the target of their addiction again, they will be cured. Even when this is possible (and it rarely is), one could still claim that a more complete treatment would also work biologically to remove pathological cravings and psychologically to help the addicted person develop and pursue a conception of a good life that they value more highly. The patient would then have more robust mental health because they would be less motivated to abuse a different drug that might remain available in their new environment and they would have the freedom to return to environments where the drug they were addicted to was available. Presumably, those processes of biological and psychological healing would eventually occur without intervention, but those changes could be made more quickly with effective biological and psychological treatments.

A more challenging counterexample is the case of the Vietnam veterans who had been addicted to opiates while serving in Vietnam but, upon returning to their lives in the United States, simply stopped using opiates (Robins, 1993). Apparently, a change in social context perfectly cured most of these people. A proponent of the conjunctive treatment claim might still insist that these recoveries would have been even swifter and more robust had the biological and psychological effects of opiate use in Vietnam been treated. No doubt there would have been some withdrawal effects that could have been ameliorated. Most of these soldiers returned to social environments where opiates were not readily available but, despite the very small chance of being offered opiates, perhaps treatment would have been better if they were trained in the psychological tools to resist such temptation. I don't think psychiatry should pursue this conception of ideal treatment even if there were sufficient resources to do so. Treatment of trivial risks and harms prioritizes mental health but prevent patients from getting on with their lives. Patients don't, typically, want mental health at any cost, they want sufficient mental health to pursue their respective conceptions of a good life. So, just as the ideal treatment pursued by the conjunctive treatment claim must be balanced with a concern for distributive justice, it must be balanced with a concern for patient autonomy.

One might wonder what it is supposed to be about the complement of biological, psychological, and social interventions that improves treatment. Perhaps it is just the case that, when all available treatments are suboptimal, more treatment is generally better than less treatment, that is, the complementary causal levels of the treatments involved might be irrelevant. In response to this, the proponent of the conjunctive treatment might point out that interventions at each causal level can have effects that cannot be achieved by interventions at the other levels. Pharmacology can influence brain chemistry in ways that psychological and social interventions cannot. Psychotherapy can make specific adjustments to mental content which biological and social interventions cannot. Social interventions can provide the patient with a supportive social context in ways that psychological and biological interventions cannot. Therefore, combinations of interventions can be more powerful than any used alone. This might be true in many cases, but it could still be the case that certain instances of mental disorder are irresponsive to the effects exclusive to, say, biological interventions. For example, our best biological interventions might be able to change brain chemistry and structure in a way that psychological or social interventions cannot but they might be completely unable to cure or mitigate a monothematic delusion (without severe side effects). The proponent of the conjunctive claim might object that this is simply because we haven't fully developed our biological interventions yet and when we do, *then* the conjunction of interventions will be the best treatment. However, once we move from designing ideal treatment based on our current technologies to designing ideal treatment using possible future technologies, then 'magic bullet' interventions are on the table and, as we have seen, they undermine the need for a conjunction of treatments.

A different kind of counterexample that would undermine the conjunctive treatment claim is any case of multimodal treatment with detrimental outcomes for some patients. To be an effective counterexample, however, it would need to be the case that the multimodal aspect of treatment was detrimental and not that one of the interventions used was detrimental. The BPS model isn't in favour of using treatments at every level even if some of them are detrimental; rather, it favours combining treatments that are effective at each of their respective levels. Harmful interactions are obviously a concern for pharmacological interventions; one shouldn't administer a patient all the drugs known to be effective at once. It seems there is less risk of harmful interactions between biological interventions, psychological interventions, and social interventions, at least, I know of no such cases. Nevertheless, I don't see why such harmful interactions couldn't occur. It is certainly possible that we haven't seen such harmful interactions because we haven't been looking for them. To the extent that harmful interactions occur between treatments at different casual levels, the conjunctive treatment claim will be undermined.

In short, the BPS model cannot claim that mental disorders are *necessarily* ideally treated with a combination of biological, psychological, and social interventions because it will be rendered false if we discover harmful interactions between treatments at different causal levels or invent 'magic bullet' treatments. Furthermore, even within the context of currently available treatments and empirical information, the conjunctive treatment claim it is still false because there are instances of mental disorders that are completely irresponsive to our best biological interventions and so should only be treated psychologically and socially. The cases that undermine the conjunctive treatment claim are, however, rare or involve speculative future cases. Therefore, we can conclude that, typically, mental disorders are ideally treated by a conjunction of biological, psychological, and social treatments but that this ideal treatment must be balanced with a concern for distributive justice and patient autonomy.

Before moving on to consider the constitution and classification of mental disorders it is worth responding to the main criticisms Ghaemi has levelled at the BPS model. Ghaemi (2010) objects that the BPS model is eclectic in its approach to treatment and research. According to Ghaemi, the BPS model cannot say why any form of treatment or direction for research would be better than any other and so recommends anything and everything. Therefore, the BPS approach is responsible for haphazard research, wastes resources, exposes patients to excessive treatment and unnecessary risk, and satisfies itself with treating symptoms rather than root causes.

These objections assume that the BPS model is disconnected from empirical evidence. It is true that without empirical evidence the BPS model would be unable to recommend treatment or research priorities with any accuracy but neither would any other theoretical framework for psychiatry. However, there is nothing in the BPS model that says one shouldn't be guided by empirical research. The BPS model should be committed to each instance of mental disorder having an objectively true aetiology and an objective best treatment and so sidesteps accusations of eclecticism. The model itself cannot provide the empirical evidence we need to discover those truths; we shouldn't expect it to because it is a theoretical framework for psychiatry. The role of the BPS model is to guide the necessary empirical work. It directs our search for the true aetiology of each mental disorder beyond a single causal level and towards the conjunction of biological, psychological, and social levels. It directs our search for the best treatment of each disorder beyond single-level interventions and towards conjunctions of biological, psychological, and social interventions. The BPS model has guided and supported much of the research cited earlier and, as this starts to pay off, we can begin to see which treatment combinations and research projects are likely to be the most cost-effective. As Essi Viding says, '[a]ny individual developmental trajectory is an emergent product of the interplay between various different levels of analyses: genetic, neural, cognitive, behavioural, and environmental ... The sheer scale of what we do not yet know becomes particularly clear when we try to think about the different levels of analyses interacting with and influencing each other ... However, exciting new data are constantly emerging that provide some pieces to the vast mental health developmental puzzle and also help focus the 'search space' for future studies' (Viding, Chapter 20, p. 164, this volume).

Constitution and classification of mental disorders

In this section I investigate the relationship between the BPS model, the constitution and classification of mental disorders, and the development of psychiatry. Although the BPS model has, arguably, paved the way for some prominent theories of mental disorder constitution, it doesn't itself provide an exact position on constitution. Therefore, the BPS model should be complemented with a plausible theory of mental disorder and the theories that would fit best either take mental disorders to be constituted by psychological factors alone or a combination of psychological and social factors. These theories of constitution lend themselves to a system of classification based on symptomatology, that is, mental disorders should be classified according to how they present psychologically (or psychosocially) since those aspects of their presentations are their only essential features. However, there is widespread concern that the current mainstream classificatory system based on the symptomatology of mental illness, the *Diagnostic and Statistical Manual of Mental Disorders* (DSM) system, is preventing psychiatry from developing into a mature form of medicine (see references in Thornton, Chapter 15, this volume). The alternative is thought to be a system that classifies mental disorders according to aetiology. Historically, the BPS model was involved in the development of the *DSM* system (Davies and Roache, 2017) and so one might think that it is complicit in the alleged stagnation of psychiatry. However, I point out that there is nothing in the BPS model that favours symptomatology over aetiology when it comes to classification but, if we do shift to an aetiologically informed classification, the BPS model recommends against the kind of bioreductive approach taken by the National Institute of Mental Health's Research Domain Criteria (RDoC) framework.

When a condition is constituted by a trait or conjunction of traits, nothing can be an instance of that condition if any of those traits is missing. Some have thought that mental disorders are constituted by their essential biological underpinnings; however, such bioreductive views face some serious objections (e.g. Bolton, 2008). The BPS model has, arguably, played a role in guiding psychiatry away from bioreductive views of constitution by insisting on the consideration of psychosocial factors. Nevertheless, the BPS model would be wrong to claim that mental disorders are constituted by combinations of biological, psychological, *and* social characteristics (Sinnott-Armstrong and Summers, Chapter 6, this volume). The problem with this conjunctive view of mental disorder constitution is that biological traits (and perhaps social traits) are not essential to mental disorders.

To generate the intuitions supporting the claim that biological characteristics are irrelevant to the constitution of mental disorders, consider the following thought experiment borrowed from Sinnott-Armstrong and Summers (Chapter 6, this volume). Imagine that 99% of people with a certain biomarker had depressed feelings, thought that life lacked meaning, and exhibited lethargy or suicide attempts *and* that 99% of people with these depressed feelings, thoughts, and actions had that biomarker. We still would think that someone without that biomarker but who genuinely had the same strong and persistent feelings, thoughts, and actions of depression would have the mental illness of depression. Conversely, a person with the biomarker but who lacked depressed feelings, thoughts, or actions would not have the mental illness of depression.[4] 'These intuitions suggest that the psychological aspects of depression—the depressed feelings, thoughts, and actions—are what constitute or define the mental illness of depression. In contrast, the biological aspects or correlates of those psychological aspects are not constitutive or definitive of depression' (Sinnott-Armstrong and Summers, Chapter 6, p. 87, this volume).

These intuitions have encouraged the most plausible views on mental disorder constitution to go one step further than the BPS model, they don't just see psychosocial factors to be as relevant as biological ones when it comes to constitution, they now reject the relevance of biological characteristics altogether (Sinnott-Armstrong and Summers, Chapter 6, this volume; Kinderman, 2005; Davies, 2016). Indeed, Sinnott-Armstrong and Summers argue that social factors are also irrelevant to the constitution of mental disorders and so the only constitutive characteristics of each mental disorder are psychological.[5] Their view is closely related to 'psychological realism' which claims that 'the level at which disorder can be identified is that of the *person*, … Whatever the technological and scientific advances we make in understanding the brain, its development and degeneration, we require psychological predicates in order to pick out instances of disorder' (Banner, 2013, p. 511; see also Broome and Bortolotti, 2009). Peter Kinderman also has a similar view which claims that, no matter the aetiology, the disruption of psychological processes is a logically necessary final step in all mental disorder (Kinderman, 2005).[6]

....

[4]Perhaps sometime in the future we will find a biomarker that occurs in every case of depression or in every case of a certain kind of depressive disorder. Then we might say that that particular disorder was constituted by that biological factor as well as its psychological presentation. However, we haven't been able to find such biomarkers despite expending much time and effort looking for them and it doesn't seem likely that we will find one any time soon.

[5]See Davies (2016) and Sinnott-Armstrong and Summers (Chapter 6, this volume) for a detailed discussion of whether social factors are involved in the constitution of mental disorders. I won't pursue this debate here since, for our purposes, it is enough to see that the BPS model cannot claim that mental disorders are biologically, psychologically, and socially constituted because biological features, at least, are inessential.

[6]Kinderman doesn't consistently distinguish aetiology from constitution and this leads to some confusion. This confusion is seen when Kinderman himself is unsure if his view is pluralist: 'Biological and social factors are properly acknowledged; one might even hope that this model might itself be seen as pluralistic. That said, the model presented here does place central

The BPS model itself cannot be the basis of a good theory of mental disorder constitution because it provides no reason to prioritize the psychological over the biological and social. However, as long as it isn't committed to the conjunctive claim about mental disorder constitution, and as far as I know nobody is claiming that it is, then it remains compatible with plausible views on mental disorder constitution, such as psychological realism. Therefore, the BPS model should be complemented with one of those views of constitution.

What does the psychological (or psychosocial) constitution of mental disorders mean for classification? One thought is that mental disorder constitutions translate straightforwardly into a classificatory system, that is, each kind of mental disorder is distinguished from the others by its distinctive psychological (or psychosocial) traits. There are two main concerns with this approach. First, how do we know we are correctly grouping symptoms together into different kinds of syndromes? Sinnott-Armstrong and Summers (Chapter 6, this volume) build their argument using examples from the current *DSM* classification of mental disorders (e.g. depression, post-traumatic stress disorder) but what if the *DSM* has incorrectly grouped symptoms into syndromes? Perhaps, for example, all instances of depressed thoughts, feelings, and actions do not form part of a single kind of mental disorder called depression and they are actually manifestations of several different kinds of depressive disorder, or perhaps some of those symptoms should be grouped with other symptoms as part of a completely different kind of disorder (Goldberg, 2010). This challenge doesn't necessarily undermine a system of classification based on symptomatology but it suggests that we might need to replace the *DSM* system with categories that better pick out the essential psychological features of each kind of disorder.

However we group symptoms into syndromes, a second problem stems from the phenomena of equifinality and multifinality. In equifinality, two cases with different aetiologies present in similar ways (Viding, Chapter 10, this volume). This entails that, if you just classify disorders according to how they present, you end up with aetiologically heterogeneous groups that are not helpfully treated in the same ways and that lead research astray (Uher and Rutter, 2012). 'If there are important causal factors that might be found in some subgroup of those with a particular *DSM* diagnosis, or in a population that cuts across current categories, these are likely to be missed by current research programmes' (Cooper, Chapter 4, p. 48, this volume). In multifinality, the same underlying causes of mental disorder might present in quite different ways depending on developmental context. When we group cases according to presentation, multifinality misleads us into dividing similar cases into different groups for the purposes of research and treatment. Equifinality and multifinality

emphasis on psychology. Although that emphasis may prevent the model from being regarded as pluralistic at present, it may well be that a pluralistic model will eventually emerge' (2005, p. 213). This ambiguity leads Gask (2018) to misunderstand Kinderman's view when she objects to him dropping consideration of biological and social factors altogether. These confusions can be resolved if we take Kinderman to be presenting a view like Sinnott-Armstrong and Summers, that is, a view that is pluralist about aetiology but holds that mental disorders are constituted by psychological factors alone.

are not just problems for the *DSM* system, they are problems for any nosology that first seeks valid classifications based on symptomatology and then moves to develop causal knowledge, for example, Ghaemi (2012), Sinnott-Armstrong and Summers (Chapter 6, this volume), and Banner (2013). Further criticisms have been levelled at the *DSM* and those criticisms are also likely to apply any system of classification based on symptomatology alone. The *DSM* system is accused of promoting overdiagnosis and the unjustified proliferation of new kinds of mental disorders because of its focus on counting symptoms (Parker, 2005). Furthermore, because the *DSM* system doesn't specify which aetiologies lead to which disorders, it is accused of allowing people to promote dubious aetiologies and treatments, for example, corporate interests promoting biological aetiologies and interventions in order to sell drugs (McHugh and Treisman, 2007).

One attempt to solve these problems is to take an aetiological approach to classification. If disorders were classified by aetiology, then diagnosis would connect the patient to a set of relevant treatments and research could more easily target aetiologically homogeneous groups. The RDoC programme is a prominent example of this approach. It aims to use neuroscience to identify dysfunctional brain circuits considered independently of diagnostic categories, for example, its target populations will not be people with schizophrenia or depression, say, but disorders of attention, anxiety, threat reactivity, or declarative memory. RDoC is not yet in a position to propose an alternative nosology but informing nosology must be a longer-term goal of the approach if it is to be useful to psychiatric practice.

This RDoC approach to classification faces the problem that two identical cases of dysfunction in a particular domain may have different clinical presentations because of differences in the developmental context of each domain. In favourable developmental contexts a dysfunction may be completely compensated for by other domains, while in less favourable contexts it may only be partially compensated for, or may even trigger dysfunction in other domains. The RDoC approach would, therefore, confront the same problem facing attempts to explain the development of mental disorders by reference to genetic risk factors. The genetic risk factors we have discovered underdetermine which disorder develops or even whether a disorder develops. Nearly all genetic risk factors for schizophrenia, for example, convey comparable risks for bipolar disorder, and other disorders such as depression, substance abuse, and epilepsy (Insel et al., 2010). One likely explanation for this is that the psychosocial context of genetic development has a significant impact on which disorder, if any, arises.

> Given that there is no systematic difference between genes or brain circuits that correlates with the difference between (say) schizophrenia and bipolar disorder, it may be that social and cultural factors play a role in explaining the difference between them, and not just the difference between, say, depression and hysterical fugue. Further, social and cultural factors may play a causal role not only in how a mental illness is expressed, but also in whether a particular individual develops a mental illness in the first place. Some sufferers from bulimia may have an underlying vulnerability to mental illness, but though some of them may have developed a *different* pathology were cultural norms different, some of them probably would not have developed a mental illness at all. (Levy, Chapter 7, p. 103, this volume; see also Holton, Chapter 13, this volume).

Not only have biologically focused causal stories failed to fully explain the development of mental disorder, empirical studies by Kendler and others have shown that, in many cases, a full aetiological picture requires that we complement biological causes with psychosocial causes. So I think that Levy is right in thinking that, if we are to build a classificatory system that is responsive to aetiology, we should 'attend to all the systematic causes of mental illness, distal and proximate, neurobiological and social' (Levy, Chapter 7, p. 107, this volume). The significance of this for bioreductive approaches like the RDoC depends on whether one accepts the conjunctive aetiological claim discussed previously—that mental disorders are always caused by a conjunction of biological, psychological, and social factors. If that claim is true, then RDoC will be unable to explain the aetiology of any mental disorder let alone classify them. However, if only some mental disorders are caused by a conjunction of biological, psychological, and social factors then RDoC could enjoy some success with disorders without psychosocial aetiological factors.

Someone defending RDoC might reply that this line of objection assumes that the categories of schizophrenia and bipolar disorder exist and this is exactly what RDoC aims to avoid. If the neurobiological aetiological story doesn't match our existing categories, so much the worse for those categories. But this response is problematic on two counts. First, the objection to bioreductive aetiological approaches needn't make any assumption about how mental disorders should be categorized, it merely claims that we shouldn't ignore psychosocial factors. It is RDoC that wrongly assumes the relevant casual factors will be exclusively neurobiological. Second, there won't be an entirely value-neutral classification of mental disorders. At the very least our classificatory system will be based on the normative distinction between mental health and mental illness. The goal of psychiatry is to help those we judge to suffer from mental illness, not to correct dysfunctional psychological domains when those dysfunctions don't happen to result in mental illness. If psychiatry investigates the aetiologies of phenomena other than what we judge to be mental illness, then psychiatry becomes disconnected from what we care about.

In order to rid ourselves as best as possible of any misleading symptomalogical categories we might allow the very general normative judgement about what counts as mental illness but then resist any further categorization on symptomalogical grounds. This would involve looking at the causal data for all mental illness to see if cases naturally fall into clusters of similar aetiological factors. Importantly, however, we should include psychosocial factors in this collection of aetiological factors, not just neurobiological ones. We would then have to make further normative judgements about which clusters of aetiological factors are sufficiently distinct from other clusters to warrant designation as particular kinds of mental disorder. The wide range of symptomology we see for mental disorders suggests that these clusters will be relatively fuzzy. It may be that members of each cluster will not have any causal factors in common that distinguish them from members of other clusters. Presumably, however, these fuzzy categories guided by aetiology will be less aetiologically heterogeneous than categories based on symptoms, and so they will be better for linking patients with treatment.

Some may still find this approach unsatisfying, however, because they believe that the familiar categories of schizophrenia, addiction, bipolar and so on, have some value.

For example, people identify as having disorders of those kinds so to say a disorder doesn't actually exist is disruptive of people's self-understandings (even if those self-understandings were, in a sense, false). It is certainly true that these categories have become entrenched in our cultures and so there are costs to making wholesale changes to them (Thornton, Chapter 15, this volume). We might, then, resist redrawing the categories of mental disorder according to aetiology and insist on finding aetiologies for the mental disorder categories we are familiar with (or something relatively similar to them). To the extent we are committed to the established categories of mental disorders, however, we will have to accept the costs of the relatively heterogeneous aetiologies within those categories.

Whatever one's position on that conflict, we currently lack sufficient aetiological knowledge to shift to a thoroughgoing aetiological classification (Frances, 2009). Therefore, even those who favour more thoroughly aetiological classifications will have to settle for a hybrid approach where an initial classification based on presentation narrows the research focus and then aetiology is used to adjust and subdivide those initial, symptom-based categories. Viding essentially articulates such a hybrid approach when she says we should:

> [U]se subtle differences in behaviour to provide clues for subsequent systematic investigation at different levels of analyses. This approach is clearly not ideal as we are still starting with behaviour and we cannot assume that the behavioural indicators we have chosen, or our ability to observe them, are always entirely accurate. But it is perhaps the best we have as a starting point and once the data accumulate, it will indicate to us how reasonable this starting point has been. We can assess whether the behavioural indicators that we have used provide meaningful differentiation at multiple levels of analyses. (Viding, Chapter 10, pp. 157–158, this volume)

This hybrid approach has already led to different categorizations, for example, researchers have distinguished neurobiologically distinct subpopulations of depression (Nemeroff and Vale, 2005) and schizophrenia (Howes and Kapur, 2009). For those, like Viding, who ultimately want to shift to a strongly aetiological classification, this hybrid approach is just a stepping stone towards a more thoroughgoing aetiological classification. For those who think there is a value in retaining the mental disorder categories we have established (or close variants of them), this hybrid approach to classification is the methodological end point.

But what does any of this have to do with the BPS model? The BPS model was influential in the development of the *DSM* which reflects the perceived importance of social, cultural, and environmental factors in accurate diagnosis and classification (Davies and Roache, 2017). Despite this, there is nothing in the BPS model that favours a symptomological classification over an aetiological classification or some hybrid view. Therefore, the BPS model doesn't stand in the way of development in psychiatric classification but it doesn't provide any guidance about which direction is best either. To the extent we pursue an aetiological classification, however, the BPS model provides some guidance on how to go about it because it specifies that the relevant aetiologies will be conjunctions of biological, psychological, and social factors. Therefore, the BPS model would recommend against the bioreductive focus of the RDoC approach. The RDoC programme might discover many interesting things about the biological processes at play in mental illness but it will fail to provide accurate aetiologies for mental disorders unless it expands its purview to consider psychosocial causal factors.

Mechanism and meaning

The final topic I will consider is the ongoing confusion over whether the BPS model is a purely scientific endeavour, one that insists on taking a scientific approach to biological, psychological, and social factors, or if it also concerns itself with subjective experience, meaning, and normative value. I argue that a plausible conception of the BPS model must be thoroughly pluralist and consider all of these factors. Psychiatry must accommodate subjective experience, meaning, and normative value, not just out of respect for the patient, but because those factors have an impact on aetiology, treatment efficacy, and nosology. Before I set out the argument for that view, however, I will briefly illustrate the present confusion with a few conflicting interpretations of the BPS model.

Engel himself was ambiguous as to whether the BPS model was strictly scientific or involved a humanist aspect (see Roache, Chapter 2, this volume, for details). This ambiguity has allowed others to develop conflicting impressions of the BPS model. Ghaemi critiques the BPS model for focusing on science to the exclusion of the humanities. Ghaemi claims that if 'one supports the BPS model on humanistic grounds … that view [is] explicitly opposed to Engel's perspective' (Ghaemi, 2010, pp. 128–129). 'Engel clearly had no patience for humanism separated from science: He wanted to show the BPS model to be a hardheaded scientific theory that incorporates psychology and sociology' (Ghaemi, 2010, p. 133). Francis Creed (2005) paints a similar picture of the BPS model when he compares it with the patient-centred model. He believes that the two models are compatible but that the BPS model does not 'explore illness experience from the patient's view point', 'regard the whole person', or aim to 'enhance doctor-patient relationships', while the patient-centred approach does (Creed, 2005, p. 194).

Fulford presents the opposite interpretation, claiming that 'from its inception the biopsychosocial model has been understood primarily in scientific terms' but that Engel 'himself urged combining the humanities with science for better patient care' (Chapter 8, p. 109, this volume). Similarly, David Pilgrim assumes the BPS model includes consideration of subjectivity and normativity, stating that:

> The BPS model mirrors the concerns of critical realists to respect both causes and meanings. Accordingly, it does not ignore either the implied expectations of the objectivism of the former or the subjectivism of the latter. Both critical realism and the BPS model have a methodological sensibility about the challenging interplay … of both interpreting meaning (verstehen) and explaining the causal antecedents of the signs and symptoms of patients (erklaren). (Pilgrim, 2015, p. 165)

What all these writers have in common is that they believe a model for psychiatry should concern itself with subjective experience, meaning, and value. I agree; in trying to formulate the best conception of the BPS model, we should reject conceptions that are strictly scientific.[7]

----

[7] I set aside the historical task of trying to work out exactly what Engel himself thought. Ghaemi

The most obvious reason that a framework for psychiatry should incorporate a humanist aspect is that psychiatric practice is primarily interpersonal. To use Peter Strawson's (2008) famous distinction, we can all take the objective stance or the participant stance towards others. The participant stance is the default stance for our ordinary social interactions where we treat others as moral equals and expect them to recognize and respond to social norms. From the objective stance, the other is seen as an object, or perhaps a problem or puzzle, 'to be managed or handled or cured or trained; perhaps simply to be avoided' (Strawson, 2008, p. 10). When engaging in science we necessarily take the objective stance; science sees everything including people as a potential object for investigation. Clearly, it would be dehumanizing to be treated exclusively as an object for investigation rather than as a participant in norm-governed social interactions. If the psychiatrist fails to switch to the interpersonal stance and consistently treats the patient as an object, they undermine the patient's status as a moral equal. This in turn erodes the patient's self-respect, self-esteem, and self-trust and is likely to exacerbate mental health problems (Kennett et al., 2018). So a concern for the patient as a person is not just a matter of meeting professional and moral obligations to others, it is relevant to therapeutic outcomes.

In fact, subjective experience, meaning and norms influence treatment efficacy in a variety of ways. First, the success conditions of treatment are set, in part, by the patient's values: 'In clinical contexts, what is important means (in part) *what is important from the perspective of the particular patient concerned*' (Fulford, Chapter 8, p. 112, this volume). Therefore, without consideration of the patient's values, the psychiatrist doesn't know with precision what the goal of treatment is or whether that goal has been hit or missed. Second, because treatment involves shared decision-making between the patient and clinicians, clinicians need to be sensitive to possible clashes in value and should try to find a framework of shared values from which to make decisions. 'The scientific perspective works well for the technical aspects of psychiatry. But a values-based perspective . . . is needed for . . . implementing biopsychosocial psychiatry in the context of the shared decision-making that underpins contemporary person-centred clinical care' (Fulford, Chapter 8, p. 125, this volume).[8] Third, some mental disorders are caused by pathological mental content, for example, where a patient finds themselves unrealistically committed to goals instilled by an overbearing parent (McConnell, Chapter 18, this volume). In such cases, treatment needs to uncover and adjust that pathological content. Assessment and treatment of pathological mental content must proceed discursively because it is a process of reinterpreting a subjective world, not finding a more accurate description of the objective world. Similarly, sometimes aspects of a specific personal narrative contribute to a person's ability to resist or overcome mental disorder. Earlier, we saw Kendler and Gyngell's

---

has claimed that we shouldn't develop the BPS model, that we should reject it given the flaws in the original version. This would allow us to make a fresh start with a new theoretical framework. However, I see no harm in trying to develop the BPS model and only abandoning it if its best version is inadequate.

[8] The preceding points about the importance of a humanist approach and the concern with values and self-understandings all equally apply to somatic medicine.

(Chapter 3, this volume) case example where Mick's childhood experiences of his alcoholic father grounds his commitment to abstinence. This entails that we could treat or prevent mental disorders by supporting the development of certain self-narratives (McConnell, 2016; McConnell and Snoek, 2018). Finally, the content of social norms will influence the form mental disorders take or even whether they manifest at all (Levy, Chapter 7; Holton, Chapter 13, this volume). For example, rates of bulimia might increase though exposure to particular ideal body images and narratives that link some body shapes to success and happiness and not others. We might then treat or prevent bulimia by reducing exposure to these ideals and narratives or by trying to adjust those ideals and narratives.

The effects of subjective experience, meaning, and norms on the development of mental disorders and treatment efficacy means that we cannot see humanism as an optional extra, a compassionate user-interface that we might tack on to empirical psychiatry (e.g. see McConnell Chapter 18, this volume) for a more detailed discussion of these issues). Rather, a humanist approach will be at the heart of effective treatment because it is the only way to engage with the patient as a person, to discover the patient's values, to share decisions, and to negotiate therapeutic changes to the patient's self-understandings and plans. Therefore, the best conception of the BPS model is one that is pluralist in a very broad sense; it doesn't just consider empirical data arising from the assessment of biological, psychological, and social targets, it also considers expressions of subjective experience, meaning, values, and social norms. This complicates the kinds of interactions that occur between the causal levels—there will be both mechanistic interactions *and* meaningful interactions. For example, events at the social level do not just influence the psychological and biological levels through things such as socioeconomic and political opportunities but also through the normative values placed on the narrative archetypes society makes available. This version of the BPS model doesn't just resist biomedical reductionism; it resists all forms of scientific reductionism.

Subjective experience, meaning, values, and norms are psychosocial phenomena par excellence so there seems nothing controversial in claiming that the BPS model should be concerned with them. In fact, we can go further and claim that a purely scientific conception of the BPS model was never really coherent. When we are doing social science and certain kinds of psychology, the targets for investigation are inherently normative so their existence and influence depend on sociopolitical dynamics. Therefore, the possible targets for much of social science and psychology are ever-changing and depend, in part, on what people value. If society changes so that, say, religious beliefs and organizations disappear, then the scientific investigation of those things is no longer possible and the data collected in the past is interesting for historical reasons only.[9] Furthermore, normatively governed psychosocial targets are only relevant to psychiatry if they influence mental health, the inherently normative value driving psychiatric practice. For example, low self-esteem, prevalence of addictive drugs, abusive families, stigma, and so on, are only relevant targets for psychiatric science, because

---

[9] At the most, it may remain scientifically relevant because the dynamic of extant beliefs and social organization share some similarities with the extinct religious beliefs and organizations.

of the impact they have on mental health. So there never really was a possibility of scientifically investigating normatively governed phenomena without consideration of the inherent normativity in both the targets of investigation and the investigation itself. Psychiatric researchers must be alert to these normative considerations if they are to helpfully direct psychosocial science research in the service of psychiatry. This is why, as discussed previously, the classification of mental disorders cannot be purely aetiological but must wait on normative judgements of what counts as mental illness. Without this normative grounding, scientific projects intended to improve psychiatry are at risk of investigating targets irrelevant to the goals of psychiatry.

Conclusion

The BPS model can uncontroversially adopt the weak claims that mental disorders are necessarily caused by biological, or psychological, or social factors, or some combination of them, and that mental disorders will necessarily be most effectively treated by biological, or psychological, or social treatments, or some combination of them. The more stronger, conjunctive claims that the BPS model might adopt are the following: mental disorders necessarily have biological, psychological, and social effects relevant to mental health; mental disorders are necessarily caused by biological, psychological, and social factors; and, mental disorders are ideally treated by a conjunction of biological, psychological, and social interventions.

I have argued that the possibility of 'magic bullet' treatments entails that the proponent of the BPS model cannot claim that mental disorders are *necessarily* caused by a conjunction of biological, psychological, and social factors or that mental disorders necessarily have biological, psychological, and social effects relevant to mental health. We should, however, expect such conjunctions of aetiological factors and effects to be relevant to the understanding of mental disorders for the foreseeable future given the poor prospect of 'magic bullet' treatments and the current empirical evidence implicating factors at all three causal levels.

The BPS model also cannot claim that mental disorders are *necessarily* ideally treated with a combination of biological, psychological, and social interventions. This claim will be rendered false if we discover harmful interactions between treatments at different causal levels or invent 'magic bullet' treatments. Furthermore, there are instances of mental disorders that are completely irresponsive to our best interventions at one casual level and so must be best treated by interventions at only one or two causal levels. That said, the cases that undermine the conjunctive treatment claim are rare or speculative, therefore, we can conclude that, typically, mental disorders are ideally treated by a conjunction of biological, psychological, and social interventions. This ideal conception of treatment must, however, be balanced with a concern for distributive justice and patient autonomy.

When it comes to the constitution and classification of mental disorders, the BPS model is somewhat limited in the guidance it can give. It would be implausible to claim that mental disorders are constituted by a conjunction of biological, psychological, and social factors. However, the BPS model is compatible with, and should be complemented with, theories that take mental disorders to be constituted by psychological or psychosocial factors. The BPS model doesn't indicate whether we should classify disorders according to symptomology, aetiology, or some hybrid view. If we pursue an aetiologically informed classification, however, the BPS model specifies that the relevant aetiologies will typically be conjunctions of biological, psychological, and social factors. Therefore, the BPS model would recommend expanding the narrow biological focus of the RDoC approach.

Finally, the best conception of the BPS model is one that is alive to both mechanism and meaning. It encourages scientific research to investigate the interactions between the biological, psychological, and social determinants of mental disorder while recognizing that normative value influences what we take to be worthy of scientific investigation and classification. It also recognizes that the intersubjective world of meaning and value generates many of the targets worth investigating with social science and psychology. This thoroughly pluralist version of the BPS model encourages us to complement our scientific knowledge with knowledge of how subjective experience, values, self-understandings, and social norms impact mental health and how treatment can be improved accordingly.

References

Banner, N.F. (2013). Mental disorders are not brain disorders. *Journal of Evaluation in Clinical Practice*, **19**(3), 509–513.

Bolton, D. (2008). *What is Mental Disorder?: An Essay in Philosophy, Science, and Values*. Oxford: Oxford University Press.

Broome, M. and Bortolotti, L. (2009). Mental illness as mental: in defence of psychological realism. *Humana Mente*, **11**, 25–44.

Craighead, W.E. and Dunlop, B.W. (2014). Combination psychotherapy and antidepressant medication treatment for depression: for whom, when, and how. *Annual Review of Psychology*, **65**, 267–300.

Creed, F. (2005). Are the patient-centred and biopsychosocial approaches compatible? In: P. White (Ed.), *Biopsychosocial Medicine* (pp. 187–200). Oxford: Oxford University Press.

Currin, L., Schmidt, U., Treasure, J., and Jick, H. (2005). Time trends in eating disorder incidence. *The British Journal of Psychiatry*, **186**(2), 132–135.

Davies, W. (2016). Externalist psychiatry. *Analysis*, **76**(3), 290–296.

Davies, W. and Roache, R. (2017). Reassessing biopsychosocial psychiatry. *The British Journal of Psychiatry*, **210**(1), 3–5.

Frances, A. (2009). Whither DSM–V? *The British Journal of Psychiatry*, **195**(5), 391–392.

Gask, L. (2018). In defence of the biopsychosocial model. *The Lancet Psychiatry*, **5**(7), 548–549.

Ghaemi, N. (2010). *The Rise and Fall of the Biopsychosocial Model*. Baltimore, MD: Johns Hopkins University Press.

Ghaemi, N. (2012). Taking disease seriously: beyond 'pragmatic' nosology. In: K.S. Kendler and J. Parnas (Eds.), *Philosophical Issues in Psychiatry II: Nosology* (pp. 42–53). Oxford: Oxford University Press.

Goldberg, D. (2010). Should our major classifications of mental disorders be revised? *The British Journal of Psychiatry*, **196**(4), 255–256.

Howes, O.D. and Kapur, S. (2009). The dopamine hypothesis of schizophrenia: version III— the final common pathway. *Schizophrenia Bulletin*, **35**(3), 549–562.

Hudson, J.I., Hiripi, E., Pope, H.G., and Kessler, R.C. (2007). The prevalence and correlates of eating disorders in the National Comorbidity Survey Replication. *Biological Psychiatry*, **61**(3), 348–358.

Insel, T., Cuthbert, B., Garvey, M., Heinssen, R., Pine, D.S., Quinn, K., Sanislow, C., and Wang, P. (2010). Research Domain Criteria (RDoC): toward a new classification framework for research on mental disorders. *American Journal of Psychiatry*, **167**(7), 748–751.

Kendler, K.S. and Baker, J.H. (2007). Genetic influences on measures of the environment: a systematic review. *Psychological Medicine*, **37**(5), 615–626.

Kendler, K.S., Gardner, C., and Dick, D.M. (2011). Predicting alcohol consumption in adolescence from alcohol-specific and general externalizing genetic risk factors, key environmental exposures and their interaction. *Psychological Medicine*, **41**(7), 1507–1516.

Kendler, K.S., Gatz, M., Gardner, C.O., and Pedersen, N.L. (2006). A Swedish national twin study of lifetime major depression. *American Journal of Psychiatry*, **163**(1), 109–114.

Kendler, K.S., Kessler, R.C., Walters, E.E., MacLean, C., Neale, M.C., Heath, A.C., and Eaves, L.J. (1995). Stressful life events, genetic liability, and onset of an episode of major depression in women. *American Journal of Psychiatry*, **152**(6), 833–842.

Kendler, K.S., Ohlsson, H., Sundquist, K., and Sundquist, J. (2014). Peer deviance, parental divorce, and genetic risk in the prediction of drug abuse in a nationwide Swedish sample. *JAMA Psychiatry*, **71**(4), 439–445.

Kendler, K.S., Sundquist, K., Ohlsson, H., Palmér, K., Maes, H., Winkleby, M.A., and Sundquist, J. (2012). Genetic and familial environmental influences on the risk for drug abuse: a national Swedish adoption study. *Archives of General Psychiatry*, **69**(7), 690–697.

Kennett, J., McConnell, D., and Snoek, A. (2018). Reactive attitudes, relationships, and addiction. In: H. Pickard and S.H. Ahmed (Eds.), *The Routledge Handbook of Philosophy and Science of Addiction* (pp. 440–452). London: Routledge.

Kinderman, P. (2005). A psychological model of mental disorder. *Harvard Review of Psychiatry*, **13**(4), 206–217.

Kitanaka, J. (2012). *Depression in Japan: Psychiatric Cures for a Society in Distress*. Princeton, NJ: Princeton University Press.

MacIntyre, A. (1984). *After Virtue: A Study in Moral Theory* (2nd ed.). New York: Oxford University Press.

McConnell, D. (2016). Narrative self-constitution and recovery from addiction. *American Philosophical Quarterly*, **53**(3), 307–322.

McConnell, D. and Snoek, A. (2018). The importance of self-narration in recovery from addiction. *Philosophy, Psychiatry, and Psychology*, **25**(3), 31–44.

McHugh, P.R. and Treisman, G. (2007). PTSD: a problematic diagnostic category. *Journal of Anxiety Disorders*, **21**(2), 211–222.

Murray, D.W., Arnold, L.E., Swanson, J., Wells, K., Burns, K., Jensen, P., Hechtman, L., Paykina, N., Legato, L., and Strauss, T. (2008). A clinical review of outcomes of the multimodal treatment study of children with attention-deficit/hyperactivity disorder (MTA). *Current Psychiatry Reports*, **10**(5), 424–431.

Nemeroff, C.B. and Vale, W.W. (2005). The neurobiology of depression: inroads to treatment and new drug discovery. *The Journal of Clinical Psychiatry*, **66**(Suppl 7). 5–13.

Parker, G. (2005). Beyond major depression. *Psychological Medicine*, **35**(4), 467–474.

Pickard, H. (2014). Stories of recovery: the role of narrative and hope in overcoming PTSD and PD. In J.Z. Sadler, B. Fulford, and C. Werendly van Staden (Eds.), *The Oxford Handbook of Psychiatric Ethics* (pp. 1315–1327). Oxford: Oxford University Press.

Pilgrim, D. (2015). The biopsychosocial model in health research: its strengths and limitations for critical realists. *Journal of Critical Realism*, **14**(2), 164–180.

Robins, L. (1993). Vietnam veterans' rapid recovery from heroin addiction: a fluke or normal expectation? *Addiction*, **88**(8), 1041–1054.

Schechtman, M. (2007). Stories, lives, and basic survival: a refinement and defense of the narrative view. *Royal Institute of Philosophy Supplement*, **82**(60), 155–178.

Strawson, P. (2008). *Freedom and Resentment and Other Essays*. London: Routledge.

Tienari, P., Wynne, L.C., Sorri, A., Lahti, I., Läksy, K., Moring, J., Naarala, M., Nieminen, P., Wahlberg, K.-E. (2004). Genotype-environment interaction in schizophrenia-spectrum disorder. Long-term follow-up study of Finnish adoptees. *The British Journal of Psychiatry: The Journal of Mental Science*, **184**, 216–222.

Uher, R. and Rutter, M. (2012). Basing psychiatric classification on scientific foundation: Problems and prospects. *International Review of Psychiatry*, **24**(6), 591–605.

Watters, E. (2010). *Crazy Like Us*. New York: Simon and Schuster.

Index